Health and Ethnicity

Published Symposia of the Society for the Study of Human Biology

39 Human Biology and Social Inequality
Edited by S. S. Strickland and P. S. Shetty

40 Urbanism, Health and Human Biology in Industrialised Countries
Edited by L. M. Schell and S. J. Uiijaszek

Numbers 1–9 were published by Pergamon Press, Headington Hill Hall, Headington, Oxford OX3 0BY. Numbers 10–24 were published by Taylor & Francis Ltd, 10–14 Macklin Street, London WC2B 5NF. Numbers 25–40 were published by Cambridge University Press, The Pitt Building, Trumpington Street, Cambridge CB2 1RP. Further details and prices of back-list numbers are available from the Secretary of the Society for the Study of Human Biology.

Society for the Study of Human Biology Series: 41

Health and Ethnicity

Edited by

Helen Macbeth

Department of Anthropology, Oxford Brookes University

and

Prakash Shetty

Public Health Nutrition Unit,
London School of Hygiene and Tropical Medicine

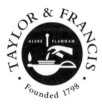

London and New York

First published 2001 by Taylor & Francis
11 New Fetter Lane, London EC4P 4EE

Simultaneously published in the USA and Canada
by Taylor & Francis
29 West 35th Street, New York, NY 10001

Taylor & Francis is an imprint of the Taylor & Francis Group

© 2001 Helen Macbeth and Prakash Shetty

Typeset in Baskerville by
Prepress Projects Ltd, Perth, Scotland
Printed and bound in Great Britain by
St Edmundsbury Press, Bury St Edmunds, Suffolk

British Library Cataloguing in Publication Data
A catalogue record for this book is available
from the British Library

Library of Congress Cataloging in Publication Data
Health and ethnicity / edited by Helen Macbeth & Prakash Shetty.
    p. cm. – (Society for the Study of Human Biology symposium
    series ; 41)
    Includes bibliographical references and index.
    1. Ethnic groups – Health and hygiene. 2. Minorities – Health
and hygiene. 3. Minorities – Medical care. 4. Social medicine. 5.
Health – Cross-cultural studies. I. Macbeth, Helen M. II. Shetty,
Prakash S. III. Series.
RA448.4. H37   2001   00-046676
613′089–dc21

ISBN 0-415-24166-9 (HB)
ISBN 0-415-24167-7 (PB)

Contents

Figures

Tables

Contributors

Sonia S. Anand
Assistant Professor of Medicine
Population Health Section
McMaster Clinic
Hamilton General Hospital
237 Barton St East
Hamilton
Ontario L8L 2X2
Canada

N. Appaji Rao
CSIR Emeritus Scientist
Department of Biochemistry
Indian Institute of Science
Bangalore 560 012
India

R. Balarajan
London School of Hygiene and Tropical Medicine
Keppel Street
London WC1E 7HT
UK

G. Baskaran
Postdoctoral Fellow
Department of Biochemistry
Indian Institute of Science
Bangalore 560 012
India

Alan H. Bittles
Foundation Professor of Human Biology
Centre for Human Genetics
Edith Cowan University
100 Joondalup Drive
Joondalup 6027
Western Australia

Raj Bhopal
Bruce and John Usher Professor of Public Health
Public Health Sciences
University of Edinburgh Medical School
Teviot Place
Edinburgh EH8 9AG
UK

Janet Cahill
Western Australian Institute for Medical Research
Medical Research Foundation Building
Rear 50 Murray Street
Perth 6000
Western Australia

George Davey Smith
Department of Social Medicine
University of Bristol
Canynge Hall
Whiteladies Road
Bristol
BS8 2PR
UK

Kevin A. Fenton
Senior Lecturer in Epidemiology and Public Health
Department of Sexually Transmitted Diseases
Royal Free and University College Medical School
University College London
Off Capper Street
London WC1E 6AU
UK

Gilbert Lewis
Department of Social Anthropology
Fellow
St John's College
Cambridge CB2 1TP
UK

Roland Littlewood
Professor of Psychiatry and Anthropology
Department of Psychiatry and Behavioural Sciences
University College London
Wolfson Building
46 Riding House Street
London W1N 8AA
UK

Paul McKeigue
Reader in Metabolic and Genetic Epidemiology
Epidemiology Unit
London School of Hygiene and Tropical Medicine
Keppel Street
London WC1E 7HT
UK

Anthony J. McMichael
Professor of Epidemiology
London School of Hygiene and Tropical Medicine
Keppel Street
London WC1E 7HT
UK

James Y. Nazroo
Senior Lecturer in Sociology
Department of Epidemiology and Public Health
University College London
1–19 Torrington Place
London WC1E 6BT
UK

Helen Macbeth
Principal Lecturer in Anthropology
Department of Anthropology
School of Social Sciences and Law
Oxford Brookes University
Headington
Oxford OX3 0BP
UK

D. Max Parkin
Chief, Unit of Descriptive Epidemiology
International Agency for Research on Cancer
150 cours Albert Thomas
69372 Lyon Cedex 08
France

H. S. Savithri
Professor of Biochemistry
Indian Institute of Science
Bangalore 560 012
India

Prakash Shetty
Professor of Human Nutrition
Public Health Nutrition Unit
London School of Hygiene and Tropical Medicine
49–51 Bedford Square
London WC1E 3DP
UK

H. S. Venkatesha Murthy
Medical Practioner
Department of Biochemistry
Indian Institute of Science
Bangalore 560 012
India

Wei Wang
Postdocroral Research Fellow
Centre for Human Genetics
Edith Cowan University
100 Joondalup Drive
Joondalup 6027
Western Australia

Ryk Ward
Professor of Biological Anthropology
Institute of Biological Anthropology
University of Oxford
58 Banbury Road
Oxford OX2
UK

David J. Weatherall
Regius Professor of Medicine
Institute of Molecular Medicine
University of Oxford
John Radcliffe Hospital
Headington
Oxford OX3 9DS
UK

Kaye Wellings
Senior Lecturer
Sexual Health Programme
Department of Public Health
London School of Hygiene and Tropical Medicine
Keppel Street
London WC1E 7HT
UK

Salim Yusuf
Professor of Medicine
Preventive Cardiology and Therapeutics Research Program
Hamilton Civic Hospital Research Centre
McMaster University
Hamilton
Canada

Preface

In multicultural societies there is increasing discussion about variations in the risk of disease and differences in the health experience of individuals from different ethnic groups. In the last two decades or more, ethnic differences in health outcomes and experiences have received more and more attention. In addition, the topic has spread to different academic disciplines, and is being researched and reported in quite distinct styles with differing objectives. This made a multidisciplinary approach to the topic of 'Health and Ethnicity' a most appropriate and timely topic for the forty-first symposium of the *Society for the Study of Human Biology*, out of which this volume arises. This edited volume is aimed at explaining the diversity in 'biomedically' measurable health conditions due to determinants that can be considered as 'ethnic'. The issue has many aspects already discussed in the literature of quite different disciplines, and yet these aspects interrelate. It is in contrast to these segregationist approaches and in an attempt to bridge the gaps caused by increasing specialisation in academic endeavour that we selected the contributors to this volume. They were chosen for their expertise and their differing perspectives on the topic while attention was paid by us to maintain the cohesion of the volume. Neither the editors nor the contributors can aspire to present the whole picture or to unite the contributions into a seamless tapestry. However, we have aspired to juxtapose chapters by specialists in quite different areas of knowledge with the hope that we may illustrate the diversity of angles significant to all who are interested in any of the perspectives on this topic.

The Society for the Study of Human Biology and the editors wish to thank Oxford Brookes University for hosting this symposium. The editors, who were responsible also for organising the symposium, wish to record our gratitude to Nestle UK and to the South Asian Association, London, for sponsorship of the organisation of the symposium and to the European Multicultural Foundation for encouragement and support. We are grateful to the team of postgraduate students from Oxford Brookes who helped in hosting this meeting. Our debt of gratitude to the contributors and to our publishers who have ensured the success of this publication.

Helen Macbeth
Prakash Shetty
October 2000

1   Introduction

Helen Macbeth and Prakash Shetty

The topic of *Health and Ethnicity* has become recognised increasingly as of relevance in modern multicultural societies. Until very recently the clinical attitude to diversity in medical histories and conditions, due to ethnic differences, was generally viewed as due either to 'racial' attributes or to the problems of migration across the globe, but there are serious problems with each of these simplifications. The problem with racial explanations is that they are based on the premise of biologically discrete races, which clinal patterns of gene frequencies show to be inaccurate. One of the difficulties with basing explanations on migration is that in Britain it is still common to hear the term 'migrant' used for people who have never migrated but were born in the United Kingdom, perhaps to parents with English birth certificates. Such people may be asked where they came from and 'Northamptonshire' is not the expected answer, but may be the reality. Yet, these descendants of earlier trans-global migrants may show some of the same medical conditions as their migrant forebears that may not be entirely genetic in aetiology. Little sensitivity was given to the complexity of the issue, for example the genetic variation within and between smaller subgroups of larger geographic categories, the many cultural differences from diet to marriage preferences, and the psychological and socio-economic aspects that are so deeply intertwined with ethnicity. When 'culture' was considered, it was generally by social anthropologists who were more likely to discuss health beliefs about diagnosis and remedy within the context of the whole cosmology of that social group than to explain how features resulting from these ideas might affect the biological condition. For these researchers, the 'Western' biomedical sciences were frequently relegated to just another belief system, and the distinctive characteristic of Western science, that it is always seeking to confirm or disprove earlier ideas, ignored. In this way those who could have provided useful insight into cultural factors affecting biology saw no point in doing so.

Within the last 25 years, gradually increasing attention has been given to the topic, but it has been spread across different academic disciplines and so researched and reported in quite distinct styles with varying theoretical goals. Two roughly contemporary books, each well known in their relevant spheres, illustrate the gap between two of the approaches. Social anthropologists and other social scientists were perhaps introduced to the topic by Helman (1984), while the collection of papers edited by Cruickshank and Beevers (1989) was aimed at a more medical readership. Not only has this dichotomy continued but also there are significant sub-disciplinary and theoretical splits either side of the primarily biomedical and the primarily socio-cultural–political divide. The latter multiplicity, mostly within social anthropology, is well described by Sargent and Johnson (1996) in their *Handbook of Medical Anthropology*, where 'anthropology' refers only to social anthropology and the words 'gene', 'genetics', 'multifactorial' and 'inheritance' do not even appear in the subject index.

It is in contrast to the above segregationist approach and in an attempt to bridge the gaps caused by specialisation into smaller and smaller units of academic endeavour, that contributors to this volume were chosen. Of course, the editors and contributors do not and cannot aspire to present the whole picture or even unite the contributions into a seamless tapestry, but by the juxtaposition of chapters by specialists in quite different areas of knowledge, we hope to demonstrate the diversity of angles significant to all who are interested in any one of the perspectives. The book is generally aimed at explaining the diversity in 'biomedically' measurable health conditions due to determinants and factors that can be called 'ethnic'.

However, the words, 'health' and 'ethnicity', are each fraught with semantic debate – a literature search on either would only show but a fraction of the library space taken up on each, but the next four chapters in this volume present viewpoints on these. Macbeth (Chapter 2) applies her enduring interest in the definition of the 'population' to the concept of the 'ethnic group' and finds it equally impossible to define. She argues, nevertheless, that for the purposes of classifications viable for clinical practice, observation and research some working definitions are important. She contrasts the simple categorisation used in much medical literature with the complexity of factors affecting health which can justifiably be described as 'ethnic'. There is a need, she argues, to research the factors themselves, or even a congruence of several factors, which may be obscured when a crude classification of ethnic or racial group is used. Bhopal (Chapter 3) acknowledges how the classification of ethnic groups based on concepts of race has become controversial, but he feels that if the concept of race is lost, acknowledgement of the effects of racism on disease patterns may be ignored. His chapter emphasises the value of simple classificatory groupings for medical assessment, but identifies how differences in the basis of grouping can be useful for different conditions and purposes, whether for clinical use or for achieving research-oriented objectives. Using the concept of 'race' can, he argues, be valuable for some purposes although a new term such as 'identifiable population' may become useful in other circumstances. What is important for science is conformity of usage both at national and international levels.

Touched upon in Bhopal's chapter but examined and emphasised more comprehensively in Chapter 4 by Nazroo and Davey Smith are the socio-economic inequalities between groups identified by racial or ethnic labels. Nazroo and Davey Smith report the patterns in the debate about the interaction of socio-economic and ethnic factors in explaining the differences in health across ethnic groups in terms of both morbidity and mortality. They discuss positions at one end of the spectrum which imply that socio-economic status makes a minimal or no contribution to ethnic inequalities in health, while the cultural and genetic elements of ethnicity play a highly significant role. At the other end of the spectrum, others argue that ethnic inequalities in health are predominantly determined by socio-economic inequalities. Using evidence on mortality and morbidity rates from both the United States of America and the United Kingdom, Nazroo and Davey Smith explore the contribution of socio-economic factors to ethnic inequalities in health, and point to the methodological and conceptual pitfalls that beset such examination.

In these three chapters, as in much of the volume, the ideas of health and ill health are firmly within the 'Western' biomedical model, but this is itself a cultural phenomenon. In the next chapter (Chapter 5), Lewis extends our perception of health and ill health by discussing how they are considered within other cultures. Consideration of the viewpoints of people from other cultures highlights that in no individual of any society is the mere absence of scientifically identifiable pathology a sufficient description of good health. This point is too frequently ignored in the biomedical literature but it has medical significance. Only when attending a clinic being observed can an individual be recorded as part of the resultant research statistics, and Carney (1989) has demonstrated the ethnic unevenness of attendance at a general practitioner's surgery. There are, of course, many other ways in which health beliefs affect both the conditions and their care with 'biomedically' measurable results. Lewis argues that concepts of health and well-being in the European medical tradition do not necessarily serve as a guide to corresponding standards and concepts in non-European societies and cultures.

That people in different societies are socialised into quite different patterns of behaviour is widely recognised now, thanks to the popularisation of social anthropology (MacClancy and McDonaugh 1996). However, this may not include the acceptance that something viewed in 'Western' society as undesirable and even medically risky for the offspring might provide important lifestyle advantages in the circumstances of some non-Western cultures. An example of this is the custom of closely consanguineous marriages. Bittles *et al.* (Chapter 6) debates the biological significance of such consanguineous marriages, explaining that first-cousin marriages are common in many societies around the world and the inbreeding disadvantages of such marriages in these societies and over time have tended to be exaggerated by 'Western' scientists. It is not surprising, therefore, that health care professionals in Europe and America view the custom of preferential first-cousin marriage as something to counsel against. Recessive conditions, such as thalassaemia, are used to exemplify the genetic disadvantage at the individual level, but Bittles *et al.* encourage a different view of the practice. They do this not so much by emphasising the socio-economic advantages, but by identifying opposing arguments about the biological consequences of inbreeding at population level.

Weatherall's consideration of the inherited disorders of haemoglobin, such as the thalassaemias (Chapter 7), continues the discussion of the evolution of gene frequencies in populations. After an introduction to the biology and the global variation in frequency of these single recessive gene characteristics he illustrates how migration and ethnic clustering of migrants affects their distribution in multicultural 'Western' societies. He discusses how these diseases have reached a high frequency due to heterozygote advantage against the infectious agent for malaria (*Plasmodium falciparum*) and explains why they occur in certain groups whose ancestors have been exposed to endemic malaria in the past. Weatherall suggests that because of demographic changes with improvements in health, as a result of economic development in developing societies, these diseases will present a major public health problem in the new millennium. After an elegant examination of the interaction of factors, geographical and temporal, genetic and non-genetic, involved in the patterns of disease risk, Ward (Chapter 8) takes forward the discussion of the consequences of genetic variability for ethnic differences in disease risk – for both communicable and non-communicable diseases. The cultural processes that maintain ethnicity have inevitably led to a certain amount of genetic differentiation, and this is discussed, but he warns against the use of an ethnic 'label' as a surrogate for genetic distinctiveness, since 'ethnic groups are as variable in their ecology as they are in their genes'.

First, detailed genetic information is provided on some monogenic diseases that show differences in frequency between ethnic groups and then the diversity of their mutational evolution is emphasised. Even with regard to the effects of single genes the topic of interaction with ecological factors is pursued. Here ecology is used in its widest sense, including all extrinsic components. Ward continues with a discussion of the polygenic conditions and their even more complex interaction with non-genetic factors. He argues that the overall extent to which genetic differences between ethnic groups influence the distribution of such multifactorial diseases as cardiovascular disease is largely unknown as both genetic and environmental factors contribute to their occurrence and distribution. Using, as a detailed example, the predisposition to hypertension in populations of African ancestry, he shows clearly how diversity between groups can be due to differences in allelic frequency and in environment. His conclusion is that within and between populations that have African ancestry, variations in risk for hypertension are primarily due to environmental causes, but that genetic explanations are more significant for the difference between these and the non-African populations. He makes the important point that research strategies to identify major genes and non-genetic factors that influence risk of complex diseases should take into account that both gene frequencies and environmental conditions tend to vary between ethnic groups.

In the following chapters of this volume emphasis is on the multifactorial conditions which manifest as disease and compromise health. The authors show how variations in health and disease risk between population groups are the result of the expression of the genetic potential under the effects of varying environmental influences and not merely due to the inherent genetic potential alone. McKeigue (Chapter 9) approaches the topic of disentangling the genetic and the non-genetic contributions to disease risk and suggests that migrant studies complemented by investigations using genetic markers in recently 'admixed' populations can help to determine whether ethnic differences in disease risk are attributable to environmental or genetic factors. He argues that the study of these populations can show genetic linkages that are valuable for identifying genetic components in complex characteristics. McKeigue suggests that in situations where recent admixture has occurred between two ethnic or racial groups with different disease risks due to genetic causes, it is in principle possible to map the genes that underlie these ethnic differences in risk. The method, which he outlines, is similar to linkage analysis of a cross between two experimental strains of animals.

McMichael pursues the theme of multifactorial causes for ethnic variations in health and argues that explanations of human population differences in disease risks are understood better by exploration of 'ancient, divergent, evolutionary paths' (Chapter 10). This idea that populations have had a past pattern of divergence provides an interesting contrast to McKeigue's approach of recently 'admixed' populations and seems to suggest that migration and admixture were not always part of our evolutionary past – a contention that would probably not be supported by either author. McMichael exemplifies his argument with non-insulin-dependent diabetes and shows how ecological components are relevant not only to contemporary non-genetic factors but also to the genetic heritage of different populations and their ancestors. This heritage, he argues, was an evolutionary adaptation to earlier environments as the ancestors migrated out of Africa and gradually changed their diets. He concludes that insights into the interplay between environment, diet and disease are a reminder of the intrinsically ecological dimension of population variations in health and disease, and that cultural development has buffered to a large extent man's relationship with the natural world. Finally, he makes two important points. The first is that we cannot discard the heritage of the long and intimate relationship that prevailed over many millennia of our evolution into the modern human species that we are. The second is that putative long-standing differences between populations are not necessarily constitutional metabolic weaknesses since, given the right dietary environment, they do not manifest as metabolic abnormalities and hence disease.

Shetty, on the other hand, examines a range of biological and disease risk factors which reveal different levels of interaction between genetic and environmental determinants, particularly those related to food and nutrition over a much shorter time span (Chapter 11). For instance, human lactation is a robust biological process such that the volume of milk produced at peak lactation is similar in women from a wide variety of racial or ethnic, cultural and nutritional circumstances. In contrast, differences in bone mineral density and risk of osteoporosis are markedly different between racial groups and cannot be simply attributed to persistent differences in nutritional, metabolic or lifestyle factors. Meanwhile, it is clear that differences in taste preferences evident in infants and children of some ethnic groups are influenced by external factors such as feeding. Rapid and dramatic changes in food, nutrition and lifestyles associated with migration or urbanisation have enhanced some disease risks, and the resultant variations have been designated as ethnic differences, but much of this variation might be more accurately described as attributable to the 'nutrition transition'. Reversion to (as in Australian Aborigines) or retention of (as in Mexican Pima Indians) traditional lifestyles reduces these risks, thereby supporting the view that these observed ethnic variations in disease risk are as much the result of 'nutrition transition' as due to any genetic differences.

Anand and Yusuf continue the theme of ethnic variations of disease risk by reviewing the global data on population variations in cardiovascular disease risk (Chapter 12). They have meticulously compared the cardiovascular disease prevalence and the risk factors among a wide range of population groups such as Europeans, Japanese, Chinese, South Asians and Africans and highlighted differences both in the disease burden and in the predisposing risk factors. They have documented the variations in these features among migrant population groups of African and South Asian origin compared with the native populations in developed societies in Europe and North America. In the case of North America, they have in addition also compared cardiovascular disease risk among the indigenous or Aboriginal tribes as well as those of Asian and Hispanic origin with those of European origin. Based on urban–rural differences and on the more recent dietary and lifestyle changes in these varied populations (both native and migrant), they illustrate the interaction between environmental and genetic factors in the manifestation of ethnic variations in cardiovascular disease risk. They emphasise the fact that conventional risk factors of cardiovascular disease risk operate in all populations and that the degree of variation at which they lead to the clinical manifestation of the disease may be attributable to differences in either protective or adverse genetic factors. Anand and Yusuf conclude by emphasising the role of socio-economic development and the urbanisation along with the consequent changes in diet and lifestyles and the increasing life expectancy in contributing to the increase in the disease burden due to cardiovascular diseases in developing countries and the need for preventive strategies to deal with this emerging problem.

Parkin tackles the topic of ethnic differences in the incidence of cancers

(Chapter 13). He starts by emphasising the need for valid incidence data for different groups and the importance of the use of such data for examining ethnic differences in cancer. Some of the global data on cancer are based on mortality, but the differential access to health care between groups can affect survival and so the comparability of such mortality data when used to study variations in disease risk. He outlines the difference between descriptive and analytical studies and examines the available information on population differences in several different types of cancers, thereby showing the success of epidemiology in identifying environmental determinants of some cancers. Macbeth's argument for greater attention to the variables relevant to ethnic self-identification should be emphasised as potentially valuable to this approach (Chapter 2). Parkin concludes by emphasising that inherited susceptibility may be due to differences in the frequency of dominant genes conferring high risk (such as in the case of breast cancer) or to genetic polymorphism in enzymes metabolising or activating carcinogens. Although ethnic differences in the prevalence of mutations of such genes are known, it is not yet clear how much of the observed differences in the incidence of cancer they explain.

So far, examination of ethnic variations in disease risk has not focused on conditions that manifest as mental or psychiatric disorders, and it is not surprising that Littlewood, who tackles these (Chapter 14), begins by clarifying some of the difficulties with vocabulary and methodology. He gives a brief history of these problems, the criticisms and the attempts to overcome them, and emphasises the significance of secular changes evident in these conditions over time. Some of the issues he tackles include, for instance, the shift in emphasis from the consequences of migration or 'racial' attributes to a greater interest in the role of cultural diversity. He also attempts to examine the current ambiguous role of 'culture', both in demands for the provision of equal and appropriate psychiatric services in psychotherapy and in the current theoretical arguments about the pathogenesis of mental illness. This is as relevant to the population at large as it is to minority ethnic populations.

Culture and ethnicity have the potential to influence sexual health in a number of ways. Fenton and Wellings (Chapter 15) examine the aspect of sexual health. They discuss the various influences that operate through a number of mechanisms which, in concert, may act to place ethnic communities at varying risk of adverse sexual health outcome, such as infection or unplanned conception, and thereby compromise the success of current risk reduction strategies. Cultural influences interact with biological mechanisms to influence the risk of these adverse health outcomes, while religion may be one feature that reinforces cultural influences on sexual behaviour. Fenton and Wellings emphasise the need for a better understanding of the complex reasons for ethnic differences and inequalities in sexual health in order to set in place appropriate health care strategies for both prevention and treatment. In the final chapter Balarajan casts a critical eye on the policy implications of ethnic variations in health and disease in a multicultural society like that found, for example, in the United Kingdom. He states that while significant strides have been made in terms of acceptance of the multicultural nature of society and of the diversity within its population, health and social care agencies face the challenge of providing a service that is equitable to all regardless of colour or creed. He believes that lack of resources may often be used as an excuse for inertia, but he argues that the provision of a service that is inclusive to all communities and responds to changing needs does not require vast expenditure but practical and innovative ways of redistributing the existing resources and the political will to see the changes through.

Readers who seek in this book straightforward answers to simple questions about the ethnic dimension in health and ill health may be frustrated, as all the issues discussed demonstrate increasingly intricate levels of complexity. Those who have considered the topic, as many have, from the populist perceptions of a simple dichotomy in the so-called 'nature nurture debate' (Macbeth 1989) will find, in these chapters, ample testimony to the intimate interaction of a multiplicity of factors and processes, genetic and non-genetic. Those who had perceived ethnic groups primarily in terms of their inherited, perhaps visible, characteristics will, we hope, learn that such definitions are insufficient, and how difficult it is to identify not only the groupings but also all the social, cultural and physical features in their differing ecologies. Yet these ecological details should be carefully studied, for some of the aspects may be considered by the people themselves as highly relevant to their self-definition as a group. This may be important in two ways. On the one hand, the aspects may be factors environmentally affecting a given health condition, in which case a link between that health condition and ethnic identity will be manifest. On the other hand, the self-definition, in turn, is likely to affect marriage patterns and so the gene frequencies in later generations, thereby linking the non-genetic bases for that self-definition indirectly to inherited tendencies. As genes are only codes for biochemical processes that develop in conjunction with internal and external environmental factors, the resultant interaction may further emphasise ethnic diversity in disease experience.

This all points to the need for as much information as possible on the social and cultural bases for self-definition. However, the bases are themselves labile; they change over time and in different ecological and socio-economic settings; they vary between individuals and are likely to be contextual for all. Furthermore, these are not variables that can be easily used in quantitative analyses, but require slower ethnographic observation. The way forward, therefore, for medical, social and political objectives, must surely be to seek a greater understanding through cross-disciplinary discussion and research. Past confrontations between biological and social scientists now appear dated, but even so real cooperation in medical research and administration remains rare. The divergence of academic objectives, philosophies and methodologies has hindered such cooperation, but the editors hope that the conjunction of the chapters in this volume will throw light on the topic of Health and Ethnicity and has exemplified the benefits of a cross-disciplinary approach.

Acknowledgements

The editors are grateful for the secretarial, clerical and editorial assistance of Diana Roberts, Eleanor McDonald, Fiona Mowatt and Sue Lawry.

References

Carney, T. (1989) 'Ethnic populations and GPs' work load', *British Medical Journal,* 299, 930–931.

Cruickshank, J.K. and Beevers, D.G. (1989) *Ethnic Factors in Health and Disease*, London: Wright.

Helman, C. (1984) *Culture, Health and Illness: an Introduction for Health Professionals*, Bristol: Wright.

Macbeth, H.M. (1989) ' "Nature/Nurture" – the false dichotomies', *Anthropology Today*, 5(4): 12–15.

MacClancy, J. and McDonaugh, C. (1996) *Popularizing Anthropology*, London: Routledge.

Sargent, C.F. and Johnson, T.M. (1996) *Handbook of Medical Anthropology: Contemporary Theory and Method* (Revised Edition), Westport: Greenwood Press.

2   Defining the ethnic group

Important and impossible

Helen Macbeth

The start to this chapter is deliberately personal to highlight some of the complexity of the topic in situations where political sensitivity may be less striking. When I was arranging research interviews of United Kingdom migrants in the western suburbs of Sydney, an Australian teenager with a smart coastal address said to me 'Oh, among the ethnics!' Is ethnicity, then, something only relating to *others*? Chapman (1993) provides a short history of derivation and use of the word. Am I not ethnic too? I confess to some discomfort that I was not allowed a vote in the recent Scottish referendum on devolution, while my brother-in-law with impeccably English ancestry and culture was able to vote simply because of his address. Even more ironically that address is in the village of my paternal grandfather and his crofter antecedents. My other grandparents were also Scottish born and I was feeling some sense of Scottish ethnicity although born and living in England. What matters, then, this self-definition or the geography of today's electoral registers? I have even been called a 'bloody Celt' by an academic supervisor who felt I was short on Lancastrian discipline – the point may have been valid, but the stereotyping within the phrasing doubtful. The self-definition and the supervisor's description clearly overlap despite my accent and current address. Is this overlap in any way due to my physical appearance or just my surname? Is the residence of myself or of my ancestors more significant, and what of the certain mobility of some of these ancestors?

If you wished to classify my ethnic group for medical purposes you might be well advised to consider my Scottish ancestry and pigmentation, as well as the culinary habits of my mother and her mother, as these might be more significant than my current address. However, even leaving aside more complicated transatlantic aspects of my personal history, my ethnicity is even harder to describe, for although I may be Scottish in England, I accept that I am considered very English when in Scotland. What is more, in both Scotland and England, lifestyle and linguistic differences between different groups, geographic and socio-economic, are many. Even in 1701, Defoe had explained how mixed is the ancestry of 'The True-born Englishman' (Defoe 1701). So, just as my own ethnicity is hard to classify, other individuals have complicated ethnicity and all ethnic groups are similarly hard to define. Exceptional groups may exist with some truly isolating features, but this is unlikely as it presumes a social homogeneity within that isolated group. Furthermore, ethnicity only becomes an issue where cultural groups are in some contact with each other. Any contact is likely to involve some individual mobility and some exchange of ideas and genes.

In the 1970s, while working on research concerned with residents of neighbouring Oxfordshire villages anecdotally referred to as 'the Otmoor population', I began wrestling with the concept of 'population' (Macbeth 1985). Steeped in the contemporary debates about village endogamy (Cavalli-Sforza and Bodmer 1971) in Palma villages or village exogamy and consequent gene flow, as shown in the marriage registers of these Oxfordshire villages (Boyce, Küchemann and Harrison 1968), I could not accept the phrase 'Otmoor population' (Macbeth 1985). It was not until the late 1980s that Gomila's (1976) paper 'Définir la population' was drawn to my attention. At about the same time I read Ardener's (1972) contribution to the concept of 'population'. From this background my ideas on 'population' and so on 'ethnic group' developed and were discussed (Macbeth 1993). While this chapter re-echoes some of the points made then, they are expanded with reference to the topic of this volume.

As might be expected of this topic, a large social anthropological and sociological literature about ethnicity exists (e.g. Barth 1969, Banks 1996, Chapman 1993, Cohen 1985, Tonkin *et al.* 1989), but it remains an elusive concept, interacting intimately with concepts of race and racism (e.g. Bhopal, this volume, Jenkins 1997) and with nationhood, nationality and nationalism (e.g. Eriksen 1993, Llobera 1989, Werbner 1996). Whatever it is, it is maintained through culture and socialisation and it affects health-related factors in many ways. Of prime importance are marriage preferences or obligations. While these are much discussed by social scientists, it has been left to the geneticists (e.g. Barbujani and Sokal 1990, Bittles and Neel 1994, Modell 1997) to link these patterns to distributions of gene frequencies. As people find mates within their cultural group, genes cluster and are passed on predominantly within that cultural group making ethnicity an independent social variable. In this way the clustering of the genes is not so much the cause of ethnicity as the outcome, the dependent variable. It is also true that situations do exist where characteristics under partial or total genetic control may be used for social classification and this can lead to a two-way process of classification and gene clustering, via stereotyping.

This early reference to genetic clustering does not imply genetic determinism of everything biological. With cultural control of so many aspects of human lifestyle, ethnicity is involved in many non-genetic factors affecting biology since conception. Ethnicity, for example, is involved in the development of food preferences (e.g. Rozin *et al.* 1986, Macbeth 1997), the cultural influences on food choices (e.g. Bourdieu 1979, MacClancy 1992, Messer 1984), the marketing and even the availability of foods, the eating patterns and so the content and timing of food intake, and, of course, the cuisine (MacClancy 1992). Cultures, including diets, however, have features which change and others which seem to withstand change. Frequently there is a recognition of change in familiar cultures but a belief that 'other' cultures endure unchanged. The latter is probably an inaccurate description of the daily activities or diet of any group. Furthermore, 'ethnic' foods need not be regularly consumed: neither haggis nor paella is consumed often by those for whom each is considered ethnic. The recent growth in the market of British cookbooks assigned to different ethnicities and localities provides delicious entertainment and reinforces stereotypes, but may poorly reflect reality in the daily lives of those presumed to eat these dishes (e.g. Macbeth 1998).

Ethnicity and culture also affect the use and abuse of other consumptions, the extent of family support or independence, male and female activities (e.g. MacCormack and Strathern 1980), exercise (e.g. MacClancy 1996) and, within the framework of society at large, even work and study routines and ethics. The role of religion and beliefs must not be forgotten, especially where these are expressly concerned with health and health care. Clearly the ways in which cultural preferences determine human biology are myriad. Furthermore, what might be considered ethnic tends to be inextricable from what is considered socio-economic in the life experiences of the so-called 'minority groups' in Western recipient countries (see Nazroo and Davey Smith, this volume).

All this does not exclude the significance of locality, the rest of the environment, both physical and social. The list can continue for pages, but the significant aspect is that despite some sophisticated statistical attempts there is no way to disentangle all these factors and their interacting effects on our multifactorial characteristics. It is not just that the genetic and the non-genetic interact, but also the ethnic and the economic, the locality and the ancestry, etc. All can be shown to affect biology.

It would be superfluous in this volume to review in detail recent medical literature about ethnic differences, but readers will be aware of the increase in reference to ethnicity in the last quarter century. There is, however, an aspect of this literature which itself deserves more attention – the categorisation of the people studied. Table 2.1 provides a few examples of classifications used. While 'White, Black and Asian', (or equivalent paraphrases) are the most common in the United Kingdom, 'White, Black and Hispanic' are more common in American articles. If 'Asians' are mentioned in the United States, Chinese and Japanese are probably referred to, while in the United Kingdom those from the Indian subcontinent are being considered. In the medical papers of other nations there are other divisions, but most are reminiscent of outdated and discredited concepts of biologically discrete racial groups. Take, for example, Steer *et al* (1995), who refer to 'White, Indo-Pakistani, Afro-Caribbean, Black African, Mediterranean, Oriental and others'. If one unites the African categories and replaces Mediterranean with American Indians, the eighteenth-century ideas of Blumenbach (Jurmain *et al.* 1999) are clearly reflected.

Table 2.1 Categories that have been used in medical literature: some recent examples

White, Black Asian
Black, White
Black, Asian
European, Asian, Afro-Caribbean
White, Indo-Pakistani, Afro-Caribbean, Black African, Mediterranean, Oriental, other
White, West Indian. Indian subcontinent
Black Caribbean, Black African
Afro-Caribbean, European
Asian, African Caribbean
Caucasian, South Asian, Afro-Caribbean
Indian subcontinent origin, European
Black and ethnic minority women
South Asians and Europeans
White, Black, Bangladeshi, Chinese and Vietnamese, other
White, Indian, Pakistani, Bangladeshi, Black, Chinese, other
South Asian, Latin American, Mediterranean, Black African
White, Indo-Pakistani, Afro-Caribbean, Oriental, other

The most powerful argument against the existence of discrete races is the clinal distributions of gene frequencies across geographic space. Yet, however much the words 'ethnic group' become the politically correct phrase, still the idea of different 'races' is deep within the concepts of our and other societies. Medical researchers are part of society, and, not surprisingly, when they seek appropriate ways and terminology to group individuals according to ethnic diversity, their categories frequently reflect the traditional ideas of 'race'. Often the grouping is as crude as that made by much less educated members of society, and in one respect that might not be so illogical, since popular attitudes impose some common life experiences on those divided and grouped along the lines perceived of as 'race'. Notably, despite legislation, access to some socio-economic activities and jobs may be affected and this in turn influences health experiences. So, as one part of ethnicity is the classification of others into a group by those *outside* that group, it may sometimes be academically defensible that the mainstream attitudes to 'race' and racial groups be used, whatever the population geneticists demonstrate about gene frequencies. However, such categories remain a very poor reflection of all the ethnic differences that affect human biology and so health.

Not only could the resultant stereotyping be risky in the diagnosis of individuals, but even more dangerous in my view is the possibility that the health differences so recorded in the research may be used to reconfirm the idea that there is biological validity in the categories first used, i.e. based on the social concepts of races. I have heard this done, and the point is revisited below.

In the United Kingdom as from 1 April (of all dates!) 1995, the Department of Health required hospitals to collect data on the ethnic group of patients. Discussions about categories to be used inevitably followed (e.g. Aspinall 1995, Hilton 1996), continue and will continue, because, as with social class, there are no clear boundaries to differentiate people into ethnic groups. There are factors, largely cultural, that bind some into social clusters, but there are overlapping contours of closeness around all such clusters. The fact that the Department of Health categories were based on census categories (Majeed *et al.* 1995) merely provides a commonality of classification, valuable perhaps for some comparisons. It does not ratify the classification. It is arguable that a freedom exists for census data and demography to use any consistent classification so long as only numbers are being considered. It is when these classifications and numbers are used for other purposes, as they will be for that is the function of census data, that problems arise. Freedom to use *any* classification certainly does not exist for medical research when the validity of the exercise is to identify trends in epidemiology that might assist in diagnosis and treatment. The point here is biology and enquiry into relationships between any lifestyle variable(s) and/or genetic characteric(s) and some aspect(s) of health and disease. The aim frequently is to illuminate aetiology, and hopefully ameliorate the condition, or the inequalities in its distribution, by searching for information that is not only descriptive but also predictive.

If ethnic classifications are only popular stereotypes suggesting an amalgamation of genetic propensities and lifestyle variables, medical advice to an individual for whom the stereotype does not apply in all aspects can be misleading or even fatal. This is as true for ethnic divisions within the so-called majority population as it is for any ethnic minority group. It is also true for other types of classification and stereotype.

Yet classifications of people into groups exist in all societies. The minimalist situation is 'our lot' and 'others', about which literature already is plentiful (Barth 1969, Cohen 1985) describing how one group's cohesion may be fostered by emphasis on what one is not. Definitions of boundaries become clearer where there is conflict. The light-hearted approach, above, to the author's Highland ethnicity can be contrasted to classificatory decisions young and elderly people today have to make in old Yugoslavia, in many parts of central Africa and in other places of conflict. A 17-year-old whose mother was English and father German was in England in the late summer of 1939 and had a stark choice to make, barely different from these classificatory decisions about ethnicity. In the European Union we are now all 'European' and the borders between nation-states are more open, but this has had an interesting corollary as the subdivisions called ethnic within nation states clamour for more attention as separate entities within this united Europe. Much of the author's current research is in an east-Pyrenean valley divided by the Franco-Spanish border, but united by its topography and, some would say, by the word 'Catalan'. Defining Catalan and Catalonia today is as difficult as defining ethnicity, but in this arena it is clear how people's ethnic affiliation can be contextual – '*our* Catalan cuisine', '*our* Catalan literature', but '*those* French' or '*those* Spanish' across the international border who act in some way that is undesirable or obtain some benefit *we* have missed out on. It is the same in any complex society. People have different roles and their ethnicity will tend to be appropriate for the context. In this way the factors relevant to biology may also vary with context. Finally, there is also change over time in people's cultures and attitudes.

Within this mosaic of inheritance, language, beliefs, loyalties, change and context lies ethnicity. We find this complexity quite comprehensible in people familiar to us, but it is equally true for people culturally distant from us, even though we may be slower to recognise this. Another corollary of this complexity is that the group within which it is appropriate to find a marriage partner may not be as clearly defined as the outsider (or the grandmother!) perceives. The fluidity of ethnic affiliation ensures that ethnic groups are not sealed containers of idiosyncratic genes. Where different definitions of the group do not coincide exactly, genes flow because of this flexibility of definition just as they do in the recognised cases of exogamy. With extremely rare exceptions, if any, ethnic groups are not isolates and gene frequencies are therefore clinal.

Such frequency distributions can be shown as contour lines in maps (Barbujani and Sokal 1990). Even such contour lines represent arbitrarily chosen quantities in the clinal situation. One could choose any series of intermediate quantities and draw the appropriate lines. One should also be hesitant to draw conclusions about gene frequencies either side of a boundary line across a clinal situation. In Figure 2.1 a hypothetical boundary is exemplified by the line x. If line x were a population boundary in a genocline, one could correctly say that the gene frequencies either side of that boundary were different. What would be incorrect, however, would be to say that this difference in gene frequencies ratified that line x is indeed a significant boundary between biological 'populations'. Any other line, e.g. line y (Figure 2.2), would similarly show genetic diversity between sectors, but the frequencies would be different. It is important, therefore, that gene frequencies either side of a boundary are not used to show that the boundary is biologically significant and that two populations are Mendelian, when a more detailed observation demonstrates a genocline. Furthermore, this misinformation about two separated Mendelian populations might subsequently be used for socio-political purposes; for this reason, geneticists should be just as aware of the problem suggested above as the epidemiologists. Clarke's (1997) criticism of the type of argument so far expressed in this chapter is that it is primarily concerned with what an ethnic group is not; this is a valid criticism by someone involved daily in clinical work. It is perhaps more useful to use Mackenzie and Crowcroft's (1996: 1054) point that 'describing the groups studied is better than trying to find a catch all name', and take note of Senior and Bhopal's (1994) bases for defining ethnic affiliation.

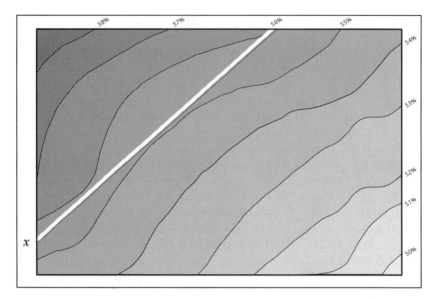

Figure 2.1 Gene frequencies either side of a hypothetical boundary line *x* . (Percentages refer to imaginary allele frequencies.)

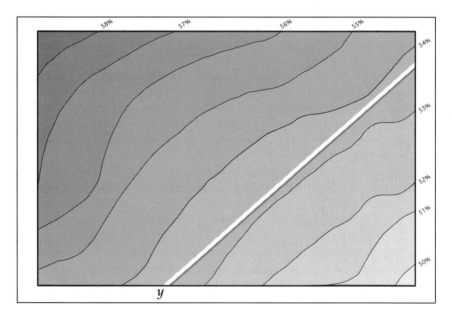

Figure 2.2 Gene frequencies either side of a hypothetical boundary line *y*. (Percentages refer to imaginary allele frequencies.)

Many of the social arguments above have been based on the emphasis people have put on to boundaries to effect group definition, even where the boundaries may have little biological significance. On the other hand Ardener (1972) argued that what binds a group is an important feature to observe. So, it would seem that one should research which cultural factors strengthen the cohesion: religious activities? commensality? sport? cuisine? dress? language or even accent? How strong are the social pressures for endogamy and how are these pressures sustained and to what extent? Does endogamy only refer to marriage, while other sexual partnerships frequently result in offspring? If so, between whom? A consideration of cultural features which foster cohesion may well prove significant in an analysis of health because of their implicit concordance with group self-definition. The social binding of an ethnic group may involve some of those lifestyle variables that affect multifactorial characteristics in our biology, and correlation of these with self-definition may be greater than the gene frequency information alone suggests. In this way, while the concordance of ethnicity with higher frequencies of some notorious monogenic diseases acts through ancestral geography and a cultural preference for endogamy, not always sustained, the correlation of ethnic self-classification with multifactorial conditions may be even greater because of the very activities which proclaim the ethnicity; one thinks of cuisine, religious practices, etc., as above. Even so the pattern is one of overlapping patches and not of boundaries enclosing discrete units.

It is clear that even the crude classifications of ethnic group used in medical literature (e.g. as shown in Table 2.1) have demonstrated biological diversity between the groups so defined. However, what seems to be needed now is much more detailed ethnographic information on the factors and activities, which bind a self-defining group as 'ethnic'. If this ethnographic information, while probably carried out by social scientists, could be aimed at illuminating the biological consequences and not just the social structure *per se*, such research might begin to have a predictive value medically. However, this is far from certain, because as soon as our knowledge reaches this level it might be too late. The dynamics of cultural change (e.g. McDonaugh 1997) create even more complexity for this quest, especially following migration and increasing assimilation into the *mores* of a recipient society, which itself would be changing. Taking a culinary example, ingredients and methods of cooking change even when those dishes, which appear to symbolise ethnic allegiance, continue (e.g. MacClancy 1992, González Turmo 1997). How many households today retain the kitchen practices (and timetable!) of the maternal grandmother? Not only do health care beliefs change as younger generations are educated for the same school curricula nationwide, but the science behind so-called 'Western' medicine is itself always progressing and being reinterpreted in different ways. Contrary to popular belief, change does occur in 'ethnic' lifestyles, even when some overt, perhaps highly visible, features, symbolising that ethnicity, apparently remain the same.

In summary, accurate definitions of ethnic groups are impossible because of the absence of meaningful boundaries. This impossibility is clearly demonstrated by the lack of concordance of definition when different people attempt to define the parameters of any group. Nevertheless, some factors, which deserve to be called ethnic, are highly significant to health experience and so are epidemiologically important. The question remains, however, can factors, which one considers to be ethnic, be studied unless one starts with some definition of the ethnic group or does one inevitably fall into a circular argument, confirming the significance of the classification one first chose in an arbitrary fashion? As self-definition tends to be contextual, it too is a chancy basis for definition, but it may be the best available, as it presumably emphasises some of those features which may be the most relevant to study. Finally, if the self-definition is allowed to be wordy and descriptive (Mackenzie and Crowcroft 1996), in the later statistics the researchers will be able to create alternative, hopefully meaningful, categories out of the variables in this descriptive information. In this way, variables, rather than ethnic labels, could be linked to the health differences observed. However, as Pringle and Rothera (1996) argue, there is a financial cost in collecting such descriptive data and the expected linkages should be clearly considered in advance. What is most needed, then, is greater public, and so political, recognition of the epidemiological importance of directing finances to such endeavours.

Acknowledgements

My thanks go to Eleanor McDonald for research and secretarial assistance and to Gerry Black for creating Figures 2.1 and 2.2.

References

Ardener, E. (1972) 'Language, ethnicity and population', *Journal of the Anthropology Society of Oxford*, 3(3): 125–132.

Aspinall, P.J. (1995) 'Department of Health's requirement for mandatory collection of data on ethnic groups of inpatients', *British Medical Journal*, 311, 1006–1009.

Banks, M. (1996) *Ethnicity: Anthropological Constructions*, London: Routledge.

Barbujani, G. and Sokal, R. (1990) 'Zones of sharp genetic change in Europe are also linguistic boundaries', *Proceedings of the National Academy of Sciences, USA*, 87, 1816–1819.

Barth, F. (ed.) (1969) *Ethnic Groups and Boundaries*, London: Allen and Unwin.

Bittles, A.H. and Neel, J.V. (1994) 'The costs of human inbreeding and their implications for variations at the DNA level', *Nature Genetics*, 8, 117–121.

Bourdieu, P. (1979) *Distinction: A Social Critique of the Judgement of Taste* (Translation R. Nice), London: Routledge and Kegan Paul.

Boyce, A.J., Küchemann, C.F. and Harrison, Biological AnthropologyG.A. (1968) 'The reconstruction of historical movement patterns', in Acheson, E.D. (ed.) *Record Linkage in Medicine*, Edinburgh: Livingstone, pp. 303–319.

Cavalli-Sforza, L.L. and Bodmer, W.F. (1971) *The Genetics of Human Populations*, San Francisco: W. H. Freeman.

Chapman, M. (1993) 'Social and biological aspects of ethnicity', in Chapman, M. (ed.) *Social and Biological Aspects of Ethnicity*, Oxford: Oxford University Press.

Clarke, A. (1997) 'Introduction', in Clarke, A. and Parsons, E. (eds.) *Culture, Kinship and Genes*, Basingstoke: Macmillan.

Cohen, A.P. (1985) *The Symbolic Construction of Community*, London: Routledge.

Eriksen, T.H. (1993) *Ethnicity and Nationalism: Anthropological Perspectives*, London: Pluto Press.

Defoe, D. (1701) *The True-Born Englishman*.

Gomila, J. (1976) 'Définir la population', in Jacquard, A. (ed.) *L'étude des isolats; Espoirs et limites*, Paris: Institut National d'Etudes Demographiques, pp. 5–36.

González Turmo, I. (1997) 'The pathways of taste: the west Andalucian case', in Macbeth, H.M. (ed.) *Food Preferences and Taste: Continuity and Change*, Oxford: Berghahn, pp. 115–126.

Hilton, C. (1996) 'Collecting ethnic-group data for inpatients: is it useful?', *British Medical Journal*, 313, 923–925.

Jenkins, R. (1997) *Rethinking Ethnicity*, London: Sage.

Jurmain, R., Nelson, H., Kilgore, L. and Trevathan, W. (1999) *Introduction to Physical Anthropology*, Belmont: Wadsworth.

Llobera, J. (1989) 'Catalan national identity: the dialectics of past and present', in Tonkin, E., McDonald, M. and Chapman, M. (eds) *History and Ethnicity*, London: Routledge.

Macbeth, H.M. (1985) 'Biological variation in human migrants', unpublished DPhil thesis, Oxford University.

Macbeth, H.M. (1993) 'Ethnicity and human biology', in Chapman, M. (ed.) *Social and Biological Aspects of Ethnicity*, Oxford: Oxford University Press, pp. 47–91.

Macbeth, H.M. (ed.) (1997) *Food Preferences and Taste: Continuity and Change*, Oxford: Berghahn.

Macbeth, H.M. (1998) 'Concepts of 'The Mediterranean Diet' in U.K. and Australia compared to food intake studies on the Catalan coast of the Mediterranean', *Rivista di Antropologia*, 76, 307–313.

MacClancy, J.V. (1992) *Consuming Culture*, London: Chapmans.

MacClancy, J.V. (ed.) (1996) *Sport, Identity and Ethnicity*, Oxford: Berg.

MacCormack, C.P. and Strathern, M. (eds) (1980) *Nature, Culture and Gender*, Cambridge: Cambridge University Press.

McDonaugh, C.E. (1997) 'Breaking the rules: changes in food acceptability among the Tharu of Nepal', in Macbeth, H.M. (ed.) *Food Preferences and Taste: Continuity and Change*, Oxford: Berghahn, pp. 155–166.

Mackenzie, K. and Crowcroft, N.S. (1996) 'Describing race, ethnicity and culture in medical research', *British Medical Journal*, 312, 1054.

Majeed, F.A., Cook, D.G., Poloniecki, J. and Martin, D. (1995) 'Using data from the 1991 census', *British Medical Journal*, 310, 1511–1514.

Messer, E. (1984) 'Anthropological perspectives on diet', *Annual Review of Anthropology*, 13, 205–250.

Modell, B. (1997) 'Kinship and medical genetics: a clinician's perspective', in Clarke, A. and Parsons, E. (eds) *Culture, Kinship and Genes*, Basingstoke: Macmillan.

Pringle, M. and Rothera, J. (1996) 'Practicality of recording patient ethnicity in general practice – descriptive intervention study and attitude survey', *British Medical Journal*, 312, 1080–1082.

Rozin, P., Fallon, A.E. and Augustoni-Ziskind, M. (1986) 'The child's conception of food: development of categories of accepted and rejected substances', *Journal of Nutrition Education*, 18, 75–81.

Senior, P.A. and Bhopal, R. (1994) 'Ethnicity as a variable in epidemiological research', *British Medical Journal*, 309, 327–330.

Steer, P., Alam, M.A., Wadsworth, J. and Welch, A. (1995) 'Relation between maternal haemoglobin concentration and birth-weight in different ethnic groups', *British Medical Journal*, 310, 489–491.

Tonkin, E., McDonald, M. and Chapman, M. (eds) (1989) *History and Ethnicity*, London: Routledge.

Werbner, P. (1996) ' "Our blood is green": cricket, identity and social empowerment among British Pakistanis', in MacClancy, J. (ed.) *Sport, Identity and Ethnicity*, Oxford: Berg, pp. 307–313.

3 Ethnicity and race as epidemiological variables

Centrality of purpose and context

Raj Bhopal

> Only when we move beyond race as a proxy and directly measure those concepts believed to be measured by race, will we make truly important advances in describing the true nature of racial variation in health.
>
> Thomas La Veist (1996: 21–29)

Introduction

Race and ethnicity are, probably, the most controversial and difficult of all commonly used epidemiological variables. They are also among the most effective in contributing to one crucial aspect of the epidemiological strategy: demonstrating population variations in disease (Polednak 1989, Smaje 1994). We are in the midst of a change of paradigm: a reconsideration of the race concept. It is a time of confusion and the need for reasoned debate is great.

Ethnicity and race are integral to much modern epidemiology and public health (Jones *et al.* 1991, Williams 1994, Ahdieh and Hahn 1996) but the historical legacy of these concepts in science is a long one. Racially orientated description and analysis was used by Hippocrates (Chadwick and Mann 1950), for whom geographical location and climate were closely linked to concepts of race. In the Hippocratic writings population characteristics such as cowardice, feebleness and mental agility were associated with differing climate and geography, and hence races. Currently, the most influential concept of race in medical research, despite its flaws scientifically (Kuper 1975, Stepan 1982, Barkan 1992), remains that of group differences due to biology. Despite all the criticisms, this remains the crux of dictionary definitions (Ellison 1998). This idea has been so powerful that societies have become *racialised*, i.e. they see race as a natural, primary (and neutral) means of grouping humans and understanding differences between them.

On the weight of 150 years of scientific analysis and popular usage, race is interpreted as the social group a person belongs to because of a mix of physical features, themselves attributable to genetic differences arising from evolution in a particular place. Physical differences, particularly skin colour, have provided an easy route for putting racism into practice. The theoretical concept of biological races has become an underpinning feature of *racialised* societies and, in turn, has created widely used social categories.

Ethnicity, by contrast, is the social group a person belongs to because of a shared culture, which means history, geographical origins, language, diet and other such features. There is no reason why physical features (i.e. biology) could not be one of these shared factors, especially when such features have influenced profoundly the history and culture of a group (as skin colour has).

In the last 50 or so years, the concept of race as a valid and important biological idea has been attacked and undermined, most effectively by advances in genetics (Kuper 1975, Osborne *et al.* 1978, Stepan 1982, Cooper 1984, Barkan 1992, Kreiger *et al.* 1993, La Veist 1994, McKenzie 1994). Social scientists are redefining race as a cultural and socio-political construct and not a biological one (Kreiger *et al.* 1993, La Veist 1994, Bennet 1997, Williams 1997). Paradoxically, the concept of ethnicity (primarily cultural) has been developed and increasingly used over the same period as a biological concept rather than a cultural one! The concept of race is changing, with greater emphasis on social, political and historical characteristics of a population. In much contemporary writing race has become virtually indistinguishable from ethnicity (Williams 1997). In practice, as race has been exposed as scientifically weak in reflecting biological differences, race is being redefined (Banton 1987). The social and political grip of race is such that scientists, whose values and beliefs, of course, reflect those of their society, prefer to redefine and re-shape the concept rather than reject it. There are also advocates for more radical action, including the outright rejection of the race concept (Ellison *et al.* 1996, Muntaner *et al.* 1996, Witzig 1996). Such criticism has caused concern and counter-argument (Walker 1997), particularly by those who see race as a means of drawing attention to inequalities (Smith 1993, Moss 1996, Bhopal 1997). A student at a seminar said to me '... race is a gigantic variable'. In her conception, race included socio-economic factors, including education, income, employment, racism and much else of importance, and encapsulated much of the idea of ethnicity.

Critique of the race variable is voluminous and growing fast. Much critique has concerned the lack of a clear definition of the concepts of race and ethnicity (Osborne *et al.* 1978, Copper 1984, Banton 1987, Kreiger *et al.* 1993, La Viest 1994, McKenzie 1994, Muntaner *et al* 1996, Witzig 1996, Ellison and De Wet 1997); lack of validity of racial and ethnic classifications (Gimenez 1989, Bhopal *et al.* 1991, *Morbidity Mortality Weekly Report* (MMWR) 1993, Special Section 1994, Hahn 1996, Bhopal 1997, Bennet and Bhopal 1998); the use of race as a confounding rather than an explanatory variable; and the failure to tackle the possibility that racism rather than race or ethnicity *per se* underlies differences in disease experience (Kreiger *et al.* 1993, McNeilly *et al.* 1995, Kreiger and Sidney 1996, Bhopal 1998).

Despite much theoretical critique, and practical experience of the harm that careless use of race does, many researchers and practitioners alike have remained convinced by the potential of race in both the population and the clinical sciences and in their applications (Rothschild 1981, Huth 1995, Walker 1997), and with the advances in genetics the interest in racial and ethnic variations is likely to grow, as illustrated in recent work to identify the genetic basis of the Black–White differences in hypertension (Baker *et al.* 1998). For many, research orientated towards race and ethnicity is self-evidently important (as it was seen to be in the past). Others have shown the difficulties of practical corrective action to ensure equity in health and health care without race and ethnicity data (Smith 1993, Moss 1996). Migration has spurred new thinking in Europe and is changing the scene in terms of both demography and disease patterns in the United States [Colledge *et al.* 1986, United States Department of Health and Human Services (USDHHS) 1985]. The quantity of race and ethnicity-orientated research continues to rise (Sheldon and Parker 1992).

We are in a period of uncertainty about the foundation of this type of research, with competing schools of thought. This state is aptly captured by the idea of paradigm change in science as proposed by Thomas Kuhn (1996). The field of race and ethnicity research is between paradigms, the biological paradigm of race having been abandoned by some scientists but with no clear successor.

La Veist (1996) (among others) has called for more and better research on race. The call is justified for the volume of race-based literature is increasing, irrespective of academic notes of caution. The challenge is to move speedily beyond critique, and towards developing, agreeing, disseminating and operationalising the best principles and practice.

The idea of this paper is to start with the observation that race and ethnicity research is perceived as important, and to develop principles to make it more effective. I also wish to move beyond the thirteen recommendations that have been summarised in Table 3.1 (Senior and Bhopal 1994, Bhopal 1997).

This analysis can be considered in the context of the questions: what are the characteristics of a good epidemiological variable? (Senior and Bhopal 1994); and do race and ethnicity exhibit these? According to Senior and Bhopal (1994) the attributes of a sound epidemiological variable are as follows.

- It should be accurately measurable.
- It should differentiate populations in some underlying characteristic relevant to health e.g. income, childhood circumstance, hormonal status, genetic inheritance, lifestyle.
- The observed differences in disease patterns should generate testable aetiological hypotheses, or be applicable to the planning and delivery of health care.

Table 3.2 lists the currently used imperfect methods of measuring race and ethnicity, and Table 3.3 shows the official classifications of race and ethnicity in the United Kingdom and United States. The recommendations in Table 3.1 and the substantial critique in the literature do not provide a route to specific action. Over 500 journals adhere to the detailed 'Uniform Requirements on Manuscripts Submitted to Biomedical Journals' issued by

Table 3.1 Recommendations on the use of ethnicity and race in health[a]

- Researchers, policy makers and professionals in the field of race, ethnicity and health should understand the history of the concept of race and the role of science.
- Ethnicity should be perceived as different from race and not as a synonym for the latter.
- Ethnicity's complex and fluid nature should be appreciated.
- The limitations of methods of classifying ethnic groups should be recognised.
- Researchers need to state their understanding of ethnicity and race, describe the characteristics of both the study and comparison populations, and provide and justify the ethnic coding.
- Investigators should recognise the potential influence of their personal values, including ethnocentricity i.e. the tendency to see matters from the perspective of their own ethnic group.
- Socio-economic differences should be considered as an explanation of differences in health between ethnic groups.
- Research on methods for ethnic classification should be given higher priority.
- Editors and researchers should develop and implement a policy on the conduct and reporting of race, ethnicity and health research.
- Ethnicity's fluid and dynamic nature means that results should not be generalised except with great caution.
- Results should be applied to the planning of health services.
- Observations of variations in disease should be followed by detailed examination of the relative importance of environmental, lifestyle, cultural and genetic influences.
- Race and ethnicity data, as for social class, have a key role in raising awareness of inequalities and stimulating policy and action.

Note
a This material is a synthesis and summary of recommendations published in two separate papers (Senior and Bhopal 1994, Bhopal 1997).

Table 3.2 Potential markers of race or ethnicity for self- or observer assignment

---

Relating mainly to concepts of race	*Relating mainly to concepts of ethnicity*
Skin colour	Name
Other physical features, such as hair texture and facial features	Language
Ancestral origin	Religion
	Diet
	Family origin
	Migration history

Table 3.3 UK 1991 census question on 'ethnic group'

Ethnic group: please tick the appropriate box

White	❑
Black Caribbean	❑
Black African	❑
Black other (please describe)	❑
Indian	❑
Pakistani	❑
Bangladeshi	❑
Chinese	❑
Any other ethnic group (please describe)	❑

If the person is descended from more than one ethnic or racial group, please tick the group to which the person considers he/she belongs, or tick the 'Any other ethnic group' box and describe the person's ancestry in the space provided.

the International Committee of Medical Journal Editors, which published in 1997 this statement on terminology for research on race and ethnicity: 'The definition and relevance of race and ethnicity are ambiguous. Authors should be particularly careful about using these categories' (International Committee for Medical Journal Editors 1997: 36–47).

The *British Medical Journal*'s (*BMJ*) recent subtle and theoretically apt guidance is based on the idea that the hypothesis should be the determining factor in racial groupings and terminology (*BMJ* 1996). However, much work on ethnicity and health is not done within an environment of generating and testing hypotheses, or by researchers with a deep knowledge about race and ethnicity as epidemiological variables.

Researchers are left with the decision either to avoid the controversy and difficulty associated with race and ethnicity variables (an action which may be socially, politically and scientifically unacceptable) or to muddle on, doing their best. New guidance, which helps to clarify when the concept of race is preferable and when ethnicity is better, is needed. Further, practitioners and researchers need guidance on when to collect detailed data, as recommended by several authors including Senior and Bhopal (1994) and La Veist (1996), and when not to.

This chapter proposes that the purpose, context and, if appropriate, hypothesis of the work at hand will dictate:

1   the underlying concept reflected by the words race and ethnicity;
2   the classification of race and ethnicity used;
3   the measurement methods; and

4   whether there is the need for direct measurement of the variables which
    are believed to be reflected by race and ethnicity as proxy measures.

Purposes and contexts

Political

The most ingrained of the purposes and contexts of race-based data collection
is political. Race-based data are needed to identify individuals and groups to
whom policies are to be applied differently, the policies themselves usually
being determined independently of scientific data, and usually on political
grounds. Examples of such policies are deciding which groups are allowed to
vote, go to a particular school, are eligible for land rights, preferential
allocation of jobs or for delivery of a service. Race-related questions have
been part of the United States census since 1790; and by counting, for the
purposes of political representation, slaves as three-fifths of a free person
and 'Indians not taxed' as no person, the issue of race was institutionalised
(Anderson and Fienberg 1995). The idea of racial superiority provided a
rationale for slavery, immigration policy and colonialism in the nineteenth
century and apartheid in the twentieth century. The history of the use of race
in politics is an unhappy one, so caution is necessary before advocating the
continued use of race in this way. One common and rational argument for
the retention of the race concept is that it is necessary to guide corrective
action to reverse the effect of past injustices.

One interesting example from the health care field is the vaccination for
children programme in the United States, where American Indians are one
of the entitlement categories for funding. To implement this policy a measure
which identifies American Indians is essential. The need here is for a quick,
simple way of identifying and counting people in different groups to plan
and deliver a service. There is no deeper need or purpose such as
understanding the costs, benefits and outcomes of vaccination. On the basis
of self-identification, or information on ancestral origins (with or without
some reliance on observation of physical characteristics), this might be
achieved. The underlying concept here is based on racial identity. Racial
classification is, here, a tool for enacting and monitoring a policy which is
itself generated in response to perceived unequal needs (or deserts, in the
sense of what one deserves). The policy is generated on political grounds, not
necessarily scientific ones. As such, the racial classification is also a socially
generated one.

For political purposes the crude division of society as White and non-White
may serve the purpose. Some advocate the idea that all discriminated minority
groups ought to describe themselves as Black, the word being a marker of a
discriminated group rather than colour (SHARE 1995). Complex
classifications may be confusing and may even defeat the purpose.

Seen this way, some academic criticism may even be unsound and inappropriate. Racial and ethnic nomenclature in the United States, for example, has been dominated by the classification of the Office of Management and Budget (OMB), adopted in 1977 and recently reviewed (OMB 1994, 1997, Bennett 1997). Table 3.4 shows the most recent 1997 classification. The classification was based on the work of a sub-committee of the Federal Interagency Committee on Education. The committee created a classification which could be used to help implement and monitor civil rights in education. The purpose of the classification was to collect data on groups which suffered from discrimination, primarily for use in monitoring civil rights legislation (Evinger 1995). With this understanding the problem is seen to lie with those who have adopted it for alternative (scientific) purposes and not with those who devised it. Indeed, the OMB document emphasises that the classification is not a scientific one.

For this type of work, e.g. to identify the number of persons eligible for a particular service, the concept of race as representing groups who are physically different, and racial classification based on the idea, is being used as a marker of eligibility and of social stratification. Arguably, the easier the marker is to measure and apply the better. In so far as discrimination is hugely influenced by the linked characteristics of skin colour and regional ancestry, the OMB's categories, based on colour and region of ancestral origin, make sense as proxy measures of discrimination.

Here, the need is for a variable and a process of classification with comparatively fixed and identifiable features. In this context ethnicity is too complex and flexible a concept. The concept of race as a physical, biological

Table 3.4 US Office of Management and Budget Classification 1997 (OMB 1997)

The minimum categories for data on race and ethnicity for Federal statistics and program administrative reporting are defined as follows:

American Indian or Alaska native
A person having origins in any of the original peoples of North and South America (including Central America), and who maintains cultural identification through tribal affiliation or community recognition

Asian or Pacific Islander
A person having origins in any of the original peoples of the Far East, Southeast Asia, the Indian subcontinent, or the Pacific Islands. This area includes, for example, China, India, Japan, Korea, the Philippine Islands, Hawaii and Samoa

Black or African American
A person having origins in any of the black racial groups of Africa

Hispanic
A person of Mexican, Puerto Rican, Cuban, Central or South American or other Spanish culture or origin, regardless of race

White
A person having origins in any of the original peoples of Europe, North Africa or the Middle East

---

indicator of the population group, the physical features themselves having been in the past the foundation for racism, works, albeit imperfectly, as a basis for the classification. The problems with race, even here, should not be glossed over – physical features do not reliably identify population groups, they vary across generations and merge imperceptibly across geographical areas. The concept of race also breaks down in respect of the offspring of mixed race. Nonetheless, it is easier to operationalise than ethnicity.

Health policy

In a policy of equality of utilisation or uptake of a particular service (say, immunisation) by race or ethnic group, a marker of race or ethnic group is needed to demonstrate whether the policy is being achieved. Similar considerations apply in ethnic monitoring to assess whether 'minority' group applicants for jobs in the health service are being considered, interviewed and employed. At such a level, and with this sole goal of surveillance or monitoring in mind, the level of detail being collected by the British National Health Service, in its ethnic monitoring exercise (in which the concept of race is actually the guiding force), may well be right (Shaw 1994). Again, race rather than ethnicity is the better concept, both because physical features are the dominant reason for the inequities to be resolved and because it is easier to collect information on. It is noteworthy, however, that such data collection exercises institutionalise racial classifications and the perception of people as members of particular racial groups. It is a small step from this to assume that group characteristics apply to an individual when they do not, i.e. stereotyping.

Race and ethnicity also figure in public health activities, such as travel health, and in policies designed to narrow, as opposed to observe, inequalities in health status. For these purposes more than a marker of race is likely to be needed, for markers do not provide understanding. For port health activities, such as screening, quarantine, segregation or exclusion from services, country of origin, travel details and immigration status, are more relevant than labels of ethnicity and race. Racial or ethnic labels can, at best, be used to focus the search for the persons to be investigated, e.g. the case for tuberculosis screening at immigration is likely to be stronger for Indians than for Norwegians, simply because the prevalence of the disease is higher in India than in Norway. Colour and self-reported or assigned race or ethnicity are therefore outward and obvious proxy markers for other more important and specific information. The race and ethnicity labels alone are at best a crude screening device, at worst a misleading distraction which can lead to error.

In other policies, such as alleviating health inequalities, colour may be a potent and visible indicator of both historical and current discrimination on the basis of race and, in so far as current policy with reversing this is concerned, colour markers will be highly relevant. It is likely, however, that the health inequality is a result of social factors including poverty, diet, employment, etc. Only for a few specific genetic diseases, the haemoglobinopathies being the best example, will biological factors be important causes. Labels of race and ethnicity are no more than markers for these other underlying factors which are the primary foci of interest but which need to be directly measured to make and implement rational policy. Clearly, group characteristics, such as high unemployment, cannot directly give information about individuals. It is equally irrational to assume that group characteristics explain an individual's susceptibility to a disease, such as diabetes or hypertension, yet there is a tendency to ascribe such diseases, in members of racial and ethnic minority groups, to genetic susceptibility.

In developing rational policy, causal understanding of the problem together with details of the characteristics of the population beyond their race will be needed. For example, in the United Kingdom rickets was demonstrated in the 1960s and 1970s to be a common problem in the recently migrating Indian, Pakistani and Bangladeshi communities (so-called 'Asian rickets'), particularly in women and children (Ford *et al.* 1972, Dunningan *et al.* 1981). Causal understanding was needed to effect policy. The national policy for solving the problem was educational. Knowing the colour of the individual and population was inadequate to help implement the policy. Country of origin was a help, but only together with knowledge of recent migration status. Language suddenly became all-important, not only to identify relevant people, but also to effect a communication strategy. Labels of race and ethnicity in these circumstances are markers of groups of people, for some of whom the policy is relevant. Race and ethnicity are a means of narrowing the search, both for populations and for generating hypotheses for understanding why the problem occurs. In this example, ethnicity is the more relevant concept to underpin research, policy-making and preventative action, because cultural factors underpin both the understanding of the cause and the successful action to deal with it. The cause was generally explained as resulting from a combination of a diet lacking in vitamin D and its precursors which contained high levels of phytates, which impaired absorption of dietary vitamin D; to behaviours and attitudes which minimised exposure to the sun (all 'ethnic' factors); and a dark skin which reduced the capacity to make vitamin D on exposure to the sun (a racial factor) (Ford *et al.* 1972, Dunningan *et al.* 1981).

Health care planning

Health care planners use race and ethnicity as a guide to assessing and meeting health care needs. They require markers to identify groups they wish to consult with, or modify services for, in accordance with health needs. In these cases ethnic or racial labels, colour labels, nationality, and migration status are usually too crude. Country of parental or grandparental birth or the racial label does occasionally help, e.g. in the management of bacillus Calmette–Guérin (BCG) immunisation at infancy, which in Britain is recommended routinely for children of Indian subcontinent origin. Here the classification Indian, Pakistani, Bangladeshi or even South Asian as an overall term will do. Another example would be in assessing the need for a haemoglobinopathy service. The size of the population which fits the racial labels 'Afro-Caribbean', 'African' and 'South Asian', together with the prevalence data, may appropriately be the starting points in making decisions. Usually, however, more detail will be needed on racial or ethnic characteristics which impinge directly on the need for, or utilisation of, a service. For example, in the planning of a breast cancer screening programme, hospice care, diabetes care service, antenatal care or screening for high blood pressure, the need is for an understanding of themes such as language proficiency, religion, dietary behaviours, and the influence of culture on health beliefs and health-related lifestyles. Sometimes needs will be the same across a number of racial or ethnic subgroups. If this is the case an umbrella term such as 'Asian', or 'Hispanic', may be applicable, as for BCG immunisation. Usually, there will be heterogeneity, in terms of language, religion, etc., making the provision of specifically targeted and appropriate services a huge challenge, for there may be substantial differences within an ethnic group, e.g. in Tanzania there were important variations among the castes of a Hindu community (Ramaiya *et al.* 1991).

Clinical care

Racial labels are sometimes used routinely to introduce the clinical history, as in 'This is a 45-year-old Indian/Caucasian/African/Chinese man', etc. This practice has been criticised (Caldwell and Popenhoe 1995). There are, arguably, some circumstances where a racial label on its own may be helpful in diagnosis or case management. For instance, in the diagnosis of abdominal and joint pain in a person of 'African' origin, the diagnosis of sickle cell crisis ought to be considered more readily than in a person of 'European' origin (even though sickle cell disease does occur in people of 'European' origin, especially in the Mediterranean area). Another example would be cough and fever, which are more likely to be due to tuberculosis in an Indian person than in a European one. In these somewhat rare circumstances, the racial label might be valuable in triggering an association between the symptoms and the diagnosis. The potential problems such as stereotyping and misdiagnosis need full acknowledgement. The association between symptoms and racial label is as likely to mislead as not. The cough with fever is much more likely to be the common cold, influenza, bronchitis or pneumonia than tuberculosis in all ethnic groups, including Indians. For these reasons, clinicians should be wary of race and ethnicity labels.

Usually in clinical care even greater detail is needed than in the above examples of health policy and planning, and colour, racial and ethnic labels, and nationality are unlikely to help. In assessing the individual patient, labels are likely to be as misleading as they are to be helpful. For example, the physician treating diabetic patients originating from the countries of the

Indian subcontinent will need to give advice on what to do during fasting. It is a common habit among Hindus, particularly women, to fast for one day per week. By contrast, fasting during daylight hours is fastidiously observed by many Muslims in the month of Ramadan (even though the religion does exempt the sick, it is common for patients to fast nevertheless). Race and ethnicity are no more than crude reminders that the patient may need to be counselled on fasting. Religion is a more accurate means of assessment than the ethnic group since Indians, in particular, are heterogeneous in religion and culture. Even so, the physician could be seriously misled by an assumption that all Muslims fast during Ramadan or that the sick have exempted themselves from the religious requirement. A detailed cultural history from each individual (Bhopal and White 1989) is needed to ensure that errors are not made. In these circumstances, clearly the concept of ethnicity is more relevant than race. In this and similar contexts ethnic labels such as 'Bangladeshi Muslim', though insufficient by themselves, are superior to racial ones such as 'Asian' or 'Asiatic' and may help to focus the clinician in taking the cultural history.

Ethnicity is often crucial to effective communication, itself the foundation of good health care, and the basis for tailoring health advice and care for a huge number of problems from the successful enrolment of a woman into the cervical screening campaign, to whether the nurses or relatives wash the dead body of a patient in hospital. While this is obvious in relation to ethnic minority groups, similar considerations apply to the 'White' ethnic groups. The London physician may need to appreciate the ethnic or cultural background of a Scottish highlander or a 'Geordie' from north-east England to manage the patient properly. For clinical work ethnicity is the key concept, but delving deeper than the ethnic label is almost always necessary. The purpose is to widen the understanding of the culture and circumstances of the individual, which is very different from the research one.

Research

It is in research that the greatest controversy has occurred. There is a conflict between the repeated claims that race and ethnicity research is of immense value, and the repeated and severe criticism of the theory, method and unsavoury applications and outcomes (Gould 1984) of the concept. Can we reconcile these conflicting positions?

First, let us recognise that there are many forms of research with distinct purposes and needs. Neither the claims that ethnicity or race research is of great value nor the criticisms are likely to apply uniformly to all forms of research. Different forms of research may apply different concepts of race and ethnicity. The racial and ethnic classifications are also likely to vary according to the type of research. Finally, the type of research will determine the depth of inquiry into the specific characteristics behind race and ethnicity, or in the words of La Veist (1996) in the quotation above, 'those concepts believed to be measured by race'. For illustration, three forms of research are considered here, surveillance, health services research and causal epidemiological research.

Surveillance

Surveillance is defined as the analysis, interpretation and feedback of systematically collected data with methods distinguished by their practicality, uniformity and rapidity, often designed to detect change (Last 1995). In the context of race and ethnicity, the main objective of surveillance is to discern and track variations in the health of populations grouped by race or ethnicity. The idea of race is a simpler one than that of ethnicity and hence might be expected to be better suited to surveillance than ethnicity. Indeed, surveillance usually uses colour (Black/White), nationality (Indian/Pakistani) or country of birth as the foundations of their classification and, when needed, as markers of population characteristics such as languages or religious origin. With respect to self-report, current classifications (see Tables 3.3 and 3.4) in the United States and the United Kingdom are primarily based on the concept of race, i.e. colour, and of region. 'Hispanic' is the apparent exception and is purportedly based on language (Spanish) but in effect is a mix of region of origin and history of living in a place under Spanish colonial rule. Hispanic is a mix of ethnic and racial concepts (Office of Management and Budget 1994, Bennett 1997).

Mostly, surveillance data systems have adopted classifications initially developed for political or health policy purposes. The OMB classification holds sway in the United States. Medicare data bases sometimes report an even cruder classification of White and non-White. Hahn and Stroup (1994) indicate that a surveillance category should be conceptually valid, measurable in a valid way, exclusive and exhaustive, meaningful to respondents, reliable, consistent and flexible. They and others have questioned the conceptual validity of racial categories such as 'Hispanic', 'Latino', 'Asian', but not the category 'White' (Hahn and Stroup 1994). Bhopal and Donaldson (1998) have pointed out the severe limitations of 'White' as a valid racial category. While the United States census has ten sub-categories for 'Asian' or 'Pacific Islanders', and five opportunities for subgrouping 'Spanish' or 'Hispanic' groupings, it has none for 'White', which accounted for 80 per cent of the population in 1990. The British census is similar, and there 94 per cent of the population are White. The focus of surveillance is therefore, necessarily, on non-White minority groups.

While surveillance needs relatively crude classifications where the race or ethnic label is an indicator of populations which may need special attention, surveillance has also been trapped by the use of classifications derived for political and policy purposes which are used in censuses and hence are the source of denominator data, essential for constructing the rates and summaries of rates, such as standard mortality rates (SMRs), which are the basis of surveillance.

People involved in surveillance should be less passive in accepting a politically derived classification, and must articulate the needs of surveillance better and compete with politically driven initiatives in developing classifications. It is likely that for reasons of cost, simplicity and stability over time the classifications used in surveillance will divide populations in a fairly crude way and continue to be based on the race concept and traditional racial classifications, rather than on the broader concepts underlying ethnicity. That said, the weaknesses of racial classification, even for surveillance, are clear – for example, as discussed earlier (p. 22), there is no objective, valid measure of a person's race, self-reporting of race varies over time, and there is no classification which copes well with those of mixed race.

Health services research

Unlike surveillance, health services research is not an easily defined activity – it takes many forms. Where health services research is examining issues of equity of access or utilisation of care or the evaluation of policy, the racial and ethnic concepts to be used and classifications needed will be driven by the questions posed, but are likely to be subject to the same needs as for surveillance and subject to the same limitations and criticisms. However, more so than for surveillance, the fact that most current racial and ethnic classifications take little account of the heterogeneity within any one category is a major limitation.

Consider the matter of uptake of breast cancer mammography. If the health services research question is '*Is* the programme being accessed by all racial or ethnic groups?' then this is akin to surveillance. There is an important difference, however, and that is of heterogeneity. Categories used in surveillance such as 'South Asian', 'Hispanic', 'Black', etc., are unreliably crude in this context. The programme may be accessed well by 'South Asians', overall, but not well by an important subgroup such as, say, 'Bangladeshi Muslim women'. Nonetheless, in terms of answering this question and tracing progress, a relatively simple racial or ethnic classification would suffice. The 'South Asian' group might be sub-divided into 'Indian', 'Pakistani' and 'Bangladeshi' and perhaps by religion and language. A mix of racial and ethnic labels could be derived, the relevant data could be collected quickly and this health services research question answered.

However, when the issue is research for the development of new policy or to effect change, or the evaluation of the quality or effectiveness of care, a much deeper understanding is likely to be necessary. The question here might be '*why* is breast mammography less well taken up by some racial and ethnic groups?' To understand why, for example if the uptake of breast cancer mammography were to be low in the 'South Asian' community, is a question which focuses on causes. Here issues such as the group's religious views, language of communication, beliefs about the importance of prevention, and views on cancer and on the service become important. In addition, the attitudes and behaviours of service providers are crucial too. In so far as racial discrimination may play a role, both the ethnicity and the race of a group will be important. In exploring this question, then, crude indicators such as religion, colour or place of birth are no more than a means of identifying a problem and a way of deriving a sample for more detailed work which will include measuring directly those concepts and population characteristics thought to be encapsulated by race and ethnicity. Here, race and ethnicity are variables which, in themselves, generate little or no understanding of the problem and hence do not serve the purpose on their own. The point in the quotation by La Veist (1996) is all-important. The 'black box' that is race and ethnicity needs to be opened to answer the question (Skrabanek 1994, Bhopal 1997). This theme is developed below.

Causes of disease

For research on causal disease paths the principles are as in health services research, those which seek to understand why something happens. Ethnicity and race may be markers or indicators of a problem which merits investigation, means of identifying relevant populations, and appropriate for sparking hypotheses but are, arguably, rarely in themselves the source of causal knowledge. Since all disease arises from the interaction of the genome and the environment, here both the race and the ethnicity concepts are of interest. Historically, the role of biology has been invoked too readily as the prime explanation for racial differences (Alper and Natowicz 1992). For example, inherited biological susceptibility was a prime explanation for syphilis, tuberculosis, conjunctivitis and nutritional disorders in African Americans (Kiple and King 1981). Unfortunately, contemporary research also gives prominence to genetic explanations and downplays environmental (and especially economic) ones. To take one example, the high rates of hypertension in populations of African origin are widely attributed to genetic factors with little attempt to test other explanations. We now confront the need to rigorously test the validity of the biological basis of race.

Definitive work can only be done by measuring directly the concepts reflected by the labels which define race and ethnicity. Again, the black box needs to be opened. This time, unlike the case of health service research, this task will necessitate genetic studies. The role of genetics in explaining hypertension in African origin populations is slowly being clarified (Baker *et al.* 1998), but, nonetheless, needs to be studied alongside environmental and social factors, including racism (Armstead *et al.* 1989, McNeilly *et al.* 1995, Kreiger and Sidney 1996).

Overall mortality rates and life expectancy differ among racial and ethnic groups in the United States and Britain. Are these differences attributable to genetic or environmental factors? Until genetic studies of the ageing process demonstrate otherwise, the differences ought to be largely, if not wholly, attributed to environmental and social factors. However, too often the allure of genetic explanations wrongly prevails (Alper and Natowicz 1992).

The mortality difference might be partly attributed to excesses of specific diseases for which the biology is better understood. To continue with the example of breast cancer, the rate of breast cancer in South Asian women differs from that in 'White' women in England and Wales (Bhopal and Rankin 1996). Since genetic factors are a demonstrated cause of breast cancer, it is important to ask whether the differences are attributable to genetic differences. It is imperative that the question is answered by direct measurement of the presence or absence of the relevant gene variants. The race and ethnicity of the population give no clue (at least to date) to their risk of possessing the causative genes linked to breast cancer, for the (few) genes which are responsible for the anatomic features which underlie the racial or ethnic classifications give no indirect clue about the distribution of breast cancer causing genes. In future years when a large number of specific disease genes are identified and the population distributions are known this may change. In that future era the widely agreed principle that the genes which underlie racial differences are not associated with the genes which cause most diseases will need to be revisited.

Equally, the difference in breast cancer might arise from social factors which vary across the two groups, e.g. diet, economic circumstances, contraception, the age at first pregnancy, etc. These are social factors which have obvious biological consequences. Again, the racial and ethnic group gives no direct information on these factors at the individual level, though the population distribution is more likely to be known than for genetic markers. Information on such social factors needs to be collected directly.

For causal analysis in this context both biological and social factors need to be directly measured, both as contributors to the causal pathway and as confounding variables.

Conclusion

The paradigm of race as a marker of fundamental genetically driven biological differences between human subgroups was deeply undermined by a combination of advances in biology showing that genetic differences between human races are small (Kuper 1975, Osborne *et al.* 1978, Stepan 1982, Cooper 1984, Barkan 1992, Kreiger *et al.* 1993, La Veist 1994, McKenzie 1994), and the moral outrage at the abuses of the concept of race, particularly by the Nazis. Nonetheless, racial and ethnic inequalities in health (and many other aspects of life) are widespread. The causes of such inequalities require detailed study. They have been caused in part by the adverse effects of racial discrimination (Kreiger *et al.* 1993, Bhopal 1998). The idea that races are different has helped develop and perpetuate racial hierarchy, which in turn has created differences and augmented differences arising from other factors. For these reasons, race and its consequences remain of utmost importance in contemporary societies.

The great political and social significance of race has meant that science, itself a socially embedded activity, has not been able to discard the concept, or to replace it with the concept of ethnicity, except partially and often as a synonym for race. Rather, many socially orientated scientists have been attempting to alter the meaning of race, from a biological one to a social one. This is an incredibly difficult endeavour in the face of popular perceptions which fix on the idea of subgroups of humans, categorised on the basis of physical differences, largely of colour and facial features, that is, on a biological view of race.

The idea that race is a social variable, and races are groups which are tied together by a common socio-political history (Banton 1987, Kreiger *et al.* 1993, La Veist 1994, La Veist 1996, President's Cancer Panel 1997), essentially of racial discrimination, is at variance with both historical and current usage as indicated, for example, in contemporary dictionaries (Ellison 1998). Most politicians, the public, scientists and health care practitioners are also unwilling to see the race concept primarily as a marker of past and current racism. The attempt to change the meaning and interpretation of race is a daunting, long-term task particularly within biomedical science.

The socio-political concept of race is close to ethnicity, which focuses on a complex of factors that groups share and that lead to group identity. Ethnicity is a much more fluid idea than race. Race could be seen as one component of ethnicity. Ethnicity, then, becomes a group identity based on a shared set of biological, cultural and socio-political characteristics.

We are in a period of controversy and confusion. The academic discourse on the concepts of race and ethnicity finds them wanting, yet most research proceeds largely unaffected by the blistering critiques of those sensitive to the failure of race as a biological concept. Researchers, practitioners and policy-makers see value in race in its traditional biological concept, even if it is no more than a crude marker, and will not discard it until a better idea replaces it.

The analysis here shows that in some respects the idea of race, even when operationalised with the crudest of classifications, e.g. Black or White, has some value in health politics, policy, planning, surveillance, some health services research and even occasionally in clinical care. In some respects the concept of ethnicity, with its emphasis on culture and change, is not necessary or even workable whereas race is. This may explain why so often the word ethnicity merely becomes a synonym for race. In other circumstances, particularly when details about cultural and social circumstances are needed (as in clinical care), the race concept does not work, so the concept of ethnicity is put into operation, sometimes under the label of race.

Sometimes the concept of race achieves its goals without any further data. Then race is not a proxy for deeper underlying characteristics of the population. More often, and particularly when there is a need to understand differences among racial and ethnic groups, data are needed on the concepts and characteristics that underlie race and ethnicity. The need for data beyond the ethnic or racial label is governed almost entirely by purpose, hypothesis and context.

Ideally, the concepts of race and ethnicity should be strictly demarcated and used precisely. In practice, this is unlikely to happen, for the terms have always had some overlapping and interactive meaning. As a new paradigm of race and ethnicity research emerges, one word may replace the two used now. This may be a new word or phrase altogether and *identifiable populations* is one idea already in the literature, or either *race* or *ethnicity* may subsume the other. An emerging practice is for the compound use of race and ethnicity, sometimes with race in inverted commas (Smaje 1994). For science the worst scenario, which is now happening and undermining the free exchange of ideas and generalising of research data, is that *race* takes this role in the Americas and *ethnicity* in Europe. The use of different concepts and vocabulary will hamper progress in this field of work and make international collaboration more difficult.

Purpose and context are the prime determinants of the way that concepts of race and ethnicity are applied, classifications are devised and employed, and data are analysed and presented. Purpose and context provide a rationale for understanding current practice and for making difficult choices. Future critique which takes purpose and context into account may be more effective in altering the practice of researchers in the future.

Acknowledgements

I am solely responsible for the views expressed here, but Dr George Ellison gave generously of his ideas and critical faculty in both shaping an early and penultimate draft. Some of the ideas were developed while I was on sabbatical in the academic year 1996/7 at the Department of Epidemiology, School of Public Health, Chapel Hill, North Carolina. I thank Drs Trude Bennett, Vic Schoenbach and other scholars there who shared their knowledge. I also thank Drs Carl Shy and David Savitz who took steps to make me welcome in that Department. My employers, Newcastle University, granted me generous study leave. I thank Lorna Hutchinson and Carole Frazer for secretarial support.

References

Ahdieh, L. and Hahn, R.A.(1996) 'Use of the terms "race", "ethnicity", and "national origins": A review of articles in the American Journal of Public Health, 1980–1989', *Ethnicity and Health*, 1, 95–98.

Alper, J.S. and Natowicz, M.R. (1992) 'The allure of genetic explanations', *British Medical Journal*, 305, 666.

Anderson, M. and Fienberg, S.E. (1995) 'Black, white, and shades of gray (and brown and yellow)', *Chance*, 8, 15–18.

Armstead, C., Lawler, K., Gorden, G., Cross, J. and Gibbons, J. (1989) 'Relationship of racial stressors to blood pressure responses and anger expression in Black college students', *Health Psychology*, 8, 541–546.

Baker, E.H., Dong, Y.B., Sagnella, G.A., Rothwell, M., Onipinla, A.K., Markandu, N.D. Cappuccio, F.P., Cook, D.G., Persu, A., Corvall, P., Jeunemaitre, X., Carter, N.D. and MacGregor, G.A. (1998) 'Association of hypertension with T594M mutation in β sub-unit of epithelial sodium channels in black people resident in London', *Lancet*, 351, 1388–1392.

Banton, M. (1987) *Racial Theories*, Cambridge: Cambridge University Press.

Barkan, E. (1992) *The Retreat of Scientific Racism*, London: Cambridge University Press.

Bennett, T. (1997) ' "Racial" and ethnic classification: two steps forward and one step back?', *Public Health Reports*, 112, 477–480.

Bennett, T. and Bhopal R.S. (1998) 'US Editors' opinions and policies on research in race, ethnicity, and health', *Journal of National Medical Association*, 90, 401–408.

Bhopal, R.S. (1997) 'Is research into ethnicity and health racist, unsound, or important science?', *British Medical Journal*, 314, 1751–1756.

Bhopal, R.S. (1998) 'The spectre of racism in health and health care', *British Medical Journal*, 316, 1970–1973.

Bhopal, R.S. and Donaldson, L.J. (1998) 'White, European, Western, Caucasian or what? Inappropriate labelling in research on race, ethnicity and health', *American Journal of Public Health*, 88, 1303–1307.

Bhopal, R.S. and Rankin, J. (1996) 'Cancer in ethnic minorities: setting priorities based on epidemiological data', *British Journal of Cancer*, 74, 522–532.

Bhopal, R.S. and White, M. (1989) 'Health promotion for ethnic minorities in Britain: past, present and future', in Ahmed, W. (ed.) *'Race' and Health in Contemporary Britain*, Milton Keynes: Open University Press.

Bhopal, R.S., Phillimore, P. and Kohli, H.S. (1991) 'Inappropriate use of the term "Asian": an obstacle to ethnicity and health research', *Journal of Public Health Medicine*, 13, 244–246.

British Medical Journal (1996) 'Ethnicity, race and culture: guidelines for research, audit and publication', *British Medical Journal*, 312, 1094.

Colledge, M., Van Geuns, H.A. and Svensson, P.G. (eds) (1986) *Migration and Health: Towards an Understanding of the Health Care Needs of Ethnic Minorities*, Geneva: World Health Organization.

Caldwell, S.H. and Popenhoe, R. (1995) 'Perception and misperceptions of skin colour', *Annals of Internal Medicine*, 122, 614–617.

Chadwick, J. and Mann, W.N. (1950) *The Medical Works of Hippocrates*, Oxford: Blackwell Scientific Publications.

Cooper, R. (1984) 'A note on the biologic concept of race and its application in epidemiologic research', *American Heart Journal*, 108, 715–722.

Dunnigan, M.G., McIntosh, W.B., Sutherland, G.R., Gardee, R., Glekin, B., Ford, J.A. and Robertson, I. (1981) 'Policy for prevention of Asian rickets in Britain: a preliminary assessment of the Glasgow Rickets Campaign', *British Medical Journal*, 288, 357–360.

Ellison, G.T.H. (1998) 'Contemporary medical definitions of "race" and "ethnicity"', *Annals of Human Biology*, 25, 555.

Ellison, G.T.H. and De Wet, T. (1997) 'Towards rational debate of "race", "population group", ethnicity and culture in South African health research. Multicultural citizenship in the new South Africa; Cape Town', *IDASA and International Sociological Association's Research Group on Ethnic, Race and Minority Relations*.

Ellison, G.T.H., De Wet, T., Ijsselmuiden, C.B. and Richter, L.M. (1996) 'Desegregating health statistics and health research in South Africa', *South African Medical Journal*, 86, 329–331, 1257–1262.

Evinger, S. (1995) 'How shall we measure our nation's diversity?', *Chance*, 8, 7–14.

Ford, J.A., Colhoun, E.M., McIntosh, W.B. and Dunnigan, M.G. (1972) 'Rickets and osteomalacia in the Glasgow Pakistani community, 1961–1971', *British Medical Journal*, 2, 677–680.

Gimenez, M.E. (1989) ' "Latino/Hispanic" – Who needs a name? The case against a standardized terminology', *International Journal of Health Services*, 19, 557–571.

Gould, S.J. (1984) *The Mismeasure of Man*, London: Pelican.

Hahn, R.A. (1996) 'Identifying ancestry: the reliability of ancestral identification in the United States by self, proxy, interviewer, and funeral director', *Epidemiology*, 7, 75–80.

Hahn, R.A. and Stroup, D.F. (1994) 'Race and ethnicity in public health surveillance: Criteria for the scientific use of social categories', *Public Health Reports*, 109, 4–12.

Huth, E.J. (1995) 'Identifying ethnicity in medical papers', *Annals of Internal Medicine*, 122, 619–621.

International Committee of Medical Journal Editors (1997), 'Uniform requirements for manuscripts submitted to biomedical journals', *Annals of Internal Medicine*, 126, 36–47.

Jones, P., La Veist, T.A, and Lillie-Blanton, M. (1991) ' "Race" in the epidemiologic literature: An examination of the American Journal of Epidemiology, 1921–1990', *American Journal of Epidemiology*, 134, 1079–1084.

Kiple, K.F. and King, V.H. (1981) *Another Dimension to the Black Diaspora*, Cambridge: Cambridge University Press.

Kreiger, N. and Sidney, S. (1996) 'Racial discrimination and blood pressure: the CARDIA study of young black and white adults', *American Journal of Public Health*, 86, 1370–1378.

Kreiger, N., Rowley, D. and Herman A. (1993) 'Racism, sexism and social class: implications for studies of health, disease and wellbeing', *American Journal of Preventive Medicine*, 9, 82–122.

Kuhn, T.S. (1996) *The Structure of Scientific Revolutions*, 3rd edn, Chicago: The University of Chicago Press.

Kuper, L. (1975) *Race, Science and Society*, Paris: UNESCO Press.

La Veist, T.A. (1994) 'Beyond dummy variables and sample selection: what health services researchers ought to know about race as a variable', *Health Services Research*, 29, 1–16.

La Veist, T.A. (1996) 'Why we should continue to study race but do a better job: an essay on race, racism and health', *Ethnicity and Disease*, 6, 21–29.

Last, J.M. (1995) *A Dictionary of Epidemiology*, 3rd edn, New York: Oxford University Press.

McKenzie, K.J. (1994) 'Race, ethnicity, culture and science', *British Medical Journal*, 309, 286–288.

McNeilly, M., Robinson, E., Anderson, N. *et al.* (1995) 'Effects of racist provocation and social support on cardiovascular reactivity in African American women', *International Journal of Behavioural Medicine*, 2, 321–338.

Morbidity Mortality Weekly Report (MMWR) (1993) 'Use of race and ethnicity in public health surveillance: summary of the CDC/ATSDR workshop', *Morbidity Mortality Weekly Report*, 42, 10–16.

Moss, K.L. (1996) 'Race and poverty data as a tool in the struggle for environmental justice', *Journal of Poverty and Race Research Action Council*, 5, 1–6.

Muntaner, C., Nieto, J. and O'Campo, P. (1996) 'The Bell curve: on race, social class, and epidemiologic research', *American Journal of Epidemiology*, 144, 531–536.

Osborne, R.T., Noble, C.E. and Weyl, N. (1978) *The Biopsychology of Age, Race and Sex*, New York: Academic Press.

Office of Management and Budget (1994) *Standards for the Classification of Federal Data on Race and Ethnicity*, Washington: Office of Management and Budget.

Office of Management and Budget (1997) *Revisions to the Standards for the Classification of Federal Data on Race and Ethnicity*, Washington: Office of Management and Budget.

Polednak, A. (1989) *Racial and Ethnic Differences in Disease*, New York: School of Medicine, State University of New York.

President's Cancer Panel (1997) *The Meaning of Race in Science – Considerations for Cancer Research*, Bethesda: National Institutes of Health, National Cancer Institute.

Ramaiya, K.L., Swai, A.B.M., McLarty, D.G., Bhopal, R.S. and Alberti, K. (1991) 'Prevalences of diabetes and cardiovascular disease risk factors in Hindu Indian subcommunities in Tanzania', *British Medical Journal*, 303, 271–303.

Rothschild, H. (1981) *Biocultural Aspects of Disease*, London: Academic Press.

Senior, P. and Bhopal, R.S. (1994) 'Ethnicity as a variable in epidemiological research', *British Medical Journal*, 309, 327–329.

SHARE (1995) 'A note on views and terminology from SHARE', *SHARE Newsletter*.

Shaw, J. (1994) *Collection of Ethnic Group Data for Admitted Patients (EL(94)77)*, Executive Quarry House, Leeds: National Health Service (NHS).

Sheldon, T.A. and Parker, H. (1992) 'Race and ethnicity in health research', *Journal of Public Health Medicine*, 14, 104–110.

Skrabanek, P. (1994) 'The emptiness of the black box', *Epidemiology*, 5, 553–555.

Smaje, C. (1994) *Health and Ethnicity: a review of the Literature*, London: King's Fund Institute.

Smith, D.B. (1993) 'The racial integration of health facilities', *Journal of Health Politics, Policy and Law*, 18, 851–869.

Special Section (1994) 'Papers from the CDC-ATSDPR workshop on the use of race and ethnicity in public health surveillance', *Public Health Reports*, 109, 4–45.

Stepan, N. (1982) *The Idea of Race in Science*, London: Macmillan.

United States Department of Health and Human Services (1985) *Report of the Secretary's Task Force on Black and Minority Health*, Washington, DC: US Government Printing Office.

Walker, A.P.R. (1997) 'Data are not now collected by ethnic group in South Africa', *British Medical Journal*, 314, 220.

Williams, D.R. (1994) 'The concept of race in health services research 1966–1990', *Health Services Research*, 29, 261–274.

Williams, D.R. (1997) 'Race and health: basic question, emerging directions', *Annals of Epidemiology*, 7, 322–333.

Witzig, R. (1996) 'The medicalization of race: scientific legitimization of flawed social construction', *Annals of Internal Medicine*, 125, 675–679.

4 The contribution of socio-economic position to health differentials between ethnic groups

Evidence from the United States and Britain

James Y. Nazroo and George Davey Smith

Introduction

Differences in health across ethnic groups, in terms of both morbidity and mortality, have been repeatedly documented in both the United States (Department of Health and Human Services 1990, Rogers 1992, Sorlie *et al.* 1992, Krieger *et al.* 1993, Rogot *et al.* 1993, Davey Smith *et al.* 1998a, Pamuk *et al.* 1998) and Britain (Marmot *et al.* 1984, Rudat 1994, Harding and Maxwell 1997, Nazroo 1997a, b). However, the factors underlying such differences remain contested. In particular, the role that socio-economic position may play is the subject of considerable debate, with some claiming that it makes minimal or no contribution to ethnic inequalities in health (Wild and McKeigue 1997); others suggesting that even if it does contribute, the cultural and genetic elements of ethnicity must also play a role (Smaje 1996); and others arguing that ethnic inequalities in health are predominantly determined by socio-economic inequalities (Navarro 1990, Sheldon and Parker 1992). In this chapter we will use evidence on mortality and morbidity rates from both the United States [the Multiple Risk Factor Intervention Trial (MRFIT) study – Davey Smith *et al.* 1996a, b, 1998a] and Britain (the Fourth National Survey of Ethnic Minorities – Nazroo 1997a, b) to explore the contribution of socio-economic factors to ethnic inequalities in health, and to point to the methodological and conceptual pitfalls that beset such work.

In Britain the possible contribution of socio-economic position to ethnic inequalities in health has, for a long time, been ignored by the majority of investigators. This may have its roots in the now classic study of immigrant mortality rates by Marmot *et al.* (1984). Published shortly after the Black report (Townsend and Davidson 1982) firmly placed inequalities in health on the research agenda, and at the same time as the Policy Studies Institute's third survey of ethnic minorities (Brown 1984) showed the poverty of ethnic minority groups living in Britain, Marmot *et al.* (1984) used a combination of British census and death certificate data to explore the relationship between country of birth and mortality rates. Central to their analysis was an assessment of the contribution that occupational class made to the differences between country of birth groups. But, given the context just described, they surprisingly found no relationship between social class and mortality for immigrant groups. These findings led them to conclude '(a) that differences in social class distribution are not the explanation of the overall different mortality of migrants; and (b) the relation of social class (as usually defined) to mortality is different among immigrant groups from the England and Wales pattern.' (Marmot *et al.* 1984: 21). It was not until 1997 that socio-economic position reappeared in published national data exploring the relationship between ethnicity and health in Britain (Harding and Maxwell 1997, Nazroo 1997a).

One of the places where socio-economic position has reappeared in data on ethnicity and health in Britain is in the most recent examination of immigrant mortality rates by Harding and Maxwell (1997). This analysis was conducted in the context of the British inequalities in health decennial supplement (Drever and Whitehead 1997) and, again used census and death certificate data to explore mortality rates by country of birth. In contrast to Marmot *et al.*'s (1984) findings, Harding and Maxwell (1997) showed clear socio-economic gradients in mortality rates for migrant groups. Despite this, like Marmot *et al.* (1984) they also found that controlling for occupational class made no contribution to the differences seen between the different country of birth groups. This led Harding and Maxwell (1997) to conclude that 'Among the non-white ethnic groups, the relationship between social class and mortality is becoming apparent in the 1990s for groups who have settled here for some time. Our overall conclusion, however, supports the earlier ones that social class is not an adequate explanation for the patterns of excess mortality observed' (Harding and Maxwell 1997: 120). So, although the most recent evidence from immigrant mortality studies suggests that there are socio-economic gradients in health for all ethnic groups, they also continue to suggest that differences in socio-economic position do not contribute to ethnic inequalities in health in Britain.

Although within the United States there is also a long tradition of investigating ethnic inequalities in health (see Trask 1916 for an early example), the relationship between this work and the investigation of socio-economic inequalities in health is quite different from that in Britain. In recent decades in the United States there has been greater interest in health differences according to 'race', than in socio-economic differentials in health *per se*. This is partly due to the limited data on socio-economic position available in routine American health statistics. Thus the USDHHS report of 1990, 'Health status of the disadvantaged', largely presents health data tabulated by 'race', rather than by socio-economic indicators. Implicit in this approach is the assumption that ethnic minority groups in the United States are disadvantaged and that their poor health status is, to some extent, due to this disadvantage. However, it also suggests that ethnic minority groups are somehow homogeneous, and therefore socio-economic differentials in health status within ethnic minority groups are not considered. Indeed, until recently (Sorlie *et al.* 1992, Davey Smith *et al.* 1996b, Pamuk *et al.* 1998) there have been few examinations of the socio-economic stratification of health within ethnic minority groups in the United States. The contribution of socio-economic factors to, in particular, Black–White health differentials in the United States has, on the other hand, been investigated in many studies (for example Rogers 1992, Sorlie *et al.* 1992, Sterling *et al.* 1993, Rogers *et al.* 1996). These studies have, however, been limited by small sample sizes or a reliance on administrative data in which information on factors other than ethnicity and socio-economic position was not available.

Methods

Data from two studies will be used here. The first is the Multiple Risk Factor Intervention Trial (MRFIT), which was conducted in the United States, where 361,662 men were screened into this study between 1973 and 1975 at twenty centres in eighteen cities, using a variety of settings, including their homes and workplaces. Full details of the MRFIT study are reported in Neaton *et al.* (1984, 1987). The men were assessed on a number of medical risk factors, such as cigarette smoking, blood pressure, serum cholesterol and previous medical history. Mortality rates over a 16-year follow-up period will be used here to assess ethnic inequalities in health, with both all cause mortality and some cause-specific rates being used. For the purposes of the analysis of ethnicity in this paper, a simple divide has been made between White and Black men. Other ethnic groups (such as Hispanic) were not included in the analysis as in total they consisted of only about 13,000 individuals. Overall, data were analysed for 300,685 White and 20,224 Black men.

No socio-economic data were collected at the time of inclusion into the MRFIT study. So income data from the 1980 United States Census have been used to determine median family income of White and Black households in the area of residence of the individual at the time of recruitment into the study (Davey Smith *et al.* 1996a, b, 1998a). Area was determined using zip code, with 4,644 zip code areas being used for the White men and 1,376 for the Black men.

The second study used here is the British Fourth National Survey of Ethnic Minorities (FNS). In 1993 and 1994 a nationally representative sample of 5,196 ethnic minority and 2,867 White people was interviewed. The sample was identified using focused enumeration (Brown and Ritchie 1981, Smith and Prior 1997) and covered those of Caribbean, Indian, Pakistani, Bangladeshi and Chinese origin. Because the Chinese sample was small (214 people), they are not included as a separate group in the data presented here.

Three health outcomes from the FNS are considered in this paper. The first was a general health question asking respondents to compare their health with that of others of the same age on a five-point scale. The responses to this question have been dichotomised into those who said their health was good or very good and those who said it was fair, poor or very poor. The second was an assessment of possible ischaemic heart disease (IHD). This included respondents aged 40 or older who said that they had had a diagnosis of heart disease or angina, or who said that they had experienced severe chest pain lasting for half an hour or more. The third was a report of a diagnosis of diabetes mellitus.

One of the great advantages of the FNS was its coverage of a range of topics related to the experiences of ethnic minority people in Britain that may be relevant to their health. These included ethnic identity, education, employment, income, household and family structure, social support, area of residence, and experiences of discrimination and harassment. These are reported in full elsewhere (Modood *et al.* 1997), although some of the relevant findings will be reported here.

Results

Socio-economic inequalities in the United States and Britain

Using income data from the 1980 United States Census, the areas in which the respondents to the MRFIT study lived were divided into five groups, based on the mean household income (in US$) in the area (less than $12,500, $12,500–$17,499, $17,500–$22,499, $22,500–$27,499 and $27,500 or more). The findings were very similar to those shown in the British data for the poorest ethnic minority groups compared with White people. More than a third of American Black men lived in an area with the lowest income category, compared with less than 1 per cent of White men in similar areas. In contrast, 30 per cent of White men were in the top income category compared with less than 5 per cent of Black men. Furthermore, 94 per cent of White men were in the top three of the five bands, while 70 per cent of Black men were in the bottom two of the five bands (see Davey Smith *et al.* 1998a for further details).

Data published from the British FNS contained a number of indicators of socio-economic position, including occupational class, unemployment rates, housing tenure and housing quality, and income (Modood *et al.* 1997). These indicators generally showed the same pattern across the ethnic groups that were included in the study, with the Indian and Caribbean groups somewhat worse off than the White group, and the Pakistani and Bangladeshi groups much worse off than the White group. These differences are, perhaps, best summed up by differences in total household income adjusted for household size. Just over a quarter of White people had less than half the average income – an indicator of poverty – compared with about two-fifths of Indian and Caribbean people and more than four-fifths of Pakistani and Bangladeshi people. In Britain the Pakistani and Bangladeshi groups are by far the poorest, and they are poorer than both White pensioners and White lone parents (see Tables 5.6, 5.7 and 5.8 in Berthoud 1997).

Inequalities in health

Figure 4.1 shows all cause mortality rates, stratified by mean family income in the area of residence, over the 16-year follow-up period in the United States MRFIT study. There is a very clear gradient for both White and Black men that is similar for both groups. The extent of the socio-economic inequality in health is shown by the twofold difference in mortality rates between those in the top and bottom income groups for both Black and White men.

Figure 4.2 contains data from the British FNS. It shows rates of reporting 'fair or poor' health for three ethnic minority groups (in order to achieve large enough sample sizes the Pakistani and Bangladeshi groups are combined), all of the ethnic minority groups combined and the comparative White sample. Each of the groups is stratified by occupational class of the head of the household, with a simple distinction drawn between manual and non-manual households and a third group, those where there was no full-time worker in the household, also included. As in the American data on all cause mortality, Figure 4.2 shows a clear relationship between reported general health and socio-economic position for each ethnic group in Britain.

Figure 4.3 also shows British FNS data, but this time each ethnic group is stratified by tenure, with owner–occupiers and renters separated. Again, for each group a very clear socio-economic gradient is evident.

The overall impression given by the one figure on the American data and the two on the British data is of clear socio-economic gradients for each ethnic

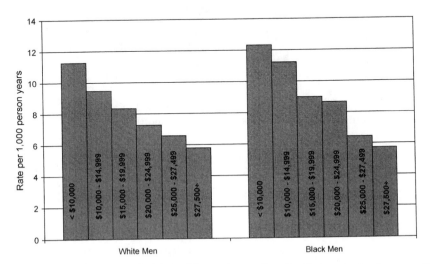

Figure 4.1 Death rates in the United States by median family income in the area of residence (MRFIT data).

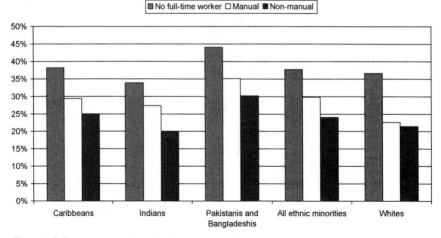

Figure 4.2 Percentage of each ethnic group who reported 'fair' or 'poor' health in the United Kingdom by ethnic group and occupational class (FNS data).

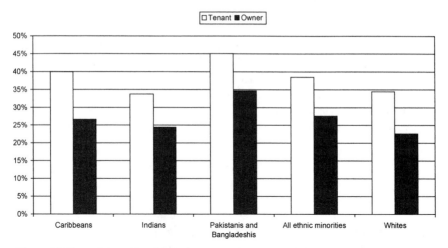

Figure 4.3 Percentage of each ethnic group who reported 'fair' or 'poor' health in the United Kingdom by housing tenure (FNS data).

group, with poorer people having poorer health and higher mortality rates. The pattern for both ethnic minority and White groups is very similar.

Standardising for socio-economic position

As in the analysis of immigrant mortality in Britain by Harding and Maxwell (1997), controlling for socio-economic position does not eliminate ethnic differences in health in the British FNS. People in the Pakistani and

Bangladeshi groups reported worse health than any other group (Nazroo 1997a) and, while Figures 4.2 and 4.3 show a clear socio-economic gradient in health for them, in each socio-economic category they continue to have much worse health than White people. For example, Figure 4.2 shows that about a third of non-manual Pakistani and Bangladeshi people reported their health as 'fair or poor', compared with less than a quarter of non-manual White people.

Although this might suggest that socio-economic factors do not contribute to ethnic inequalities in health, it is important to recognise that the process of standardising for socio-economic position when making comparisons across groups, particularly ethnic groups, is not as straightforward as it might at first sight seem. As Kaufman *et al.* (1997, 1998) point out, the process of standardisation is effectively an attempt to deal with the non-random nature of samples used in cross-sectional studies – controlling for all relevant 'extraneous' explanatory factors introduces the *appearance* of randomisation. However, attempting to introduce randomisation into cross-sectional studies by adding 'controls' has a number of problems. These have been summarised by Kaufman *et al.* (1998) as follows, 'When considering socio-economic exposures and making comparisons between racial/ethnic groups ... the material, behavioral, and psychological circumstances of diverse socio-economic and racial/ethnic groups are distinct on so many dimensions that no realistic adjustment can plausibly simulate randomization.' (Kaufman *et al.* 1998: 147).

Indeed, an analysis of ethnic differences in income within class groups in the FNS emphasises this point. Table 5.2 in Nazroo (1997a) showed that while total household income adjusted for household size followed the class gradient for each ethnic group, within each class group ethnic minority people had a smaller income than White people. The differences were particularly large for the Pakistani and Bangladeshi group, who, as was shown earlier, are the poorest group and also the group with the poorest health. Within each class group they had, at most, half the income of the White group and those in social classes I and II had a lower average income than White people in social classes IV and V. Nazroo (1997a) also showed that a similar pattern exists for other indicators of socio-economic position. For example, unemployed White people had been unemployed for a shorter period than their ethnic minority equivalents, and within tenure groups White people had better housing than some ethnic minority groups.

Similarly, census data in the United States show that while median family income increases with increasing number of years of education for both White and Black people, within each education group Black men and women have a substantially lower income than their White equivalents. Indeed, Black men and women had a household income equivalent to that of White men and women in the education group below them (Pamuk *et al.* 1998).

One way of addressing this problem is to use alternative indicators of socio-economic position that more accurately reflect ethnic differences to adjust for socio-economic differences when making comparisons across ethnic groups. However, most studies do not contain sufficient material on socio-economic circumstances to do this. Fortunately, as described earlier (p. 43), we were able to add income data to the MRFIT study and the FNS contained considerable detail on socio-economic position. The rich material in the FNS was used to construct an index of 'standard of living'. Full details of this index can be found in Nazroo (1997a), but it was based on the following items:

- number of people per room;
- absence of, or shared, basic amenities in household, including bath or shower; bathroom; kitchen; inside toilet; hot water from a tap; central heating;
- possession of consumer goods, including TV; video; fridge; freezer; washing machine; tumble drier; dishwasher; microwave; CD player; PC; phone;
- number of cars.

Figure 4.4 uses data from the FNS to illustrate the effect of adjusting for alternative indicators of socio-economic position. It shows the relative risk of reporting 'fair or poor' health, for Pakistani and Bangladeshi people, compared with the White group. The value for the White group is represented by the *x*-axis, which is drawn at the value of '1'. The vertical lines represent relative risks, with the mid-point of the lines showing the actual relative risk and the end-points representing 95 per cent confidence limits. So, if the line does not cross the value of '1', the differences are statistically significant, and the further they are from the *x*-axis the greater the difference.

The first vertical line shows data that have only been standardised for age and gender. The next two lines show the effect of standardising for occupational class and housing tenure, and shows that adjusting for these standard indicators makes little or no difference. The final bar shows the effect of adjusting for the index of standard of living and shows that this leads to considerable attenuation of the increased tendency of Pakistani and Bangladeshi people to report 'fair or poor' health compared with the White group.

Figure 4.5 does the same for the possible IHD outcome and shows a similar pattern to that for general health. Adjustments for occupational class and tenure have little effect, while adjusting for the standard of living indicator leads to a considerable attenuation in the increased risk seen in Pakistanis and Bangladeshis.

Returning to the United States MRFIT data, Figure 4.6 shows the effect of standardising for mean household income in the area of residence on the relative risk for Black compared with White men for all cause mortality and mortality for all cardiovascular disease (CVD) outcomes. Like the figures using British data, it shows that socio-economic position makes a major

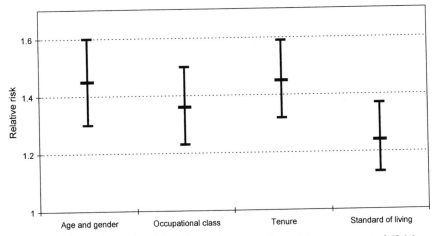

Figure 4.4 Effect of standardising for socio-economic position on reported 'fair' or 'poor' health by the Pakistani and Bangladeshi population compared with White people (RR = 1.0) in the United Kingdom (FNS data).

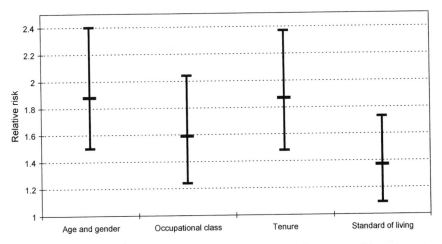

Figure 4.5 Effect of standardising for socio-economic position on possible ischaemic heart disease among Pakistani and Bangladeshi people compared with White people (RR = 1.0) in the United Kingdom (FNS data).

contribution to the outcomes shown. Adjustment for income reduced the age-adjusted relative risk from 1.47 to 1.19; however, about two-thirds of the elevated mortality risk among Black men was statistically explained by this income measure. Conversely, adjusting the Black–White mortality differential for a number of other risk factors – diastolic blood pressure, serum cholesterol, cigarette smoking, existing diabetes and prior hospitalisation for coronary heart disease – only decreased the relative risk from 1.47 to 1.40. This demonstrates that socio-economic position – as indexed by income of area of

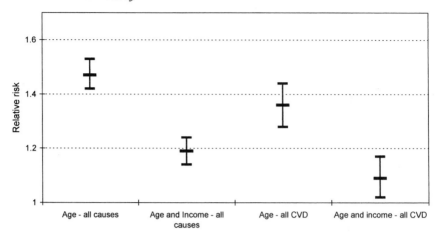

Figure 4.6 Effect of standardising for socio-economic position on all cause and all cardiovascular disease mortality in the United States (MRFIT data).

residence – is a considerably more important determinant of Black–White differentials in mortality than biological markers of risk and behavioural factors, such as cigarette smoking or diet (to the extent to which the diet influences serum cholesterol and blood pressure). However, this does not mean that biological and behavioural risk factors are unimportant as determinants of mortality risk *within* ethnic groups. Even though they do not contribute to Black–White differences, they are strong predictors of cardiovascular and cancer mortality for both Black and White people, and considerable improvements in life expectancy could be produced if they were modified.

The last three figures have suggested that differences in socio-economic position make a key contribution to ethnic inequalities in health, particularly if we consider seriously Kaufman *et al.*'s (1997, 1998) caution on the difficulties associated with making effective adjustments for socio-economic position.

However, a consideration of some of the specific health outcomes within the MRFIT and FNS data suggests that this is not the only conclusion that can be drawn. Figure 4.7 shows the effects of standardising for income on the relative risk of mortality for prostate cancer and myeloma among Black men compared with White men. While this adjustment made a big difference to the all cause relative risk, as Figure 4.7 shows it made no difference in the outcomes of the two cancers. This is to be expected, since these causes of death are not strongly associated with socio-economic position among either Black or White men (Davey Smith *et al.* 1996a, b).

Figure 4.8 shows a similar pattern in the British data for the relative risk of diabetes mellitus in Pakistani and Bangladeshi populations compared with White people. Although making an adjustment for the more sensitive indicator of socio-economic position, i.e. standard of living, does lead to a

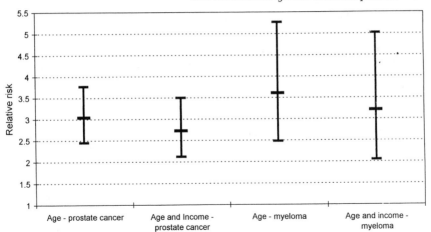

Figure 4.7 Effect of standardising for socio-economic position on prostate cancer and myeloma mortality in the United States (MFRIT data).

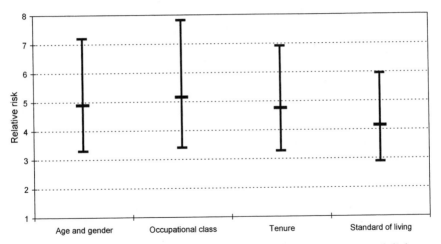

Figure 4.8 Effect of standardising for socio-economic position on reported diabetes in Britain (FNS data).

reduction in the relative risk, the much higher risk of diabetes mellitus among the Pakistani and Bangladeshi group persists.

Discussion

We have used mortality data from the United States and morbidity data from Britain to describe the contribution of socio-economic factors to ethnic inequalities in health. Both sets of data have produced similar findings. Within both the American and the British populations, ethnic minorities are on average poorer than White people. In particular, Black people in the United

States and Pakistani and Bangladeshi people in Britain are likely to be living in very poor circumstances. Not surprisingly, for both White and ethnic minority groups there is clear evidence of socio-economic inequalities in health. For example, in the United States Black and White men living in the poorest areas had twice the mortality rates of their counterparts in the richest areas.

Despite this, an initial examination of the British data suggested that socio-economic differences do not contribute to ethnic inequalities in health. However, statistically adjusting for socio-economic position when making comparisons across ethnic groups is not as simple as it may at first seem (Kaufman *et al.* 1997, 1998). The indicators of socio-economic position that are available in most studies do not adequately account for ethnic differences in socio-economic position. For example, in Britain the income of Pakistani and Bangladeshi people in particular social class groups is below half that of their White equivalents (Nazroo 1997a). Similarly, in the United States within given categories of socio-economic indicators, Black people suffer more disadvantages than White people. For example, within education categories Black men and women have considerably lower household incomes than their White equivalents (Pamuk *et al.* 1998), within occupational groups White people have higher incomes than Black people (Oliver and Shapiro 1995) and among those below the poverty line Black people are more likely to remain in this situation much longer than White people (Oliver and Shapiro 1995). Even within income strata, Black people have considerably lower wealth levels than White people and are less likely to be home-owners (Oliver and Shapiro 1995).

These are just a few examples of the considerable volume of data demonstrating that within any given band of socio-economic status, the social circumstances of ethnic minorities in Britain and the United States are less favourable than those of White people. There are, therefore, serious problems with crude attempts to adjust for socio-economic factors using conventional socio-economic indicators. In the parlance of epidemiology there will be a considerable amount of 'residual confounding' (Davey Smith and Phillips 1992) when adjustment is made for indicators that are measured with error and that have systematically different connotations in different ethnic groups. This is of particular concern if any persisting residual difference in health following an attempted 'adjustment' for socio-economic factors is then attributed to being a consequence of cultural or genetic differences through a process of elimination.

In this chapter, by using more and adequate indicators of socio-economic position we were able to demonstrate that socio-economic factors make a large contribution to ethnic inequalities in health. Although this leads us to conclude that ethnic inequalities in health are largely determined by inequalities in socio-economic position, a consideration of some specific forms of mortality and morbidity suggest that other factors may also be important and that the relative importance of particular factors in determining ethnic inequalities in health might vary according to the type of morbidity examined and also on the ethnic group actually being considered. For example, the indicators of socio-economic position used here made a large contribution to ethnic differences in all cause mortality and CVD mortality in the United States, as well as the reported general health and probable IHD in Britain, but they made no contribution to the differences in mortality from myeloma and prostate cancer between American Black and White men, and little contribution to differences in reported rates of diabetes among Pakistani and Bangladeshi people compared with White people in Britain.

A more nuanced approach to the factors underlying ethnic differences in health is required than simply considering them to be socio-economic, or cultural/behavioural or racial/genetic (Hummer 1996). Racism is of central importance here. First, the socio-economic differences between ethnic groups should not be considered as somehow autonomous (a likely danger associated with an approach which attempts to examine the extent to which socio-economic differentials 'explain' ethnic differentials in health). As Oliver and Shapiro (1995) demonstrate, the socio-economic disadvantage of Black people in the United States is the outcome of a long history of institutional racism and discrimination that has produced the current levels of disadvantage which are seen. Similarly, while the post-war migration of ethnic minority people into Britain was driven by a shortage of labour, this process and the socio-economic disadvantages faced by ethnic minority migrants in Britain was, and continues to be, structured by racism that has its roots in colonial history (Miles 1982, Gilroy 1987).

Besides producing socio-economic disparities, racism will also have other effects. Findings from the FNS data suggested widespread experiences of racial harassment among ethnic minority people in Britain, with more than one in eight respondents reporting having experienced at least one incident over the preceding year (Virdee 1997). Virdee (1997) points out that the mechanistic approach to counting incidents necessary for survey work is likely to underestimate the hostility ethnic minority people face. It ignores the context in which harassment operates and how it can become a pervading part of the experience of the lives of ethnic minority people, for example through the repeated harassment of an individual or family, or the way in which the harassment of one person in a community sends clear messages to the others in the community.

In addition, assessments of harassment neither cover experiences of discrimination nor the extent of prejudice felt by White people. For example, the FNS showed that among ethnic minority respondents there was a widespread belief that employers discriminated against ethnic minority applicants for jobs, together with a widespread experience of such discrimination (Modood 1997). Furthermore, when White people were asked about their opinions, one in five said that they were racially prejudiced against Caribbeans and one in four said they were racially prejudiced against Asians (Virdee 1997).

Experiences of harassment and discrimination might affect health in a number of ways, although there have only been limited explorations of this. In addition to being directly discriminated against, ethnic minority people know that they are disadvantaged and excluded compared with others, and hence have a clear perception of their relative disadvantage, which, as Wilkinson (1996) has argued, may well have a significant impact on health. This may be particularly important if the unfair treatment is not challenged (Krieger and Sidney 1996).

We also know that ethnic minority people are concentrated in particular geographical locations that are quite different from those where White people are more likely to live and are also likely to be more deprived areas (Massey and Denton 1989, Owen 1994). There is a growing body of work suggesting that characteristics of areas of residence may influence health over and above socio-economic characteristics of the people living within these areas (Townsend *et al.* 1988, Macintyre *et al.* 1993, Geronimus *et al.* 1996, Anderson *et al.* 1997, Davey Smith *et al.* 1998b). However, it is also possible that the concentration of ethnic minority people in particular areas may be protective of health, allowing the development of a strong community that enhances social support, reduces the sense of alienation, increases the group's access to political power and protects against the direct effects of racism (Halpern 1993, Smaje 1995).

Of course, there remains the possibility that cultural and biological differences contribute to ethnic inequalities in health. Here it is important to recognise that neither cultural practices nor biology are static. Ethnic identity changes over time and is dependent on social context; and other elements of identity also contribute to cultural practices (Nazroo 1998). Over time, environmental factors also become reflected in current biological measures. So biological differences may be a consequence both of genetic and of environmental determinants.

Many important determinants of health are physiological characteristics that are strongly influenced by socio-economic and other environmental factors, and in turn have a long-lasting influence on health. For example, low birth weight, which is strongly influenced by adverse material circumstances acting over the lifetime of the mother, is associated with high rates of diabetes mellitus, coronary heart disease, respiratory disease and hypertension in adult life. Similarly, short stature, influenced by nutrition in early life, is related to an increased risk of respiratory and cardiovascular mortality. Birth weight, growth in childhood, achieved stature and lung function are aspects of bodily *habitus*, which are at the same time socially influenced and biologically determined (Kuh and Ben-Shlomo 1997). The role of such parameters in explaining differentials in health status between ethnic groups, or socio-economic differentials within ethnic groups, therefore reflects explanations that are at the same time social and biological. An understandable tendency to reject any form of explanation presented in biological terms fails to recognise the extent to which socio-economic and environmental forces become embodied and, through this embodiment, influence the health of people throughout their lives, and may even influence the health of subsequent generations (Geronimus 1992, Davey Smith *et al.* 1997a).

To understand adequately ethnic inequalities in health, both interactive effects and the development of advantage and disadvantage over a lifetime need to be considered (Davey Smith *et al.* 1997b, Kuh and Ben-Shlomo 1997). The early-life socio-economic circumstances of ethnic minority adults may have been less favourable than those of White adults and there is growing evidence that socio-economic conditions in early life can influence mortality, in particular from cardiovascular disease and some cancers (Davey Smith *et al.* 1998c). The manner in which socio-economic disadvantage accumulates across the life-course to influence health has been referred to as 'weathering' with respect to the health of Black women in the United States (Geronimus 1992). The life-course perspective may be particularly important for migrants who will have been through a number of life-course transitions, and whose childhood might have involved significant deprivation, but this approach illustrates the complexity inherent in attempts to explain differences in health. However, it remains the case that the strongest evidence implicates socio-economic inequalities as the key determinant of ethnic inequalities in health.

Acknowledgements

The mortality follow-up of the men screened for the Multiple Risk Factor Analysis Trial was supported by a National Institutes for Health research grant, RO1 HL28715. The principal investigators and senior staff of the clinical, coordinating and support centres; the National Heart, Lung, and Blood Institute project office; and members of the Multiple Risk Factor Intervention Trial Policy Advisory Board and Mortality Review Committee are listed in a previous report (*JAMA* 1982, **248**, 1465–1477). Our comparative work on socio-economic differentials in health within and between ethnic groups has been helped by support to J. Nazroo 'Ethnic variations in health: assessing the role of class, gender and geography' Economic and Social Research Council grant, L128251019, and G. Davey Smith, H. Lambert, W. Ahmad, S. Fenton 'Comparative methods for studying socio-economic position and health in different ethnic communities' Economic and Social Research Council grant, L128251007. We thank Anne Rennie for help in preparation of the manuscript.

References

Anderson R.T., Sorlie, P., Backlund, E., Johnson, N. and Kaplan, G.A. (1997) 'Mortality effects of community socioeconomic status', *Epidemiology*, 8, 42–47.

Berthoud, R. (1997) 'Income and standards of living', in Modood, T., Berthoud, R., Lakey, J., Nazroo, J., Smith, P., Virdee, S. and Beishon, S. (eds) *Ethnic Minorities in Britain: Diversity and Disadvantage*, London: Policy Studies Institute, pp. 150–183.

Brown, C. (1984) *Black and White Britain: the Third PSI Survey*, London: Heinemann.

Brown, C. and Ritchie, J. (1981) *Focussed Enumeration: the Development of a Method for Sampling Ethnic Minority Groups*, London: Policy Studies Institute/SCPR.

Davey Smith, G. and Phillips, A.N. (1992) 'Confounding in epidemiological studies: why "independent" effects may not be all they seem', *British Medical Journal*, 305, 757–759.

Davey Smith, G., Neaton, J.D., Wentworth, D., Stamler, R. and Stamler, J. (1996a) 'Socioeconomic Differentials in mortality risk among men screened for the Multiple Risk Factor Intervention Trial: Part I – results for 300,685 White men', *American Journal of Public Health*, 86, 486–496.

Davey Smith, G., Wentworth, D., Neaton, J.D., Stamler, R. and Stamler, J. (1996b) 'Socioeconomic differentials in mortality risk among men screened for the Multiple Risk Factor Intervention Trial: Part II – results for 20,224 Black men', *American Journal of Public Health*, 86, 497–504.

Davey Smith, G., Hart, C., Ferell, C., Upton, M., Hole, D., Hawthorne, V., and Watt, G. (1997a) 'Birth weight of offspring and mortality in the Renfrew and Paisley study: prospective observational study', *British Medical Journal*, 315, 1189–1193.

Davey Smith, G., Hart, C., Blane, D., Gillis, C. and Hawthorne, V. (1997b) 'Lifetime socioeconomic position and mortality: prospective observational study', *British Medical Journal*, 314, 547–552.

Davey Smith, G., Neaton, J.D, Wentworth, D., Stamler, R. and Stamler, J. (1998a) 'Mortality differences between black and white men in the USA: contribution of income and other risk factors among men screened for the MRFIT', *Lancet*, 351, 934–939.

Davey Smith, G., Hart, C., Watt, G., Hole, D. and Hawthorne, V. (1998b) 'Individual social class, area-based deprivation, cardiovascular disease risk-factors, and mortality: the Renfrew and Paisley study', *Journal of Epidemiology and Community Health*, 52, 399–405.

Davey Smith, G., Hart, C., Blane, D. and Hole, D. (1998c) 'Adverse socioeconomic conditions in childhood and cause-specific adult mortality: prospective observational study', *British Medical Journal*, 316, 1631–1635.

Department of Health and Human Services (1990) *Health Status of the Disadvantaged: Chart Book 1990*, Washington: DHSS.

Drever, F. and Whitehead, M. (1997) *Health Inequalities: Decennial supplement No. 15*, London: The Stationery Office.

Geronimus, A.T. (1992) 'The weathering hypothesis and the health of African-American women and infants: evidence and speculations', *Ethnicity and Disease*, 2, 207–221.

Geronimus, A.T., Bound, J., Waidmann, T.A., Hillemeier, M.M. and Burns, P.B. (1996) 'Excess mortality among blacks and whites in the United States', *New England Journal of Medicine*, 335, 1552–1558.

Gilroy, P. (1987) *There Ain't No Black in the Union Jack*, London: Hutchinson.

Halpern, D. (1993) 'Minorities and mental health', *Social Science and Medicine*, 36, 597–607.

Harding, S. and Maxwell, R. (1997) 'Differences in mortality of migrants', in Drever, F. and Whitehead, M. (eds) *Health Inequalities: Decennial supplement No. 15*, London: The Stationery Office.

Hummer, R.A. (1996) 'Black-white differences in health and mortality: a review and conceptual model' *The Sociological Quarterly*, 37, 105–125.

Kaufman, J.S., Cooper, R.S. and McGee, D.L. (1997) 'Socioeconomic status and health in blacks and whites. The problem of residual confounding and the resiliency of race', *Epidemiology*, 8, 621–628.

Kaufman, J.S., Long, A.E., Liao, Y., Cooper, R.S. and McGee, D.L. (1998) 'The relation between income and mortality in U.S. Blacks and Whites', *Epidemiology*, 9, 147–155.

Krieger, N., Rowley, D.L., Herman, A.A., Avery, B. and Philips, M.T. (1993) 'Racism, sexism, and social class: implications for studies of health, disease, and well-being', *American Journal of Preventive Medicine*, 9 (Suppl.), 82–122.

Krieger, N. and Sidney, S. (1996) 'Racial discrimination and blood pressure: the CARDIA study of young black and white adults', *American Journal of Public Health*, 86, 1370–1378.

Kuh, D. and Ben-Shlomo, Y. (1997) *A Life Course Approach to Chronic Disease Epidemiology*, Oxford: Oxford University Press.

Macintyre, S., MacIver, S. and Sooman, A. (1993) 'Area, class and health: should we be focusing on places or people?', *Journal of Social Policy*, 22, 213–234.

Marmot, M.G., Adelstein, A.M., Bulusu, L. and Office for Population Census and Surveys (OPCS) (1984) *Immigrant Mortality in England and Wales 1970–78: Causes of Death by Country of Birth*, London: HMSO.

Massey, D. and Denton N. (1989) 'Hypersegregation in US metropolitan areas: Black and Hispanic segregation along five dimensions', *Demography*, 26, 373–392.

Miles, R. (1982) *Racism and Migrant Labour*, London: Routledge and Kegan Paul.

Modood, T. (1997) 'Employment', in Modood, T., Berthoud, R., Lakey, J., Nazroo, J., Smith, P., Virdee, S. and Beishon, S. (eds) *Ethnic Minorities in Britain: Diversity and Disadvantage*, London: Policy Studies Institute, pp. 83–149.

Modood, T., Berthoud, R., Lakey, J., Nazroo, J., Smith, P., Virdee, S. and Beishon, S. (1997) *Ethnic Minorities in Britain: Diversity and Disadvantage*, London: Policy Studies Institute.

Navarro, V. (1990) 'Race or class versus race and class: mortality differentials in the United States', *Lancet*, 336, 1238–1240.

Nazroo, J.Y. (1997a) *The Health of Britain's Ethnic Minorities: Findings From a National Survey*, London: Policy Studies Institute.

Nazroo, J.Y. (1997b) *Mental Health and Ethnicity: Findings from a National Community Survey*, London: Policy Studies Institute.

Nazroo, J.Y. (1998) 'Genetic, cultural or socio-economic vulnerability? Explaining ethnic inequalities in health', *Sociology of Health and Illness*, 20, 714–734.

Neaton, J.D., Kuller, L.H., Wentworth, D. and Borhani, N.O. (1984) 'Total and cardiovascular mortality in relation to cigarette smoking, serum cholesterol concentration and diastolic blood pressure among black and white males followed for up to five years', *American Heart Journal*, 108, 759–769.

Neaton, J.D., Grimm, R.H. and Cutler, J.A. (1987) 'Recruitment of participants for the Multiple Risk Factor Intervention Trial (MRFIT)', *Controlled Clinical Trials*, 8, 415–535.

Oliver, M.L. and Shapiro, T.M. (1995) *Black Wealth/White Wealth: a New Perspective on Racial Inequality*, New York: Routledge.

Owen, D. (1994) 'Spatial variations in ethnic minority groups populations in Great Britain', *Population Trends*, 78, 23–33.

Pamuk, E., Makuc, D., Heck, K., Reuben, C. and Lochner, K. (1998) *Socioeconomic Status and Health Chartbook. Health, United States, 1998*, Hyattsville, MD: National Center for Health Statistics.

Rogers, R.G. (1992) 'Living and dying in the USA: socio-demographic determinants of death among blacks and whites', *Demography*, 29, 287–303.

Rogot, E., Sorlie, P.D., Johnson, N.J. and Schmitt, C. (1993) *A Mortality Study of 1.3 Million Persons by Demographic, Social and Economic Factors: 1979–1985. Follow-up, US National Longitudinal Mortality Study*, Washington: National Institutes of Health.

Rudat, K. (1994) *Black and Minority Ethnic Groups in England: Health and Lifestyles*, London: Health Education Authority.

Sheldon, T.A. and Parker, H. (1992) 'Race and ethnicity in health research', *Journal of Public Health Medicine*, 14, 104–110.

Smaje, C. (1995) 'Ethnic residential concentration and health: evidence for a positive effect?', *Policy and Politics*, 23, 251–69.

Smaje, C. (1996) 'The ethnic patterning of health: new directions for theory and research', *Sociology of Health and Illness*, 18, 139–171.

Smith, P and Prior, G. (1997) *The Fourth National Survey of Ethnic Minorities: Technical Report*, London: Social and Community Planning Research.

Sorlie, P., Rogot, E., Anderson, R., Johnson, N.J. and Backlund, E. (1992) 'Black-white mortality differences by family income', *Lancet*, 340, 346–350.

Sterling, T., Rosenbaum, W. and Weinkam, J. (1993) 'Income, race and mortality', *Journal of the National Medical Association*, 85, 906–911.

Townsend, P. and Davidson, N. (1982) *Inequalities in Health (the Black Report)*, Middlesex: Penguin.

Townsend, P., Phillimore, P. and Beattie, A. (1988) *Health and Deprivation: Inequality and the North*, London: Routledge.

Trask, J.W. (1916) 'The significance of the mortality rates of the coloured population of the United States', *American Journal of Public Health*, 6, 254–260.

Virdee, S. (1997) 'Racial harassment', in Modood, T., Berthoud, R., Lakey, J., Nazroo, J., Smith, P., Virdee, S. and Beishon, S. (1997) *Ethnic Minorities in Britain: Diversity and Disadvantage*, London: Policy Studies Institute.

Wild, S. and McKeigue, P. (1997) 'Cross sectional analysis of mortality by country of birth in England and Wales, 1970–92', *British Medical Journal*, 314, 705–710.

Wilkinson, R.G. (1996) *Unhealthy Societies: the Afflictions of Inequality*, London: Routledge.

5 Health

An elusive concept

Gilbert Lewis

'Health' is not a specialist's word; its everyday use is obvious. 'How do you do?' 'How are you?' – ideas of health are implicitly applied in daily life and liable to mean different things to different people. Precisely what it means may come to mind rarely, except when someone feels ill or notices a change. Indeed, in many cultures, it might not be possible to find a single term closely corresponding to our word 'health', but even so the people of those cultures would have a great variety of ideas and actions to discuss which they see as relevant to health. A number of elements recur in general ideas about health, despite the diversity of the societies. This chapter will point out some of them, especially with reference to health as an attribute of the person and the question of accepting that there must be a social or cultural component in ideas of health.

'Health' is the unmarked member of a linguistic pair, with 'illness' the marked concept. So 'health' may include 'illness' (indeed 'health' statistics usually turn out to be findings about the distributions of different diseases, disabilities and causes of death); but not the reverse – 'illness' does not include 'health'. The markedness fits the way we tend to take health for granted, while illness makes us stop and think. Is health, then, merely the absence of identifiable disease or infirmity?

Health as an ideal

This was not the view taken by the World Health Organization (WHO) at its foundation in 1948: the chosen definition expresses an ideal, 'Health is a state of complete physical, mental and social well-being, and not merely the absence of disease and infirmity' (WHO 1992). But that definition is of an aim which puts health beyond everyone's reach. Who is perfect in such terms? Saracci (1997) points out that such a state of complete physical mental and social well-being corresponds perhaps more to happiness than to health. Happiness and health are not identical. An improvement in health may be had but sometimes only at the cost of control and self-restraint [he quoted Sigmund Freud on the experience of stopping smoking cigars – 'I am better than I was, but not happier' (Freud 1930)].

The quest for happiness is open-ended, boundless even. The WHO's 1948 definition was meant both as an idea and as an ideal to inspire and to go beyond the merely negative definitions of health. It states an aspiration, a global ideal, and affirms the positive sense which many cultures have wanted to give to the idea of health. In antiquity, for example, the story of Pandora's box, of Hesiod's Golden Race or the expulsion from the Garden of Eden in the Bible all present ideas of a time without illness, a place of perfect health. Health and happiness, immortality and lack of toil came together in images of what was lost. A vision of health, ease and nature in harmony, which is also to be found in other myths of a world lost or of one to gain, an Arcadia or a Utopia. 'Physical mental and social well-being' spell out the components of a much later, but rather similar, holistic vision. Certainly, if health requires social well-being, it must depend also on values and must vary by culture and ethnicity. People in many societies have conceived of health in generally holistic ideal terms.

Criteria for distinguishing health: fact, variation or bias

The diversity of standards for health is evident: they may differ by species, populations, cultures, individuals, environments, time-frames for judgement, lifestyles and values. Social anthropologists have not tried to compare and analyse concepts of health in the way they have ideas about illness, but similar issues of cultural relativity would lie in wait for them.

One early and penetrating sociological examination of the concept of health is embedded in Durkheim's 'The Rules of Sociological Method' (1964, first published 1895). His chapter on 'Rules for distinguishing between the normal and the pathological', although really concerned with society, deviance and crime, proceeds by comparison and analogy and dissects the concept of health. Health is generally taken to be something good and desirable: he asks whether it has objective criteria. He associates health with normality. He argues that we should take the average as the normal because, if we do not, we shall only expose our personal values or prejudices when we select certain attributes to serve as signs of health. He implies that nature guarantees that the average should be healthy. It would follow from the idea of selection of the fittest. 'One cannot without contradiction, even conceive of a species which would be incurably diseased in itself and by virtue of its fundamental constitution. The healthy constitutes the norm *par excellence* and can consequently be in no way abnormal' [Durkheim 1964 (1895): 58].

The problems for this view come with questions about the complex relationships between an organism or species and its present environment, the time-frame, the interactions between present circumstances and constitutions inherited, evolved in the past: especially for human populations and individuals who make plans, devise new rules and now modify their living conditions so fast.

Durkheim [1964 (1895)] reached his conclusion after rejecting two possible criteria: (1) perfect adaptation of an organism to its environment and (2) survival. The first was rejected because he could find no way to distinguish completeness or perfection of adaptation. Health might of course be defined in relative rather than absolute terms. Standards would then be variable and must be related both to the environment and to the individual: old age and infancy are both accompanied by special risks and susceptibility to illness. But we should not want to argue along absolutist lines that only the young adult, never the infant, can be healthy. In some respects (e.g. over body size and dietary requirements) individuals set their own standards for normality. If health standards certainly vary by species, in which circumstances should they be adjusted for population, ethnic group, caste or culture? Some of the answers (e.g. a 'proper' diet) might seem to depend on questions of fact, others on questions of value.

The second criterion Durkheim [1964 (1895)] questioned was survival (life): it was impracticable. He was looking for objective criteria (effects on mortality, morbidity, fertility), but we cannot calculate the effect on survival of some of the abnormalities we take to be signs of illness or unhealthy. The events and afflictions are too varied in severity, unclear in timing and causal links, to disentangle and calculate. Certain maladies may, in the long run, increase chances of survival – for example, through effects on future resistance or immunity. (Durkheim's examples were inoculations with vaccines – ours might include genetic factors such as those associated with the sickle cell trait or non-insulin-dependent diabetes mellitus.) Circumstances may change. What is found to be normal may depend on the current environment and living conditions of the population measured, but also of course it depends on the past. Durkheim recognised that there might be special difficulties in identifying the healthy with the normal under conditions of rapid change.

By advocating statistical normality as he does in the quotation cited above, Durkheim [1964 (1895)] appears to put his trust in nature. But, of course, some human populations have characteristics which are very common yet regarded as undesirable (e.g. obesity, blood pressure rising with age, dental caries), and other characteristics are rare yet desirable (great strength, great intelligence). Do selection for fitness and adaptation to environment work on human populations differently from populations of animals and plants? Perhaps so, in the sense that people can evade some of the pressures because they alter their environments to suit themselves, according to their desires or wants and needs. When people change their environments and activity levels (as they do with towns, machines, medical technology, etc.) and change the conditions in which they live, they may escape some of the constraints and much of the harshness of natural selection. Trial involves error. Things unwanted and the errors judged by human selection do not necessarily mirror or match those which would be condemned by natural selection.

The old view of health was freedom from discomfort or disability and from any objective disturbances of function. For most of history (and still for many people in the world), the subject's view has been decisive: there were no X-rays or laboratory tests to look inside the body while someone was alive. The subject's view could scarcely be challenged. Now the subject's feelings of health or illness may be contradicted by the results of laboratory or clinical investigations. The old view was generally consistent with experience. Now subtle tests at the minute levels of cellular and sub-cellular pathology or chemistry may come to confuse the boundaries between perceived health and sickness. Someone may be infected or have abnormal results without feeling discomfort or showing objective disturbance. The contrast between health and illness is not a simple matter of yes or no when someone has inherited a particular gene, a potential for illness, a particular risk that may depend on other contributing factors. Epidemiology, genetics and the molecular biology of the cell provide information of a different sort and scale from that previously used by people to make their own decisions about health. Health and illness are clear conceptual opposites but the middle ground of the continuum between them is in practice far less clear.

Commitments to cultural ideas about health

People in every society learn their own culture's accepted ideas about behaviour, diet and risk, the nature and constitution of the body, the uses, properties and dangers of the environment. Health in the sense of life, well-being and survival is bound to be a basic matter of concern even though the subject of health is so basic and pervasive that it may be difficult to know how to circumscribe it, where to start and where to stop. Many of the ideas are likely to be deeply rooted and resistant to change. Ideas on proper diet, or theories of conception, often are customary taboos and there are local beliefs about certain risks or dangers, the normal course of a child's development, preferences or prohibitions on marriage. They have passed the test of time for they enabled the particular people's forefathers and ancestors to survive; the customs belong to them and tradition legitimates them (Horton 1982).

The Huli live in the Southern Highlands of New Guinea. Stephen Frankel (1986) gives careful attention to their ideas on health as well as on illness. He draws a striking picture of their sense of environment, health and adaptation. The Huli have no single term for 'health', instead a constellation of ideas and actions indicate their views. They recognise health in various frames:

- as the *absence* of disease;
- as *resilience* – they seek to resist the intrusion of illness by prophylactic rituals, e.g. to strengthen the child in preparation for birth of a sibling, to bind the soul within the body, to remove the taint of pollution; they see individuals as more or less resilient to illness, e.g. the vulnerability of the old and young, the variation in some people's skill in caring for their health; at root the view that life is fragile, illness a danger of living;

• they also associate *health and social effectiveness* – make health seem as much a social as a physical state. They express deep concern for their bodies and the achievement of an ideal state of physical resilience and social distinction. The skin which shines and gleams with health is linked in their view to social effectiveness, particularly the attraction of wealth and influence. They take responsibility for it by preparation in the bachelor cult and observance of elaborate rules to avoid pollution from women. The special actions and events associated with rites of passage, rules about diet, daily activities contain a cluster of ideas and images about growth, successful development, the normal course of human life, the means to health and the dangers to avoid.

Above I quoted from Durkheim: 'One cannot, without contradiction, even conceive of a species which would be incurably diseased in itself and by virtue of its fundamental constitution' [Durkheim 1964 (1985): 58]. His sentence is consistent with a common attitude to illness in which health is conceived as natural, given by nature, innate or intrinsic, something belonging to the self; illness, as the enemy, is something which comes from outside. In many traditions, there are myths that pose questions about the origins of sickness; why death must come; whether illness is part of human nature or comes from forces or things outside, or as punishment for fault or sin. Is health, then, natural and illness not? Or is my illness also part of me? Theories about the causes of illness are often extremely complex in terms of the messages they contain about implied responsibilities for health and illness. New or foreign ideas of germs, bacteria, or inherited disease may be assimilated at first in traditional terms of blame and responsibility (Lewis 1993). These may be given by ideas about invisible spirits, or sorcery, or pollution, or through particular beliefs about fate or destiny, or come from ideas about kinship and the transmission of parental substance or potential.

Health from inside: illness without

Although it is clear that ideas of health and illness differ by culture, they are not fixed. A conspicuous amount of borrowing of ideas and exchange has gone on (Leslie 1976) and goes on, for example, most notably in the global spread of biomedicine. Contemporary medicine in urban Japan includes influences from various sources including Shintoism, Chinese medicine, ideas deriving from Taoism and Confucian philosophy, as well as Western medicine (Lock 1980, Kuriyama 1992). The lack of uniformity is striking. Japan at the time of Lock's study had high standards of health (life expectancy for men in 1973 was 71 years, for women 76). Despite the mixture of ideas and sources, some Japanese ideas and attitudes are strongly marked and distinctive. Lock (1980) and Ohnuki-Tierney (1986) describe the Japanese concern about purity and protection of the inside from defilement: a practical code – contemporary but also one with deep, old roots. Ohnuki-Tierney (1986) quotes the following instructions stuck inside books from a local public library, 'Before and after reading, wash your hands well.' 'Do not lick your fingers to turn the pages'. The duty to avoid contamination and dirt, especially outside foreign dirt, is taught early. As a cultural theme of concern, it is based on ancient but sharp dualisms of thought about inside–outside, clean–dirty, safe–dangerous and good–bad. To prevent the risk of defilement by dirt from outside, they follow an elaborate code of hygiene; it affects attitudes to the body, shoes, clothing, house space, times to bathe, the treatment of waste, strangers, animals; it is an ethic of purity.

Chinese medical thought brought into Japan a collection of elaborated ideas classifying elements and relationships of the macrocosm and microcosm, correspondences between the body, seasons, substances, ideas about the structure and relationships of organs in the body. It provided a basis for theories about energy, ideas about health, harmony and balance, about diet and activities. Although many people who use it may not know of its Chinese medical origins, the Japanese concept of *ki* appears in many everyday words associated with emotions, well-being and changes in feeling. 'Change in a person is seen as transient, oscillations about a hypothetical norm, which is a state of balance. The image of a human being is of a relatively fixed container, a body type, largely determined by hereditary constitution, around and in which a dance of the exchange of energy is ceaselessly enacted – a view influenced by and close to East Asian medical beliefs. Health and ill health are both normal, the body continually moves in and out of both states, which are intimately related to a dynamic image derived from *ki*' (Lock 1980: 85).

Despite their persistent emphasis on hygiene, Ohnuki-Tierney (1984) draws attention to the curious point that the Japanese do not see themselves as clean and healthy. Rather the opposite is true. Many people feel they are often slightly ill – 'down' – their state of health is not constant but fluctuates between health and illness. They associate it with a susceptible or weak (in other words, sensitive) constitution; they talk openly about their illnesses and have little hesitation about taking sick leave if they feel the need to, a readiness that might surprise the Westerner 'overshadowed by the image of the 'workaholic' Japanese' (Ohnuki-Tierney 1984: 52). The type of constitution (*taishitsu*) one is born with makes one susceptible to particular kinds of infirmity – it is a kind of chronic mild illness (*jibyo*) or susceptibility one carries round with one for life. The weaknesses of constitution must be offset with appropriate food and behaviour. From the individual's point of view, the constitutional weakness is normal. Health and ill health can both be normal, depending on the individual.

Holism and health

In commenting on these ideas of health, I have assumed that the individual is the significant unit on which the ideas are focused. But in many biological views of health and survival, it would be the species, the population or the environment (Dubos 1968). Indeed balance, nature and adaptation have been at the heart of many concepts of health and well-being. Holism is commonly associated with health, and this should hardly be surprising since the word itself, 'health', derives from 'hale' or 'whole'.

Apart from particular explanations of illness by the effects of pollution, strong emotions, sorcery, spirits, the Huli in the Southern Highlands of New Guinea also have a body of lore and ritual about the environment in which they live, and their place in it, their common health and future (Frankel 1986). It guides a set of major rituals performed at certain sacred sites concerned with the fertility of the earth and the people. It involves a holistic view of health depending on their relationship to the land, their neighbours and each other.

They say that the earth, mountains and rivers are responsive to human deeds and misdeeds. Should men of the wrong groups meet, the earth would deteriorate. They conserve traditions of a time of darkness (*mbingi*) when a great fall of black ash destroyed houses, trees and crops, but after it came rain, followed by a time of black earth and great fertility (Frankel ibid.). There is geological evidence of a fall of volcanic ash in soil layers dated to about 1700 (Frankel ibid.). The Huli think that since the great fertility following the time of darkness, there has been a gradual deterioration in the fertility of earth, pigs and people, the earth desiccating and ageing as the human body does, an upsurge of illness, and moral decline, loss of respect for custom, promiscuity, European changes (Frankel ibid.).

The rituals of *dindi gamu* that they were performing at their sacred sites (linked, they say, by giant subterranean liana-like roots) were attempts to bring the *mbingi* time of darkness back to restore fertility. They tell a myth about the mistaken killing of a child *Bayebaye* (whose name means 'perfect'): his mother's curse at his killing which would, for them, account for why things got worse. The *dindi gamu* rites and beliefs transmit a holistic sense of the interconnectedness of geological and human affairs, served to explain their sense of physical and moral decline. The ideas lay behind many aspects of their relationships with neighbours, their response to the coming of White people and to Christianity, the story of the Crucifixion, and the reasons for their large-scale, abrupt conversion (Frankel ibid.).

A holistic idea of health combining elements of balance and adaptation has appeared in many distinct theories and cosmologies. The health and adaptation of different peoples to their particular environments was the theme of the Hippocratic book on 'Airs Waters and Places' (Lloyd 1976). Harriet Ngubane (1977) describes the thought of the Nyuswa Zulu, beginning her account by explaining about the special relationship a person has with his or her environment – a view of belonging. According to the Zulu, the people of a particular region are adjusted to their surroundings – its plant and animal life, the environment and atmosphere. Strangers may leave invisible tracks and foreign elements when they travel through a place. Others, passing by, can pick up harm from these tracks. Although normally people establish and maintain themselves in balance and harmony with their surroundings, an environment may become polluted by undesirable tracks or by harmful substances discarded in healing.

A critical theme in Zulu thought is the notion of 'balance' (of 'things being in order') *vis-à-vis* other people and the environment. 'For a Zulu conceives good health not only as consisting of a healthy body, but as a healthy situation of everything that concerns him. Good health means the harmonious working and co-ordination of his universe' (Ngubane 1977: 27–28).

Despite the diversity in detailed views about the causes and significance of signs of illness, I think there would be a good measure of agreement about unwelcome departures from physical health, but perhaps less agreement about the signs of departure from mental health, and less still over what should be regarded as departures from social health.

The social or cultural component in health

On the question of whether health must inevitably be granted a social dimension or be reserved as a medical concept, Barbara Wootton's (1959) observations are still cogent. All ways of life are not equally good. 'Adjustment' cannot be accepted as a criterion of health unless we face the question: Adjustment to what?

> Fine phrases cannot, however, obscure the fact that adjustment means adjustment to a particular culture or to a particular set of institutions; and that to conceive adjustment and maladjustment in medical terms is in effect to identify health with the ability to come to terms with that culture or with those institutions – be they totalitarian methods of government, the dingy culture of an urban slum, the contemporary English law of marriage, or what I have elsewhere called the standards of an 'acquisitive, competitive, hierarchical, envious' society.
>
> (Wootton 1959: 218)

She was writing with the question of mental health in mind. If we cannot find objective terms to define mental ill health and health, then the road is wide open to classify all forms of anti-social behaviour as symptoms of illness or mental disorder, in other words to obliterate the distinction between criminality and illness altogether. It was very clear, she concluded, that we have a long way to go to reach a definition of physical-cum-mental health that is objective and wholly free of social value judgements.

References

Dubos, R. (1968) *Man, Medicine and Environment*, Harmondsworth: Penguin.
Durkheim, E. (1964) *The Rules of Sociological Method*, translated by G. Catlin, New York: Free Press. First published as *'Les Règles de la méthode sociologique'* (1895), Paris.

Frankel, S. (1986) *The Huli Response to Illness*, Cambridge: Cambridge University Press.

Freud, S. (1930) Letter to Lou Andreas-Salome, May 8, 1930. Cited in Loike and Wogenstein (1975) *Sigmund Freud, House Catalogue*, Vienna.

Horton, R. (1982) 'Tradition and modernity revisited', in Hollis, M. and Lukes, S. (eds) *Rationality and Relativism*, Oxford: Blackwell Publishers.

Kuriyama, S. (1992) 'Between mind and eye: Japanese anatomy in the eighteenth century', in Leslie, C. and Young, A. (eds) *Paths to Asian Medical Knowledge*, Berkeley: University of California Press.

Leslie, C. (1976) *Asian Medical Systems: a Comparative Study*, Berkeley: University of California Press.

Lewis, G. (1993) 'Double standards of treatment evaluation' in Lindenbaum, S. and Lock, M. (eds) *Knowledge, Power and Practice*, Berkeley: University of California Press.

Lloyd, G.E.R. (1976) *The Hippocratic Writings*, Harmondsworth: Penguin.

Lock, M. (1980) *East Asian Medicine in Urban Japan: Varieties of Medical Experience*, Berkeley: University of California Press.

Ngubane, H. (1977) *Body and Mind in Zulu Medicine*, London: Academic Press.

Ohnuki-Tierney, E. (1984) *Illness and Culture in Contemporary Japan: an Anthropological View*, Cambridge: Cambridge University Press.

Saracci, R. (1997) 'The World Health Organization needs to reconsider its definition of health', *British Medical Journal*, 314, 1409–1410.

Wootton, B. (1959) *Social Science and Social Pathology*, London: Allen and Unwin.

World Health Organization (1992) *Basic Documents*, thirty-ninth edition, Geneva: WHO.

6   Human inbreeding

A familiar story full of surprises

Alan H. Bittles, H. S. Savithri,
H. S. Venkatesha Murthy, G. Baskaran,
Wei Wang, Janet Cahill and N. Appaji Rao

Introduction

In most Western countries, especially those located in Northern Europe, North America and Australasia, marriages between close biological relatives generally are regarded as both highly undesirable from a social perspective and dangerous in terms of the physical and mental well-being of their progeny. By comparison, in North and sub-Saharan Africa, and West, Central and South Asia consanguineous unions are widely contracted, and in some communities they account for a majority of marital unions in the current generation (Bittles 1994).

There appears to be no particular rationale for this sub-division of human populations into opposing forms of marriage preference and, as illustrated in Table 6.1, even within the major religions there are quite marked differences in attitude to close-kin marriage. Thus, in Christianity, the Orthodox churches prohibit consanguineous marriage, and the Roman Catholic church requires Diocesan permission for marriages between first cousins, and until early in the present century this ruling included second- and third-cousin unions. According to the Venerable Bede (731), the basis for the Latin church's guidance on acceptable levels of consanguinity within marriage was originally stated in a communication by Pope Gregory I to St Augustine in 597, 'experience shows that such unions do not result in children, and "sacred law forbids a man to uncover the nakedness of his kindred" ', the latter comment being derived from the book of Leviticus 18:6. However, following the Reformation, the Protestant denominations opted to use as their guidelines a restricted version of the detailed Judaic regulations established in Leviticus 18: 7–18 and to sanction marriages up to and including unions between first cousins, equivalent to a coefficient of inbreeding in the progeny (F) of 0.0625.

A similar degree of non-uniformity exists in Hinduism. The Aryan Hindus of north India impose a prohibition on marriage with biological kin that extends back approximately seven generations on the male side and five generations on the female side (Kapadia 1958). By comparison, for the Dravidian Hindus of south India marriage between first cousins of the type

Table 6.1 Religious attitudes to consanguineous marriage

Buddhism	Permissive
Christianity	
Orthodox	Proscribed
Roman Catholic	Approval required
Protestant	Permissive
Hinduism	
Aryan	Proscribed
Dravidian	Permissive
Islam	
Sunni	Permissive
Shia	Permissive
Judaism	
Askenazi	Permissive
Sephardi	Permissive
Sikhism	Proscribed

mother's brother's daughter (MBD) is strongly favoured and, particularly in the states of Andhra Pradesh, Karnataka and Tamil Nadu, uncle–niece marriages ($F = 0.125$) also are widely contracted.

In general, Muslim regulations on marriage parallel the Judaic pattern prescribed in Leviticus, but, although uncle–niece unions are permitted in Judaism, a form of marriage that was not adopted by the Reformed Protestant churches, they are forbidden by the Koran. Yet double first-cousin marriages ($F = 0.125$) are recognised within Islam. In South Asia, Buddhism sanctions marriage between first cousins whereas the Sikh religion, which also originated in north India, follows the Aryan Hindu marital tradition and forbids consanguineous marriage, although in some minority Sikh groups there may be a relaxation of this proscription.

There is a similar lack of coherence in the legislation that has been enacted in different countries to govern permitted types of marital relationships. Thus while first-cousin marriages are legal in the United Kingdom and Australia, they are criminal offences in eight of the states of the United States and illegal in a further twenty-two states (Ottenheimer 1990). Exceptions can be incorporated into state laws, for example, to permit uncle–niece marriage within the Jewish community of Rhode Island (Bratt 1984). Legislation approved and adopted at the national level may also prove to be inoperable in practice, as exemplified by the Hindu Marriage Act of 1955, which includes a ban on uncle–niece marriage (Kapadia 1958). Yet in a study conducted between 1980 and 1989 in Bangalore and Mysore, the two major cities of the state of Karnataka in south India, 21.3 per cent of Hindu marriages were uncle–niece unions (Bittles *et al.* 1992).

The prevalence of consanguineous unions

An estimate of the current global prevalence of consanguineous unions can be derived from national population projections [Population Reference Bureau (PRB) 1998] and collated reports on the prevalence of consanguineous marriage at national, regional and local levels (Bittles 1998). For this purpose, a consanguineous marriage is defined as a union between individuals related as second cousins or closer, equivalent in their progeny to $F = 0.0156$. As shown in Table 6.2, populations can be sub-divided into four main categories: those in which the level of consanguinity is unknown, either because it has not been reported or the data are of insufficient reliability and depth to predict the percentage consanguinity with any real degree of confidence, and populations in which consanguineous unions account for less than 1 per cent, 1–10 per cent and 20–50+ per cent of marriages.

In compiling these data a deliberately conservative approach has been adopted, and so the numbers recorded can reasonably be regarded as lower bound estimates. It is apparent that with the exception of a country such as Japan, which has undergone rapid industrialisation and urbanisation since World War II (Schull 1958, Imaizumi *et al.* 1975, Imaizumi 1986), past predictions of a rapid global decline in the prevalence of consanguineous unions have proved to be invalid. In fact, the recorded numbers of consanguineous unions appear to have grown at least in tempo with the increasing global population, and in some communities the proportion of marriages contracted between close biological kin also has expanded. The simplest explanation for this observation is that because greater numbers of children have been surviving to marriageable age in virtually all economically less developed countries during the course of the last generation, the prevailing social preference for consanguineous unions is more readily accommodated.

Migrant communities now permanently resident in Western countries may represent a special case, especially where they practice a religion not followed by the majority indigenous population. In such communities, the available evidence suggests that the prevalence of consanguineous unions is increasing, in many cases from an already high level, examples being the Pakistani community in the United Kingdom (Darr and Modell 1988), the Moroccan

Table 6.2 Global prevalence of consanguineous marriage

	Millions
Unknown	1,064
< 1%	1,061
1–10%	2,811
20–50+%	991
Global population	5,926

Sources: Bittles (1998) and PRB (1998).

and Turkish communities in Belgium (Reniers 1998) and the Lebanese community in Australia (de Costa 1988). Various reasons can be advanced to explain this finding, including the desire to find a marital partner from within the community, which itself may be numerically small and composed of a restricted number of kindreds, and the wish to maintain community traditions in a new and unfamiliar environment. However, explanations of this type tend to underestimate the very real belief that marriage within the family, as opposed simply to community endogamy, is both the most desirable and the most reliable marital option (Bittles *et al.* 1991, Hussain and Bittles 1998). As noted above, the current increase in the numbers of persons of marriageable age within these communities in effect facilitates the fulfilment of this belief.

Applying similar logic, at some future time a decline in the prevalence of consanguineous unions can be predicted, concomitant with the expected reduction in family sizes. Nevertheless, this decline probably will not be uniform in extent across populations but principally be observed in urbanised populations and among couples who share higher educational standards and later ages at marriage. Indeed, there already is evidence of such a change occurring in Pakistan (Hussain and Bittles 1998). The specific type of consanguineous union contracted may also prove to be an important determining factor and, as family sizes reduce, double first-cousin and uncle–niece marriages predictably will become increasingly difficult to arrange within the accepted norms of spousal age difference at marriage. Where there is a specific type of consanguineous union favoured within a community, for example MBD first-cousin marriage in Hindu south India, it will be interesting to observe whether greater emphasis is placed on the requirement to marry within the prescribed marriage pattern or to contract marriage with a family member irrespective of the precise type of cousin union.

Assessing the outcomes of consanguineous marriages

As mentioned in the introduction to this chapter, in Western societies there is a strong belief that the progeny of close kin unions will exhibit elevated levels of physical and/or mental defect, the implication being that these adverse outcomes are caused by the expression of detrimental recessive genes which have accumulated in the kindred and/or community because of inbreeding over multiple generations, i.e. the phenomenon of inbreeding depression. The evidence produced to support this contention often has been vague and largely anecdotal in nature, with little or no proof that the claimed pattern(s) of ill health stemmed specifically from the expression of specific recessive genes. An opposite and ultimately beneficial genetic perspective on consanguinity also has been advanced, suggesting that in communities in which close-kin unions were traditionally preferential there would have been a gradual but significant elimination of detrimental recessive genes from the gene pool through generational time (Sanghvi 1966). According to this scenario, in communities with an unbroken history of strict endogamy and preferential consanguinity, a lower incidence of disorders with a recessive mode of inheritance would be expected.

Unfortunately, since most communities in which consanguinity is preferential are poorly developed in socio-economic terms, until quite recently data of appropriate quality were not available to test these opposing hypotheses. In a meta-analysis of thirty-eight surveys conducted in seven countries, it was estimated that the progeny of first cousins had a 4.4 per cent increased risk of mortality from the late prenatal to reproductive phases (Bittles and Neel 1994). Using this estimate, it could then be calculated that in a country such as Pakistan with 50.3 per cent consanguineous marriage (Bittles *et al.* 1993), equivalent to a mean coefficient of inbreeding (α) = 0.0280, the practice of consanguineous marriage was associated with 19.7 out of 1,000 deaths in the pre-reproductive years.

A potential problem with this type of calculation is that, in the majority of surveys on which the meta-analysis was based, control for the possible contributory effects of socio-demographic variables was minimal, and in many less developed countries it has been shown that factors such as maternal illiteracy, young maternal age and short birth interval may be significant adverse influences on infant and/or childhood survival. Further, the majority of consanguineous marriages are contracted in communities with low socio-economic status in which these types of factors would be operating (Bittles 1994).

In an attempt to overcome this problem, the comparative influences of socio-demographic variables and consanguinity on survival up to 5 years of age were simultaneously examined using retrospective data abstracted from the 1990/1991 Pakistan Demographic and Health Survey (PDHS). The PDHS was designed as a nationally representative study based on household interviews of 6,611 women who had delivered 26,408 offspring during the previous 18 years, and in the survey 60.2 per cent of women reported that they were married to a first or second cousin (α = 0.0326). The PDHS data confirmed that non-genetic variables have a significant negative effect on early survival with, for example, a birth interval of less than 18 months principally associated with deaths in the first month of life whereas maternal illiteracy mainly affected mortality in the 2–5 year age group. But, even after controlling for these variables, consanguinity demonstrably exerted a significant adverse effect on both neonatal and post-neonatal survival (Grant and Bittles 1997).

A more intensive local study in squatter settlements in Karachi reached a similar conclusion (Hussain and Bittles 1998). In the Karachi study, which included all the main ethnic groups in the country and with Hindus and Christians as well as Muslim subjects recruited, 58.7 per cent of marriages were consanguineous (α = 0.0316). The study also demonstrated differing family histories of inbred unions, although it is unclear whether this pattern mainly reflected the level of preference for close kin marriage within each family or the past availability of appropriate family members of marriageable age. A possible additional variable in Pakistani communities is membership of the *bradari* (literally translated as brotherhood) to which each of the families belonged, as an earlier study in Punjab had revealed significant inter-*bradari* differences in terms of preference for consanguineous unions (Shami *et al.* 1993).

The effects of consanguinity at the genome level

The findings of a number of studies from south India on the relationship between consanguinity and mortality have been interpreted as support for the hypothesis that consanguineous marriages contracted over many generations had resulted in the purging of recessive lethals from the gene pool (John and Jayabal 1971, Rao and Inbaraj 1977, Govinda Reddy 1985). In each case, however, the authors appeared to have assumed unrealistically high consanguinity-associated death rates and there was little or no control for the possible contributory effects of socio-demographic variables. In fact, studies in Karnataka on sick children (Radha Rama Devi *et al.* 1987) and neonates screened for amino acidopathies (Appaji Rao *et al.* 1988) indicated the presence of a wide range of genetic disorders in the overall gene pool, with confirmation of the expected positive relationship between consanguinity and the incidence of recessive disorders. Similar findings have been reported in prospective studies on the British Pakistani community in Birmingham, with elevated levels of serious malformations and chronic disease/disabilities observed (Bundey 1992, Bundey and Alam 1993). In some Pakistani families in Bradford, more than one recessive lethal gene was segregating which, for example, resulted in the birth of children who either were diagnosed with cystic fibrosis or β-thalassaemia, or like their parents were carriers of mutations at the loci responsible for both cystic fibrosis and β-thalassaemia (Darr and Modell 1988).

To investigate further the relationship between consanguineous marriage and homozygosity at the genome level, a study was initiated in the Sankethi community resident in Shimoga district in the state of Karnataka, south India. The Sankethi are a Hindu Brahmin community who practice agriculture, with the areca nut as an important cash crop, and they have a major reputation as Vedic scholars. Many members of the community, which globally totals some 11,000 persons, are now employed in the academic and medical professions. Their recorded history can be traced back to the fourteenth century when the community migrated from the district of Shengottai at the southernmost tip of India into Karnataka, and in 1524 AD a group of twenty Sankethi families was granted land in Shimoga district by the Vijayanagara Emperor, Krishna Deva Raya. The two villages that were founded by these families, Mathur and Hosahalli, continue to thrive and remain an important home residence of the community to the present day. Throughout their history the Sankethi were strictly endogamous and consanguineous marriages have been frequent, thus they offer an excellent opportunity to assess directly the effects of long-term consanguinity on residual heterozygosity at the genome level.

Finger-prick blood samples were obtained from members of the Sankethi community, the DNA in each sample was obtained by proteinase K digest and chloroform–phenol extraction; the samples were analysed on an ABI 373 automated sequencer using fluorescence detection. Ten dinucleotide microsatellite markers selected from the Stanford panel for chromosomes 13 and 15 were run on each sample. Microsatellites are repeat DNA sequences that are found throughout the genome and, since they are believed to be selectively neutral, they have been widely applied to studies of genomic variation across and within human populations.

The resultant data for the three initial families tested are summarised in Table 6.3, with the mean levels of residual heterozygosity observed in the Sankethi families compared with published results obtained from the Centre de Polymorphisme Humain (CEPH) panel compiled from subjects of outbred, European origin. As would have been expected in such an endogamous community, the levels of heterozygosity at the various microsatellite loci were on average lower in the Sankethi than in the control CEPH sample, with mean values of 70 per cent, 61 per cent and 76 per cent for families A, B and C at loci on chromosome 13, and 73 per cent, 65 per cent and 79 per cent heterozygosity at loci on chromosome 15 respectively. By comparison, mean heterozygosity in the CEPH samples was 81 per cent for loci on chromosome 13 and 75 per cent for those located on chromosome 15. Given the history of the community, with their small founding population, strict endogamy over at least 450 years and the continuing tradition of consanguineous unions, the actual levels of residual heterozygosity as measured at these dinucleotide loci appears to have remained surprisingly high.

Table 6.3 Microsatellite heterozygosity levels in the Sankethi community and reference population

	Mean heterozygosity (%)	
	Chromosome 13	Chromosome 15
Sankethi		
Family A	70 (range 53–85)	73 (range 61–83)
Family B	61 (range 34–83)	65 (range 56–72)
Family C	76 (range 61–99)	79 (range 59–95)
Reference population	81 (range 67–90)	75 (range 57–86)

Discussion

Contrary to prevailing expectation, consanguineous marriage is still the preferred form of marital union for a large proportion of the world's population, and our understanding of the outcomes of such unions is far from complete. The inadequacy of the available pedigree data has been a major stumbling-block in attempts to investigate the effects of inbreeding and, as the large majority of consanguineous unions are contracted in less developed countries with low levels of literacy, to a great extent this remains the case. However, the situation is very different among migrant communities now resident in Western countries, and it manifestly would be to the benefit of these communities if our understanding of their marital preferences were adequately understood, especially given the greatly increased emphasis now placed on the role of genetics in medicine.

There has been a tendency to overestimate the adverse genetic effects of human inbreeding, due at least in part to the flawed design of many early studies and, as has been indicated in the present chapter, this defect remains in much of the current biological research on the topic. At the same time, the past omission of consanguinity as a possible explanatory factor in assessing causes of mortality and morbidity has seriously blighted the conclusions reached in a majority of the demographic studies conducted in less developed countries since, as indicated by the results of the PDHS, there is considerable overlap between consanguinity and non-genetic variables as determinants of fertility, mortality and morbidity (Grant and Bittles 1997, Hussain and Bittles 1998, 1999).

It would appear that some downward revision of the precise role(s) played by non-genetic variables as determinants of health is now in train. For example, a recent re-examination of the widely assumed causal relationship between maternal education and childhood mortality indicated that when other explanatory factors, such as husband's education, and piped water and toilet facilities, were added into the analysis, the impact of maternal education was significant in only a minority of the countries investigated (Desai and Alva 1998). Although all such findings may be subject to further reassessment, it does reinforce the need for genuinely multidisciplinary studies into the outcomes of consanguineous marriage, and an approach of this nature could go a long way to meeting the criticism that too much emphasis has been placed solely on the role of consanguinity in explaining the poor health outcomes experienced by the British Pakistani community (Ahmad 1994).

It should also be stressed that as the socio-economic status of a country or immigrant community changes through time, so conclusions drawn at an earlier stage in their economic development may need to be substantially revised to allow for the influence and effects of these underlying changes. In this respect, while the retrospective data collected in the PDHS showed that consanguinity exerted a lesser effect on early survival than the non-genetic variables examined, a current assessment could well reveal an alteration in the weighted ranking order of each contribution. Equally, it could be argued that given superior access to high-quality health care, the adverse health outcomes experienced by the British Pakistani community arising from the expression of detrimental recessive genes will more probably result in infant and childhood morbidity, in some cases even extending into adulthood, rather than the elevated neonatal and post-neonatal mortality that has been reported in Pakistan (Bittles *et al.* 1993, Grant and Bittles 1997).

From a genetic perspective, the multiple pathways of consanguineous marriage that often are encountered in communities with a long history of endogamy can cause difficulties with data assessment, since it usually is impossible to determine the precise level of cumulative inbreeding beyond a span of four or five generations (Bundey and Alam 1993, Nelson *et al.* 1997). The use of microsatellite analysis to directly achieve this goal offers obvious advantages but, as with any relatively new technique, the results obtained will need to be interpreted with appropriate caution.

On the assumption that ongoing studies in the Sankethi community reveal a similar pattern to those briefly summarised in Table 6.3, the question arises why the observed levels of residual heterozygosity at microsatellite loci are higher than might intuitively have been predicted. Undisclosed genetic admixture is a possible explanation, and current microsatellite studies on the Y chromosome should provide a definitive answer to this topic. A second possibility is that the levels of mutation occurring at the microsatellite loci investigated are much higher and more variable than have been reported to date. A third possibility, and perhaps the most intriguing, is that excessive homozygosity at loci involved in early prenatal human development may result in spontaneous fetal loss, which has a much higher prevalence than generally has been recognised (Bittles and Matson 1999).

Continuing studies on the Sankethi, and concurrent investigations conducted with other communities in Pakistan and the People's Republic of China, which practise consanguineous marriage, should assist in the solution of this question. In the interim, it is interesting to note that among infertile consanguineous couples enrolled in assisted reproduction programmes, there is evidence of an elevated rate of miscarriage (Egbase *et al.* 1996). Whether this denotes the early expression of specific detrimental recessive genes or is associated with a more general consanguinity-influenced effect again is a topic that merits further research.

Acknowledgements

The invaluable cooperation of the Sankethi community is acknowledged with gratitude. The work was made possible by generous financial assistance from The Wellcome Trust, grant number 037709/Z/93, the Australian Research Council, grant numbers A350312 and A350363, and the Department of Biotechnology, India. During the preparation of the manuscript, AHB was Visiting Senior Research Associate in the Morrison Institute for Population and Resource Studies, Stanford University.

References

Ahmad, W.I.U. (1994) 'Reflections on the consanguinity and birth outcome debate', *Journal of Public Health Medicine*, 16, 423–428.

Appaji Rao, N., Radha Rama Devi, A., Savithri, H.S., Venkat Rao, S. and Bittles, A.H. (1988) 'Neonatal screening for amino acidaemias in Karnataka, South India', *Clinical Genetics*, 34, 60–63.

Bede, The Venerable (731) Book 1, Chapter 27, Question 5 in *Ecclesiastical History of the English People* [1990], London: Penguin Books, pp. 79–81.

Bittles, A.H. (1994) 'The role and significance of consanguinity as a demographic variable', *Population and Development Review*, 20, 561–584.

Bittles, A.H. (1998) *Empirical Estimates of the Global Prevalence of Consanguineous Marriage in Contemporary Societies*. Morrison Institute for Population and Resources Studies Working Report 74, Stanford: Stanford University.

Bittles, A.H. and Matson, P. (1999) 'Genetic influences on infertility', in Bentley, G. and Mascie-Taylor, C.G.N. (eds) *Infertility in the Modern World: Present and Future Prospects*, Cambridge: Cambridge University Press.

Bittles, A.H. and Neel, J.V. (1994) 'The costs of human inbreeding and their implications for variations at the DNA level', *Nature Genetics*, 8, 117–121.

Bittles, A.H., Grant, J.C. and Shami, S.A. (1993) 'Consanguinity as a determinant of reproductive behaviour and mortality in Pakistan', *International Journal of Epidemiology*, 22, 63–67.

Bittles, A.H., Mason, W.M., Greene, J. and Appaji Rao, N. (1991) 'Reproductive behavior and health in consanguineous marriages', *Science*, 252, 789–794.

Bittles, A.H., Shami, S.A. and Appaji Rao, N. (1992) 'Consanguineous marriage in Southern Asia: incidence, causes and effects', in Bittles, A.H. and Roberts, D.F. (eds) *Minority Populations: Genetics, Demography and Health*, London: Macmillan, pp. 102–118.

Bratt, C.S. (1984) 'Incest statutes and the fundamental right of marriage: is Oedipus free to marry?', *Family Law Quarterly*, 18, 257–309.

Bundey, S. (1992) 'A prospective study on the health of Birmingham babies in different ethnic groups, with particular reference to the effect of inbreeding', in Bittles, A.H. and Roberts D.F. (eds) *Minority Populations: Genetics, Demography and Health*, London: Macmillan, pp. 143–155.

Bundey, S. and Alam, H. (1993) 'A five-year prospective study of the health of children in different ethnic groups, with special reference to the effect of inbreeding', *European Journal of Human Genetics*, 1, 101–114.

Darr, A. and Modell, B. (1988) 'The frequency of consanguineous marriage among British Pakistanis', *Journal of Medical Genetics*, 25, 186–190.

de Costa, C. (1988) 'Pregnancy outcomes in Lebanese-born women in Western Sydney', *Medical Journal of Australia*, 149, 457–460.

Desai, S. and Alva, S. (1998) 'Maternal education and child health: is there a strong causal relationship?', *Demography*, 35, 71–81.

Egbase, P.E., Al-Sharhan, M., Al-Othman, S., Al-Mutawa, M. and Grudzinskas, J.G. (1996) 'Outcome of assisted reproduction technology in infertile couples of consanguineous marriage', *Journal of Assisted Reproduction and Genetics*, 13, 279–281.

Govinda Reddy, P. (1985) 'Effects of inbreeding on mortality: a study among three South Indian communities', *Human Biology*, 57, 47–59.

Grant, J.C. and Bittles, A.H. (1997) 'The comparative role of consanguinity in infant and child mortality in Pakistan', *Annals of Human Genetics*, 61, 143–149.

Hussain, R. and Bittles, A.H. (1998) 'The prevalence and demographic characteristics of consanguineous marriages in Pakistan', *Journal of Biosocial Science*, 30, 261–275.

Hussain, R. and Bittles, A.H. (1999) 'Consanguinity and differentials in age at marriage, contraceptive use and fertility in Pakistan', *Journal of Biosocial Science*, 31, 121–138.

Imaizumi, Y. (1986) 'A recent survey of consanguineous marriages in Japan', *Clinical Genetics*, 30, 230–233.

Imaizumi, Y., Shinozaki, N. and Aoki, H. (1975) 'Inbreeding in Japan: results of a nation-wide study', *Japanese Journal of Human Genetics*, 20, 91–107.

John, T.J. and Jayabal, P. (1971) 'Foetal and child loss in relation to consanguinity in southern India', *Indian Journal of Medical Research*, 59, 1050–1053.

Kapadia, K.M. (1958) *Marriage and the Family in India*, Calcutta: Oxford University Press.

Nelson, J., Smith, M. and Bittles, A.H. (1997) 'Consanguineous marriage and its clinical consequences in migrants to Australia', *Clinical Genetics*, 52, 142–146.

Ottenheimer, M. (1990) 'Lewis Henry Morgan and the prohibition of cousin marriage in the United States', *Journal of Family History*, 15, 325–334.

Population Reference Bureau (1998) *World Population Data Sheet*, Washington, DC: Population Reference Bureau.

Radha Rama Devi, A., Appaji Rao, N. and Bittles, A.H. (1987) 'Inbreeding and the incidence of childhood genetic disorders in Karnataka, South India', *Journal of Medical Genetics*, 24, 362–365.

Rao, P.S.S. and Inbaraj, S.G. (1977) 'Trends in human reproductive wastage in relation to long-term practice of inbreeding', *Annals of Human Genetics*, 42, 401–43.

Reniers, G. (1998) *Post-migration Survival of Traditional Marriage Patterns: Consanguineous Marriage among Turkish and Moroccan Immigrants in Belgium*. IPD Working Paper 1998–1, Gent: Universiteit Gent.

Sanghvi, L.D. (1966) 'Inbreeding in India', *Eugenics Quarterly*, 13, 291–301.

Schull, W.J. (1958) 'Empirical risks in consanguineous marriages: sex ratio, malformation and viability', *American Journal of Human Genetics*, 10, 294–343.

Shami, S.A., Grant, J.C. and Bittles, A.H. (1993) 'Consanguineous marriages within social/occupational class boundaries in Pakistan', *Journal of Biosocial Science*, 26, 91–96.

7 The inherited disorders of haemoglobin

David J. Weatherall

Introduction

The inherited disorders of haemoglobin, comprising the structural haemoglobin variants and the thalassaemias, are the commonest monogenic diseases in man. Their study, though they are relatively rare diseases in richer Western countries, has greatly increased our understanding of the nature and control of genetic disorders in general. Paradoxically, however, these conditions are likely to pose an increasing world health problem in the new millennium by developing in transition countries, as rates of neonatal and childhood mortality decline because of better sanitation, nutrition and control of infection. Babies with serious genetic diseases like the haemoglobinopathies will then survive the first few months of life; throughout Africa, the Middle East, the Indian subcontinent and Southeast Asia, thousands of children will be born annually with these conditions, many of whom will live long enough to require treatment (Weatherall and Clegg 1996).

The effects of these demographic changes were graphically illustrated in Cyprus, a country that underwent such a demographic transition shortly after World War II (Fawdry 1944, Weatherall and Clegg 1981). Thalassaemia was not recognised on the island until 1944, when, as the result of a malaria eradication programme and related improvements in public health, it became clear that among the children there was a common form of anaemia with enlargement of the spleen that was not due to infection. This turned out to be thalassaemia. By the early 1970s it was reckoned that, if steps were not taken to reduce the prevalence of the disease, in about 40 years the blood required to treat these children would amount to 78,000 units per year, about 40 per cent of the population would need to be donors and the total cost of treatment would equal or exceed the island's health budget.

Because of major population movements over the second half of the twentieth century, the inherited disorders of haemoglobin have become disseminated widely in the richer countries of the West (Weatherall and Clegg 1996). In the United Kingdom, for example, they now constitute the second commonest genetic diseases and affect a wide range of the immigrant population. In this chapter I shall outline the major clinical problems posed by these diseases and how their control is being envisaged, and to what extent these measures have been successful to date. In the context of this volume on ethnicity and health, thalassaemias represent largely genetic variations in disease between subgroups within a multicultural Western population. This chapter also highlights how monogenic diseases in man, such as thalassaemias, are quite heterogenous in their clinical presentation and manifestations.

Normal human haemoglobin synthesis

Human adult haemoglobin is a mixture of proteins consisting of a major component, haemoglobin A, and a minor component, haemoglobin A_2, the latter making up about 2.5 per cent of the total. In intrauterine life, the main haemoglobin is haemoglobin F. The structure of these haemoglobins is similar; each consists of two separate pairs of identical globin chains. Except for some of the embryonic haemoglobins, which will not be considered here, all the normal human haemoglobins have one pair of α-chains: in haemoglobin A these are combined with β-chains ($\alpha_2\beta_2$), in haemoglobin A_2 with δ-chains ($\alpha_2\delta_2$), and in haemoglobin F with γ-chains ($\alpha_2\gamma_2$). After the decline of embryonic haemoglobin synthesis, haemoglobin F is the main oxygen carrier of fetal life. Its synthesis starts to decline shortly before term, and by the end of the first year after birth it is almost entirely replaced by haemoglobins A and A_2.

The structure of the α- and non-α-globin chains is directed by two gene clusters, the α-gene cluster on chromosome 16 and the β-gene cluster on chromosome 11. These clusters and the genes that they contain have been completely sequenced and much is known about the regulation of individual globin genes, but less is known about the control of the transition from embryonic to fetal and fetal to adult haemoglobin synthesis (Grosveld *et al.* 1993).

The haemoglobinopathies

The inherited disorders of haemoglobin fall into two groups. First, there are over 700 structural haemoglobin variants, most of which result from single amino acid substitutions in the α- or β-globin chains. The only variants, which reach polymorphic frequencies, are haemoglobins S, C and E. Second, there are the thalassaemias, disorders which result from a reduced rate of synthesis of either the α-, β-, or δ- and β-globin chains; hence they are subdivided into the α-, β- and $\delta\beta$-thalassaemias. There are over 170 different mutations that underlie β-thalassaemia (Thein 1993). The bulk of them are point mutations, which result in premature chain termination, frameshifts or defects in splicing. Another set involves the promoter regions of the β-globin genes.

The genetics of the α-thalassaemias is more complex (Higgs 1993). There are two α-globin genes per haploid genome, written $\alpha\alpha/\alpha\alpha$. There are two major classes of α-thalassaemia, called α⁺- and α°-thalassaemia. The α⁺-thalassaemias result from either deletions of the α-globin genes, written in the heterozygous and homozygous states as $-\alpha/\alpha\alpha$ or $-\alpha/-\alpha$, respectively, or from point mutations which inactivate these genes, which are designated $\alpha^T\alpha/\alpha\alpha$ or $\alpha^T\alpha/\alpha^T\alpha$. The α°-thalassaemias result from long deletions, which either remove both α-globin genes, or key regulatory regions upstream from the α-globin gene cluster.

Clinical features

The sickling disorders

The sickling disorders consist of the homozygous state for the sickle cell gene, SS, and the compound heterozygous states for the sickle cell and haemoglobin C genes, SC, or β-thalassaemia, S-β-thalassaemia.

The homozygous state for the sickle cell gene, sickle cell anaemia, is characterised by chronic anaemia and tissue damage resulting from blockage of small blood vessels. The glutamic acid to valine substitution at position 6 in the β-globin chain results in the formation of stacks of haemoglobin molecules, which cause the sickling deformation of the red cell in the deoxygenated state. The pathophysiology of sickling is extremely complex and has been the subject of several extensive reviews (Bunn and Forget 1986, Weatherall *et al.* 1995). One of the problems with this condition is its extraordinary clinical heterogeneity. In the steady state patients are anaemic but adapt well because of the right shift in their whole-blood oxygen dissociation curves associated with sickle cell haemoglobin. However, they are prone to severe infections because their spleens atrophy as a result of repeated minor infarction and to a variety of acute episodes called 'sickling crises'. These include widespread bone pain, sequestration of sickle cells into the lungs with respiratory failure, strokes, and massive sequestration of sickle cells into the spleen with profound anaemia.

There is remarkable variation in the severity of sickle cell anaemia among different racial groups. In Africa the disease still kills large numbers of infants early in life, whereas in the Caribbean it seems to run a less severe course. The reasons for this discrepancy are unknown. There is an even milder form of the disease, which occurs in Saudi Arabia and parts of India, which is associated with unusually high levels of fetal haemoglobin production. Fetal haemoglobin protects against sickling and this, together with the high frequency of α-thalassaemia, which is also known to ameliorate the disease, may be at least partly responsible for the mild phenotypes in these populations. However, this is only a partial explanation for its clinical heterogeneity and much remains to be learnt whether this reflects predominantly genetic or environmental factors.

α-*Thalassaemia*

The severe forms of α^o-thalassaemia, in their homozygous state, are associated with stillbirth and the clinical picture of hydrops fetalis. Milder forms are compatible with survival into adult life. Since the α^o-thalassaemias are only found in parts of South-East Asia and the Mediterranean, these are the only regions where their homozygous states are associated with a high frequency of stillbirth. The α^+-thalassaemias, which occur widely across Africa, the Middle East and throughout South-East Asia, produce a mild hypochromic anaemia in the homozygous states, while their heterozygous states are clinically silent.

β-*Thalassaemias*

The β-thalassaemias are also clinically heterogeneous. At the severe end of the spectrum they cause profound anaemia, which leads to transfusion dependence; at the other end of the scale, in the homozygous or compound heterozygous states they may be associated with only a moderate degree of anaemia. This heterogeneity reflects a number of factors including the nature of the underlying mutation, the inherent ability to synthesise haemoglobin F after birth and the co-inheritance of α-thalassaemia (Weatherall 1994).

The severe forms of β-thalassaemia are all associated with profound anaemia and require regular transfusion. Children treated in this way accumulate iron and if it is not removed by chelation they die of the effects of iron overload involving the liver, pancreas, endocrine glands and, ultimately, the myocardium. If well transfused and given adequate chelating agents to remove iron, they can now live in good health to reproductive age and are able to have their own children.

Combinations of thalassaemia and structural haemoglobin variants

The two most important interactions of this type are sickle cell β-thalassaemia, and haemoglobin E β-thalassaemia. The former, in its more severe forms, is associated with a clinical picture similar to that of sickle cell anaemia. Haemoglobin E thalassaemia is widespread throughout the Indian subcontinent, Burma and South-East Asia and will be one of the most important clinical forms of thalassaemia in the twenty-first century (Weatherall and Clegg 1981). Haemoglobin E is synthesised at a reduced rate and produces the clinical picture of a mild form of β-thalassaemia. In the homozygous state it causes only mild hypochromic anaemia but when it is inherited together with β-thalassaemia it results in a disorder with a remarkable clinical spectrum ranging from a picture similar to severe homozygous β-thalassaemia to a mild non-transfusion-dependent condition. Very little is known about its natural history and why some patients run such a severe course.

World distribution and population genetics

The sickling disorders

The sickling disorders are distributed throughout tropical Africa, parts of the Mediterranean region, the Middle East, and in parts of India. Studies of associated restriction fragment length polymorphisms (RFLPs) indicate that the gene has arisen at least twice, once in India or the Middle East and once in Africa (reviewed by Flint *et al.* 1993, Weatherall *et al.* 1995). There is some, though less convincing, evidence that the disease may have arisen several times in Africa. Early work suggesting that it has reached its high frequency as a result of heterozygote advantage against *Plasmodium falciparum* malaria has been confirmed recently by studies suggesting that heterozygotes have somewhere in the region of 80 per cent protection against the more severe complications of this form of malaria.

As mentioned earlier (p. 81), sickle cell anaemia is extremely heterogeneous in its clinical manifestations and much of this probably reflects the environment, general level of nutrition and exposure to infection, and availability of medical resources. However, it is clear that genetic factors play an important role, particularly the level of haemoglobin F. This explains, at least in part, the difference between the disease in Africa compared with Saudi Arabia and the Indian subcontinent.

Haemoglobin E

This is probably the commonest structural haemoglobin variant and has an extremely high frequency in eastern parts of the Indian subcontinent, Burma, Thailand, Cambodia, Vietnam, and parts of Malaysia and the Indonesian islands (Flint *et al.* 1993). It seems likely that this has also reached its high frequencies by heterozygote protection against malaria, although there is little formal evidence in favour of this hypothesis.

The thalassaemias

As mentioned earlier (p. 82) the α^0-thalassaemias reach high frequencies in southern China, Thailand and Vietnam, and in some of the Mediterranean islands. The α^+-thalassaemias are widely distributed across Africa, the Middle East and throughout South-East Asia. Each region has different varieties, indicating that they have arisen locally and come under selection. Recent work has provided clear evidence for the protective effect of the homozygous and probably heterozygous states for α^+-thalassaemia against both *Plasmodium vivax* and *P. falciparum* malaria (Williams *et al.* 1996, Allen *et al.* 1997). Interestingly, the α^+-thalassaemias seem to protect against other infections, although whether this is secondary to their protective effect on malaria is not yet clear.

The β-thalassaemias are distributed widely throughout the Mediterranean region, parts of Africa, the Middle East, the Indian subcontinent and in South-East Asia in a line stretching from southern China through Thailand, Vietnam, Malaysia and to the Indonesian islands. Each high-frequency population has a few common mutations that are unique to that region, suggesting that the disease has arisen locally and been expanded by selection. There is some evidence that the selective factor is, again, *P. falciparum* malaria, although the evidence is far less conclusive than that for α-thalassaemia.

Haemoglobinopathies in migrant populations

The major routes of migration of populations with the haemoglobin disorders are outlined in Figure 7.1. Thalassaemia has come to Europe and the United Kingdom from several regions, including South-East Asia, the Indian subcontinent, either directly or via East Africa, and the Mediterranean region. Thus in the United Kingdom, because of the heterogeneity of its immigrant population, there are many different varieties of thalassaemia. This disease has also been imported into the United States directly from the Mediterranean region and is now being seen with increasing frequency on the West Coast owing to the recent spate of immigrants from Vietnam and Cambodia; haemoglobin E is also being imported from the same source.

The sickling disorders have come to the United Kingdom from Africa, either directly or via the Caribbean populations. They are also seen in Mediterranean and Indian immigrants.

Because these diseases are so common they are producing an increasing

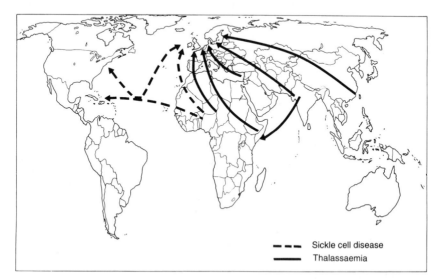

Figure 7.1 Different routes by which the haemoglobin disorders have reached the United Kingdom.

health load for countries with a large immigrant population from high-incidence regions. For example, in the United Kingdom the haemoglobin-opathies are probably, after cystic fibrosis, the commonest inherited diseases. The distribution of these diseases within the recipient nations in generations to come will depend on the marriage and mobility patterns of the offspring of the immigrants and their attitudes to ethnic affiliation in the future.

Future problems for the control and management of the haemoglobin disorders

As mentioned earlier (p. 79), with increasing social, economic and nutritional improvements, and with the use of better sanitation and the control of neonatal and early childhood infections, there is no doubt that these genetic anaemias will pose an increasing health problem in the twenty-first century.

Although in the richer Western countries, parts of the Caribbean, and some parts of the Middle East many patients with sickle cell anaemia are now surviving to adult life, the situation is different in sub-Saharan Africa, where the disease is still killing many patients in infancy or early childhood. There is no doubt that many of these early deaths could be prevented by better socio-economic conditions combined with screening programmes at birth and the use of prophylactic penicillin and pneumococcal vaccines. However, there is still a high frequency of other complications and the disease requires sophisticated medical services. It can easily be identified in the carrier state, and prenatal diagnosis is an option, but because of the remarkable clinical heterogeneity, and the fact that some patients run an extremely mild course, many populations have not yet taken this up.

The situation with the thalassaemias is even more challenging. Although the α-thalassaemias are commoner than the β-thalassaemias, because the more severe forms lead to intrauterine death they do not pose a major burden on health care. It is the β-thalassaemias and haemoglobin E that present the major problem. The high-frequency regions, described earlier (p. 82), are also those which the 1993 World Bank Report describes as already having seen a major decrease in death rates in the first 5 years of life, and where the greatest population increases for the next 20 years are predicted. Although, because of the patchy distribution of these diseases, it is difficult to obtain accurate population data, enough is known to give some indication of the magnitude of the problem that will be faced. For example, in a small country like Thailand, where as early as 1969 it was estimated that there were more than sixty different varieties of thalassaemia and over a quarter of a million symptomatic children, it has been shown recently that, over the next 30 years, approximately 100,000 new cases of haemoglobin E thalassaemia alone will be added to the population; if the World Bank's estimate of a population increase in this country between 1991 and 2025, of 57 million to close to 100 million, is correct, this figure may be a gross underestimate. In larger countries like Indonesia, in which the World Bank estimates a population increase from about 180 million to close to 300 million, the situation may be even more serious, although there is an uneven distribution of β-thalassaemia and haemoglobin E among the different island populations. Preliminary surveys from the author's laboratory indicate that, in some, up to 10 per cent of the population are carriers for either haemoglobin E or β-thalassaemia. Hence many thousands of children homozygous for β-thalassaemia or with haemoglobin E thalassaemia will require expensive treatment. Similar gene frequencies exist in parts of India, which could double its population by 2025, and from what is known of the frequency in Malaysia and Vietnam it is clear that there will also be a major increase in the population of children requiring therapy.

Community screening and prenatal diagnosis, which have been applied successfully for the control of thalassaemia in the Mediterranean islands and in some of the richer Western countries, may be difficult to establish in the vast mainland populations of the Indian subcontinent and South-East Asia. Apart from organisational problems, there are religious issues that may make them unacceptable to some ethnic groups among which thalassaemia is very common. In addition, while there are some encouraging developments in the management, orally active chelating drugs for example, the increased costs of blood products, because of the necessity to screen them for infectious agents, will make long-term, symptomatic treatment extremely expensive. Bone marrow transplantation, while it is effective in the management of sickle cell anaemia and β-thalassaemia, is not available to everybody because of lack of suitable donors, and when available it is extremely expensive.

In the richer countries these disorders can be controlled. This requires screening during pregnancy or in the neonatal period backed up by careful and sensitive genetic counselling. Many patients wish to undergo prenatal diagnosis, at least for the more severe forms of β-thalassaemia, and neonatal diagnosis of sickle cell anaemia is extremely important because the early use of penicillin and a suitable vaccination programme can undoubtedly reduce the number of deaths during the first few years of life. Thus the technology is all available and all that is needed is good organisation backed up with sensitive counselling, directed particularly at avoiding any hint of discrimination for those who are carriers of the genes for the haemoglobinopathies.

The situation in the developing world is more complex. It is vital therefore that the WHO, World Bank and other international agencies realise that these diseases will soon produce a major public health problem. Their client governments need to be properly informed, and adequate surveys of the frequency of the disease established, together with advice about setting up centres for their control and management.

Each country will have to decide on the way that it wishes to approach this problem, either by counselling, marital advice or prenatal diagnosis, or by evolving adequate facilities for treatment. These national decisions may well need to incorporate different approaches where ethnic diversity within a multicultural society exists.

References

Allen, S.J., O'Donnell, A., Alexander, N.D.E., Alpers, M.P., Peto, T.E.A., Clegg, J.B. and Weatherall, D.J. (1997) 'α^+-thalassaemia protects children against disease due to malaria and other infections', *Proceedings of the National Academy of Sciences, USA*, 94, 14736–14741.

Bunn, H.F. and Forget, B.G. (1986) *Haemoglobin: Molecular, Genetic and Clinical Aspects*, Philadelphia: W.B. Saunders.

Fawdry, A.L. (1944) 'Erythroblastic anaemia of childhood (Cooley's) anaemia in Cyprus', *Lancet*, 1, 171–176.

Flint, J., Harding, R.M., Boyce, A.J. and Clegg, J.B. (1993) 'The population genetics of the haemoglobinopathies', *Clinics in Haematology*, 6, 215–262.

Grosveld, F., Dillon, N. and Higgs, D. (1993) 'The regulation of human globin gene expression', *Clinics in Haematology*, 6, 31–55.

Higgs, D.R. (1993) 'α-Thalassaemia', *Clinics in Haematology*, 6, 117–150.

Thein, S.L. (1993) 'β-Thalassaemia', *Clinics in Haematology*, 6, 151–175.

Weatherall, D.J. (1994) 'Thalassaemia', in Stamatoyannopoulos, G., Nienhuis, A.W., Majerus, P.W. and Varmus, H. (eds) *The Molecular Basis of Blood Diseases*, Philadelphia: W.B. Saunders, p. 157.

Weatherall, D.J. and Clegg, J.B. (1981) *The Thalassaemia Syndromes*, Oxford: Blackwell Scientific Publications.

Weatherall, D.J. and Clegg, J.B. (1996) 'Thalassaemia – a global public health problem', *Nature Medicine*, 2, 847–849.

Weatherall, D.J., Clegg, J.B., Higgs, D.R. and Wood, W.G. (1995) 'The haemoglobin-opathies', in Scriver, C.R., Beaudet, A.L., Sly, W.S. and Valle, D. (eds) *The Metabolic and Molecular Bases of Inherited Disease*, New York: McGraw-Hill Book Co., p. 3417.

Williams, T.N., Maitland, K., Bennett, S., Ganczakowski, M., Peto, T.E.A., Newbold, C.I., Bowden, D.K., Weatherall, D.J. and Clegg, J.B. (1996) 'High incidence of malaria in α-thalassaemia children', *Nature*, 383, 522–525.

World Bank (1993) *Annual Report*, Washington, DC: World Bank.

8   Genetic variation and ethnic variability in disease risk

Ryk Ward

Spatial and temporal variation in disease risk: the role of ethnicity

It is almost trite to note that risk of disease varies by time and place. From John Snow onwards, the perceptive investigation of spatial and temporal variability in disease risk has helped uncover the aetiology of disease. This premise underpins the science of epidemiology. By applying this principle, epidemiological studies have succeeded in identifying the causal factors for a great many diseases with varied aetiologies. As a consequence, this discipline has made a substantial contribution to worldwide public health. However, the ability to transform epidemiological findings into successful public health policy requires more than identifying the underlying aetiology of disease. Development of public health policy is substantially influenced by whether causal factors are perceived to be intrinsic or extrinsic in nature.

At the biological level, the distinction between intrinsic and extrinsic is necessarily blurred by the complexities of pathophysiology. Even so, the perception of aetiological dichotomy can exert a considerable impact on how modification of disease risk is approached. Appropriate manipulation of *extrinsic* risk factors, whether environmental or behavioural, offers the promise of disease prevention. By contrast, while disease due to *intrinsic* factors may be susceptible to treatment, it will be much harder to prevent its initial occurrence. Since prevention is usually cheaper and more effective than treatment, the perception of whether disease risk is intrinsic or extrinsic has important implications for public health policy.

In this context, understanding and interpreting the aetiological foundation of 'ethnic-specific' disease risk can influence the way strategies are developed to reduce the burden of disease. As a consequence, the public health implication of identifying ethnic differentials in disease risk transcends the etymological arguments over the meaning of 'ethnicity'. Communities and individuals are increasingly classified in terms of their ethnic identity – whether self-defined or administratively imposed. In the epidemiological context, ethnicity is frequently regarded as important a clue to aetiology as was Snow's identification of the company that supplied water to the Broad Street pump. If disease distributions vary by ethnicity, as they surely do, it matters a great deal how the factors contributing to ethnic-specific risk are perceived. If ethnic-specific risk is considered to be the consequence of intrinsic factors, approaches to prevention are likely to be muted. This is particularly so when *'ethnicity'* is equated to *'genetic'* – as is all too frequently the case. The perception of how ethnic differences influence disease risk, and the extent to which these differences are perceived to be genetic in origin, have important implications for both the population and the individual.

Characteristics of the external environment are universally regarded as risk factors that are unambiguously extrinsic in nature. In this case, the distinction between temporal variation and spatial variation can be used as a surrogate indicator of the relative importance of extrinsic factors. Variation in disease risk over time is best interpreted as a consequence of the temporal variation of aetiological factors that are external to the population. Such extrinsic agents can range from physical factors, such as changing climatic patterns, to socio-demographic changes that influence population density and nutritional profiles. Except in a rather superficial sense, temporal variation in disease risk does not reflect changes in the intrinsic properties of the population. This is particularly true for infectious disease.

While there are notable differences in the prevalence of infectious disease among ethnic groups, the primary reason is attributable to external factors that influence the ecology of pathogens and their vectors. Consequently, temporal variation in risk of infectious disease is attributed to changes in the external environment. An example is the dramatic reduction in the burden of infectious diseases since the turn of the century, brought about by a general rise in living standards. These striking changes, which occurred throughout the developed world, were not confined to a subset of ethnically defined populations, and there is no evidence that intrinsic biological differences among populations played a role. The substantial differences in infectious disease risk that remain, including the re-emergence of infectious disease as a significant public health threat, are due to ecological and economic differentials. Similarly, although less dramatic, the secular changes in risk of non-infectious disease can also be attributed to the changing distribution of external risk factors. The reduction in cardiovascular mortality essentially occurs at the national level, rather than at the level of ethnic groups. Differential rates of change are far more likely to be due to aspects of the macro-social environment than differences in genetic heritage.

Spatial variability in disease risk can be more problematic to interpret. While extrinsic factors resulting from spatial variation of the physical and biological environment contribute to disease risk, intrinsic attributes of the population are also implicated. Since communities tend to be spatially constrained, this includes ethnicity. At a global scale, much of the geographic and ecological variation in disease is frequently perceived to result from 'ethnic-specific risk distributions' (Polednak 1989). Indeed, it is not uncommon to find that much of the spatial variation in disease risk is simply attributed to ethnic differences in risk, as if this constituted an adequate explanation of aetiology. This is particularly true for non-infectious disease. For example, the epidemiological literature is replete with discussions concerning the increased susceptibility of (US) Black people to hypertension and other cardiovascular disease. For over 50 years, there has been a persistent tendency to attribute this major public health problem to 'African genes' (Cooper and Rotimi 1994). This is despite the pioneering work of Scotch (1963), Akinkugbe and Ojo (1969) and Shaper *et al.* (1969), which clearly implicated environment, rather than genes, as the root cause of differential risk of hypertension. In similar fashion, even anthropologists have entered the fray by coining the 'New World Syndrome' (Weiss *et al.* 1984) as an appellation for increased susceptibility to a myriad set of diseases (not just one) presumed to characterise all Amerindians.

Unfortunately, such labels provide little insight about the real factors that predispose to disease risk. Even worse, their all too frequent use is likely to divert attention from the underlying complexity of interactions that lead to disease. To believe that the dramatic elevation in diabetes prevalence among some Native American groups is simply a consequence of Amerindian genes can turn attention from other, even more important, factors. Since Chinese, Asian Indians, African Americans and Micronesians can also display similarly elevated rates of diabetes, it should be clear that the critical risk factors transcend ethnic background and genetic heritage. This is not to gainsay that genes play a role. They surely do, especially at the individual level. It is also important to recognise that even quite general changes in the environment can interact with underlying variation in genetic susceptibility to cause substantial changes in the risk of non-infectious disease. However, by failing to recognise that ethnicity defines community ecology, as well as genetic heritage, epidemiological studies run the risk of not only focusing on the less relevant risk factor but also on the risk factor that is most resistant to change.

Ethnic variability in disease risk: risk differentials in ecology and genetic heritage

Although attributing variation in disease risk to ethnic differences explains little, it is important to recognise that ethnic groups do exhibit characteristic profiles of disease. This suggests more attention should be paid to what is presumed to be encompassed by the label 'ethnic differences'. Moving beyond the recognition of ethnic differences in disease risk to a considered analysis of the underlying factors that contribute to these differences will help identify the relative contribution of both extrinsic and intrinsic factors. This could lead to advances in both treatment and prevention. While the interpretation of 'ethnicity' is fraught with difficulty (Macbeth, Chapter 2), the implicit meaning of the term can range from a definition of the macro-social environment to an indication of genetic constitution. Within the epidemiological literature, where ethnic identity is often equated with racial classification (Polednak 1989), the label is frequently used as a surrogate for 'genetic distinctiveness'. In reality the situation is much more complex. By and large, it is true that ethnic groups tend to differ in their genetic composition (to a greater or lesser degree). These genetic differences can influence the distribution of disease risk. However, with the exception of the classical Mendelian disorders, environmental factors also influence disease risk, and ethnic groups are as variable in their ecology as they are in the genes.

In many respects, ethnicity has the greatest relevance for the distribution of non-infectious disease. While the prevalence of certain infectious diseases exhibits associations with ethnicity, this is essentially due to the geographic constraints on the distribution of infectious pathogens and their vectors. This was especially true before the advent of large-scale human migrations, when the geographic structure of populations meant ethnicity was tightly linked to a local ecosystem. Five thousand years ago, the geographic demarcation of many infectious diseases tended to coincide with ethnic boundaries. Since then, the impact of empire and conquest has disrupted the demographic integrity of local populations. This uncoupled the formerly tight relationship between individual communities and their local environment. In today's world, being *in* Africa rather than being *an* African is the relevant risk factor for contracting falciparum malaria. However, because of its effect on the contemporary pattern of genetic factors that influence disease risk, the historical correlation between ecological habitat and local genetic differentiation still has importance today.

The ecological factors that differentiate ethnic groups are many and varied. There are a number of ways in which this ecological variation can lead to the characteristic distribution of disease risk among ethnic groups. It is transparent that whenever ethnic groups occupy distinct geographical localities they will differ in their immediate physical and biological environment. Such variation in the external environment not only has a major impact on the risk of infectious disease but also can influence the risk of a multitude of non-infectious diseases. More relevant, and certainly more challenging for the epidemiologist, is the impact of what might be termed the 'ethnic macro-social environment', which exerts a major influence on the risk of disease. Ethnic distinctiveness is partly a function of cultural ecology and of social ecology, and each of these aspects of the ethnic macro-social environment can play a critical role in the risk of disease. Cultural ecology, which can influence everything from house style to the availability of basic foodstuffs, can have a significant impact on both infectious and non-infectious disease. The social ecology of the group, which will affect the distribution of high-risk behaviours, not only influences risk of transmission of infectious disease but is critically important in determining exposure to adverse environmental factors.

To a large extent, it is the interaction between cultural ecology and social ecology, rather than geographic locality, which determines the ethnic-specific distribution of environmental risk factors. It is against the profile of the ethnic macro-social environment that any genetic propensity to disease will act. Since every ethnic group is defined by its characteristic macro-social environment, as well as by its unique genetic history, it follows that 'ethnicity' must also incorporate a distinctive pattern of disease risk. A unique pattern of disease risk is thus just as important a marker of ethnic identity as is outward appearance or cultural custom. For this reason, 'ethnicity' is frequently used as a critical descriptor when analysing the complex diseases that are such a burden for contemporary societies. However, it needs to be stressed that no single component dominates this consequence of ethnicity. Consideration of the extensive tabulation by Polednak (1989) indicates that genetic heritage *and* socio-cultural environment, or a combination of both, can lead to substantial fluctuations in disease risk among ethnic groups. For some diseases socio-cultural factors play the dominant role [e.g. risk of sexually transmitted diseases (STDs) and human immunodeficiency virus (HIV)], in others genetic heritage is the more important (e.g. sickle cell disease in African populations and Tay–Sachs disease in Ashkenazi Jews). However, for the vast majority of diseases, both genetic heritage and socio-cultural environment play a role, albeit with differing magnitudes. The rest of this chapter examines how underlying differences in genetic heritage can influence the ethnic-specific distribution of disease risk.

Distribution of genetic variation in human populations: some consequences

The relationship between genetic differentiation and ethnicity is one that has to be squarely faced if we are to make sense of the way in which genes may influence ethnic variability in disease risk. Irrespective of how the term *'ethnicity'* is interpreted, there is an almost universal presumption that genetic distinctiveness is somehow involved. This is partly because of a tendency to interpret cultural differences as if they had a biological basis. Nevertheless, this perception has some validity because many of the processes that lead to the establishment of culturally distinct traits also lead to genetic differences. At the most fundamental level, the social perception of ethnic differences between communities tends to impede gene flow between them. Cultural divergence is usually enhanced by population sub-structure and by isolation between populations. The same factors inevitably result in genetic differentiation. Conversely, those demographic and ecological factors that accelerate, or retard, the rate of genetic drift will also influence the degree of cultural divergence. Certainly, this seems to hold for linguistic divergence. It is also likely to be true for many other cultural attributes, even though the tempo of cultural differentiation may be very different from the rate at which genetic differences accumulate (Ward *et al.* 1991).

The factors that influence the rate of genetic differentiation include the degree of isolation among populations, the size of founding populations, the amount of demographic expansion or contraction they experienced, plus the amount of contact with surrounding populations. However, the interaction between mutation and drift means that genetic variants are not static over time. The most common and widely distributed genetic variants tend to be oldest, while more recent variants are rarer and have a more restricted distribution. As Thompson and Neel (1996) have emphasised, the demographic processes that result in the formation of tribal groups ensure that each different group exhibits its own, characteristic, distribution of specific genetic variants. The most common variants will be shared among many groups, although the frequency will vary from one group to another. Less common variants will be restricted to cultural groups within a given region, and the least frequent variants will tend to be restricted to a single cultural entity. More detailed analyses, based on the coalescent model, also emphasise the primacy of demographic processes in shaping the local distribution of genetic variants (Slatkin and Rannala 1997). Thus, otherwise rare variants can display a markedly elevated frequency within a local group, or a geographic region, without needing to invoke the action of natural selection. Since the social correlates of human reproductive behaviour only serve to magnify the effects of genetic drift (Austerlitz and Heyer 1998), the effect of cultural divergence on the extent of local genetic differentiation is likely to be more universal and more profound than is usually realised.

In terms of human history, the most pertinent time frame for these processes is unlikely to extend beyond 20,000 years ago. The demographic and ecological processes within this period of human history led to the formation of local populations that are recognisably distinct in both the cultural and genetic sense. More ancient historical events, such as those associated with the early expansions out of Africa, will have had more widespread effects such as the association of common polymorphisms with a regionally defined attribute, such as a common language family. However, it is critical to recognise the degree of demographic relativity embodied in the measure and interpretation of genetic differentiation among human groups. Over a quarter of a century ago, the detailed analysis of Amerindian tribal groups indicated that allelic variation among villages within a single tribe represented a considerable fraction of the genetic diversity observed at the continental level (Neel and Ward 1970). At the global level, analysis of the existing data indicated that 70 per cent to 85 per cent of human genetic diversity was contained within ethnic groups, rather than among them (Lewontin 1972). A more recent analysis of mtDNA sequence variation has reaffirmed these conclusions, by demonstrating a single Amerindian tribe contains appreciable amounts of molecular variability (Ward *et al.* 1991). Thus, irrespective of how 'ethnicity' is defined, genetic differentiation within ethnic groups will be at least as important an influence on the genetic distribution of disease risk, as the genetic differences among them. However, since it is precisely the cultural consequences of the demographic and sociological history of a population that defines its 'ethnicity', it also follows that populations that are ethnically distinct are also likely to have their own distinct set of monogenic disorders.

Ethnic variation in disease risk: monogenic disease

Since populations vary genetically, any contribution that genetic factors make towards risk of disease will result in population-specific differentiation of disease risk. This is most obvious for monogenic diseases, which are inherited as Mendelian variants. Even before the advent of the molecular revolution, it was recognised that some Mendelian disorders were constrained to a specific population group. Perhaps the most clear-cut example is the geographic distribution of cystic fibrosis. While this is the most frequent recessive disorder in Caucasians of Northern European extraction, it is relatively uncommon in other major population groups. With the increased resolution provided by the molecular dissection of the *CFTR* gene, it is now possible to be more precise about the genetic basis for the ethnic variation in disease risk. The accumulated data suggest that spatial variation in the incidence of cystic fibrosis is largely attributable to underlying differences in the frequency of a single mutant allele, the *ΔF508* mutation. This allele, which may have originated as far back as 40,000 years ago, is common in Europe but rare elsewhere. Further, the relative contribution of the *ΔF508* mutation to cystic fibrosis varies considerably within Europe, accounting for 80 per cent of disease chromosomes in Sweden, but only 50 per cent in Spain. More detailed analysis of mutant chromosomes indicates that the geographic variation of this mutation is unlikely to be the result of a simple clinal pattern. In particular, analysis of linkage disequilibrium across the *ΔF508* haplotype indicates that the overall genetic affinities among populations do not account for the relative frequency of this mutation within regional populations (Bertranpetit and Calafell 1996). The situation appears far more complex, with each local population displaying a characteristic frequency of the *ΔF508* mutation, and a slightly different mix of the other mutant alleles.

One explanation for the observed distribution of cystic fibrosis is that ancient environmental variation led to differing selective forces that gave rise to local increases in the frequency of the *ΔF508* allele. These local differences might then have been frozen by a subsequent population expansion, perhaps that associated with the introduction of agriculture. Since the *CFTR* gene is intimately involved with regulating the flux of chloride ions, a series of epidemics of diarrhoeal disease represents a plausible selective regime. It is thought that mutant forms of the *CFTR* gene might reduce the amount of intestinal fluid loss and hence increase survival. Intriguingly, recent *in vitro* studies indicate that *Salmonella typhi*, the causative agent for typhoid, requires an intact *CFTR* product to enter cells efficiently (Pier *et al.* 1998). This provides a putative selective mechanism to account for the geographically constrained distribution of the *ΔF508* mutation.

Hence, the ethnic differences in risk of cystic fibrosis observed among contemporary populations may represent the consequences of past ethnic differences in socio-demographic structure. Different population sizes and variation in the time when agriculture was adopted could have resulted in differing intensities of typhoid epidemics and, hence, a differential selective force on the gene. A strikingly similar geographic pattern is observed for the C282Y mutation in the haemochromatosis gene (Merryweather-Clarke *et al.* 1997). This mutation, which accounts for about 80 per cent of cases in Caucasian populations, appears to have arisen quite recently (about 2,000 years ago) and spread rapidly throughout north-western Europe. Again, it is tempting to speculate that past epidemics have played a role in the distribution of this disease, though the evidence here is far more circumstantial. However, as noted above (p. 91), the demographic processes that led to the formation of ethnic groups within Europe are also capable of giving rise to the complex pattern of genetic differentiation observed for these two Mendelian disorders.

The relationship between ethnic identity and risk of genetic disease is perhaps most clearly seen in the instance of religious isolates. For well over a quarter of a century it has been recognised that diseases such as Tay–Sachs disease (TSD) occur in high frequency in Ashkenazi Jews, with one in thirty individuals carrying a TSD mutation. This knowledge has been used to establish effective targeted screening programmes in many United States communities, in a way that would not have been practical if applied to the general population. However, it would be a mistake to presume that ethnic distinctiveness in risk of genetic disease is confined to only a small handful of monogenic disorders. Within Europe, comprehensive investigation of the distribution of Mendelian disorders at the population level indicates that Finns are characterised by an extensive set of genetic diseases that are rare, or absent, from other European populations (Peltonen *et al.* 1995). Conversely, other genetic diseases, which are common elsewhere in Europe, tend to be absent from the Finnish population. This highlights the fact that definition of a genetic isolate can, in some instances, be commensurate with perception of national identity. In the case of the Finns, their striking constellation of unique genetic disorders can be attributed to a major demographic expansion that occurred only a few thousand years ago, but which left an indelible trace in the genetic record (Sajantila *et al.* 1996). Thus, the socio-demographic processes that led to the present-day distribution of the cultural attributes that define the contemporary 'Finnish' population also resulted in a distinct pattern of genetic diseases that characterises this population.

In all the above instances, the increased frequency of Mendelian disease within a particular population group is simply a reflection of the unique evolutionary patterns that shaped that group. Past selective differentials are frequently presumed to underlie major differences in allele frequencies between groups. The attractiveness of the selective argument is in large part due to the indisputable importance of differential selection in shaping the global distribution of the haemoglobinopathies (Flint *et al.* 1993), still the most dramatic example of an ethnically constrained pattern of genetic disease. However, the vagaries of demographic history represent an equally likely explanation. Analysis of tribally specific 'private polymorphisms' in South American populations provides a model of how genetic differentiation at the tribal level, followed by demographic expansion, can lead to elevated frequencies of a particular allele within a culturally defined group (Thompson and Neel 1996). Thus, the consequences of demographic expansion in a series of relatively isolated tribal populations, characterised by a high degree of local correlation between uniting gametes, can lead to variable frequencies of genetic disease among populations. In particular, there is no need to invoke selection as a cause for common disease entities, such as cystic fibrosis (Thompson and Neel 1997). This logic applies with even greater force for rarer mutations of more recent origin. Hence, in general, the particular history that shaped each ethnic group has also led to the ethnic-specific distribution of monogenic disease. Cultural heritage (which embodies genetic history), not natural selection, was probably the more important process in determining contemporary patterns of monogenic disease among different ethnic groups.

Molecular dissection of Mendelian disease: one disease, many lesions

With the increased resolution afforded by detailed molecular analysis of individual loci that cause Mendelian disease has come the recognition that 'single gene disorders' are not caused by a single mutation, as formerly believed. Instead, each individual Mendelian disorder is frequently the result of tens, if not hundreds, of individual mutations. Literally hundreds of mutations are now known to underlie the occurrence of common recessive disorders: over 850 for cystic fibrosis and in excess of 400 for phenylketonuria (PKU) (Scriver *et al.* 1996). Similarly, a very large number of individually distinct mutations are now known to be involved in the dominantly inherited susceptibility to familial hypercholesterolaemia [multiple mutations in the low-density lipoprotein (LDL) receptor gene] or familial breast cancer (multiple mutations in the *BRCA1* and *BRCA2* genes).

There are two important consequences to these observations. First, and most obvious, is that each distinct mutation has the potential to result in a slightly different phenotype. Whether acting alone, in concert with 'background modifier genes' or in combination with environmental factors, every individual mutation adds variability to the clinical spectrum of disease. Initially, it was anticipated that clinical prognosis could be clarified by determining the specific molecular lesion. However, the detailed analysis of a large number of PKU mutations indicates that reality is not so simple. In general, it is impossible to obtain a definitive relationship between a specific mutation and the clinical course of disease (Scriver and Waters 1999). For PKU, the barriers to defining a clear-cut relationship range from the impact of the environment (amount of dietary phenylalanine), to the modifying effects of complex multifactorial traits (physiology of the blood–brain barrier). The complexity is increased by the varied molecular consequences of individual mutations (e.g. their influence on protein folding and hence *in vivo* protein stability). Nevertheless, despite these complications, increased molecular characterisation of individual mutations that underlie each Mendelian disorder is starting to refine the spectrum of disease. Eventually, this will have some predictive value for the individual patient, as well as for populations in which a particular mutation has an elevated frequency.

The second consequence is that each mutation necessarily has its own evolutionary history. While less obvious, this is arguably more important. In essence, the hundreds of individual mutations that collectively give rise to a monogenic disease like cystic fibrosis represent hundreds of independent evolutionary histories. Each genetic variant has its own time depth, resulting in a population distribution that is constrained in inverse proportion to the age of the mutation. Relatively recent mutations will be constrained to local population groups, in analogous fashion to private polymorphisms (Thompson and Neel 1996), and will exhibit a very low frequency on a global basis. Such mutations, of which theory predicts a great number, will tend to be restricted to a single ethnic group and may reach an appreciable frequency within that group. Cogent examples are the characteristic 'founder' mutations of the *BRCA1* and *BRCA2* genes that are found in the French Canadian (Tonin *et al.* 1998) and Ashkenazim (Hartge *et al.* 1999) populations respectively. Older mutations, though exhibiting a higher frequency at the global level and likely to have a broad regional distribution, will be fewer in number. Such mutations will be found in many different, though related, ethnic groups, as is the case for the *ΔF508* mutation in cystic fibrosis (Bertranpetit and Calafell 1996). The net result of these multiple independent evolutionary histories is that each distinguishable mutation will have its own population-specific distribution: recent mutations largely constrained to an individual ethnic group, older mutations shared by many different ethnic groups.

The overall consequence is that the mutational spectrum of monogenic disease will differ from one ethnic group to another. To the extent that different mutations lead to distinguishable phenotypes, the clinical presentation of each monogenic disease will also tend to be ethnic specific. Further, as a consequence of their unique evolutionary history, most mutational lesions will reside on a chromosome, or haplotype, that is largely constrained to a single ethnic group. Thus, each ethnic-specific mutation will be surrounded by a unique constellation of polymorphic markers. This implies that individual ethnic groups will require a different set of markers to screen for the presence of disease alleles.

Failure to recognise the practical implications of the individual evolutionary histories of individual mutations will compromise the provision of efficient genetic services to individual ethnic groups. Because most detailed information about Mendelian disorders comes from populations of European ancestry, the provision of genetic services to minority ethnic groups is considerably less cost-effective than it could be. While the practical consequences of these theoretical consequences are still largely unexplored, there are already discouraging examples where screening for genetic disease, such as familial breast cancer (the *BRCA1* and *BRCA2* genes) is much less effective than originally anticipated (Devilee 1999). This has even turned out to be the case when screening for three 'founder' mutations presumed to exist in elevated frequencies within Ashkenazi Jews (Hartge *et al.* 1999). It seems clear that, to develop effective screening programs, detailed knowledge about the aggregation of individual mutations within specific ethnic groups will be more important than enumerating the total mutational spectrum. Given the growing tendency for genetic medicine to be integrated into modern health care, failure to recognise the ethnic specific distribution of individual mutations will only add to the existing disadvantages experienced by minority groups.

Single genes and more complex ethnic diseases: infectious disease

The genetic differentiation that correlates with the social identification of ethnic groups can lead to significant associations between ethnicity and genetic response to infectious disease. The most obvious examples are also the oldest. It is well known that the haemoglobinopathies, which confer some degree of protection against malaria, tend to be associated with specific ethnic groups. This association reflects the historical geography of past ecosystems within which selection operated. Nonetheless, it results in an ethnic specific distribution of susceptibility and resistance to infection. Conversely, high frequencies of an erstwhile protective allele can exert a significantly deleterious effect on populations that inhabit environments from which malaria has been eradicated. As a consequence, there are many developed countries, especially those which have substantial populations derived from the African diaspora, which require the establishment of public health and community health programmes to address this problem. The spectrum of different evolutionary histories that led to contemporary populations has resulted in ethnic groups that differ in their response to existing pathogens. These ethnic groups may be burdened with the adverse consequences of an ancient evolutionary struggle between pathogen and host.

The same evolutionary processes can lead to ethnic-specific differences with respect to the risk of infectious diseases. This includes the response to totally new pathogens. A telling example is how HIV infection is modulated by allelic variation at the *CCR5* gene. The protein produced by this particular chemokine receptor gene, part of a multi-gene family located on the short arm of chromosome 3, happens to be the site by which the human immunodeficiency virus gains entry into certain target cells (Dragic *et al.* 1996). Deletion of a thirty-two-nucleotide segment alters the structure of the receptor protein and denies HIV entry. As a result, individuals homozygous for the *CCR5–Δ32* allele are essentially resistant to HIV infection, while infected heterozygotes display a much slower progression to full blown acquired immune deficiency syndrome (AIDS). Initial surveys indicated that, while the *CCR5–Δ32* allele was absent in African and Asian populations, it was most frequent in northern European populations, especially Ashkenazi Jews (Martinson *et al.* 1997). More recent surveys have confirmed the absence of this allele from African, Asian and Native American populations. They have also identified a wide geographic cline across north-west Europe into Eurasia. Scandinavian populations exhibit the highest frequencies of around 14 per cent, while Mediterranean populations have much lower frequencies of around 5 per cent. In central Asian populations, the frequency diminishes even further to 2–3 per cent (Stephens *et al.* 1998).

The high frequency of the *CCR5–Δ32* mutation in north-western European populations, coupled with the distribution of its associated haplotypes, suggests it occurred a relatively short time ago (2,500–4,500 years ago) then spread rapidly across northern Europe into central Asia (Libert *et al.* 1998, Stephens *et al.* 1998). Such a scenario has been interpreted as the footprint of a strong bout of selection that swept across northern Eurasia some 2,000 years ago. One possibility is an ancient plague, now long extinct. Alternatively, as already discussed (p. 96), such a distribution might simply be the consequence of the differential demographic expansion of subdivided populations.

Irrespective of the specific evolutionary processes that caused the variable distribution of the *CCR5–Δ32* mutation, the outcome is that susceptibility to HIV infection varies by ethnic group. This finding is likely to be repeated for HIV as additional gene products that influence pathogenesis are identified. Moreover, these observations indicate a general principle. The impact of infectious disease, both new and old, will tend to vary from one ethnic group to another as a consequence of their different genetic heritages. Overall, ethnic groups will vary not only in their total burden of infectious disease, but also in the spectrum of factors that influences outcome. In part this is due to the correlation between geography and ethnicity. The former defines the biological ecosystem that constrains the distribution of pathogens and their vectors. The latter defines the community macro-social environment of the community that modulates probability of infection. To this latter must also be added the way in which the genetic heritage of the community influences susceptibility and resistance.

Multifactorial disease: more complex aetiologies

Multifactorial diseases, such as hypertension or non-insulin-dependent diabetes mellitus (NIDDM), are essentially the consequence of interaction between susceptible genotypes and deleterious environments. While the strength of the contribution of each component varies by disease, the essential feature is that adverse components in both genetic background and surrounding environment are required before manifestation of disease. Hence, no single factor is either uniquely necessary or uniquely sufficient. This is particularly true of genetic factors, because evolutionary pressure for functional homeostasis, for individuals and populations, necessarily imposes constraints on genetic variation. For complex physiological processes that involve multiple interacting components, only so much variation can be compatible with long-term survival. Environmental variability is subject to no such constraints. This is especially true for those aspects that are modified by human intervention, such as nutritional profiles. Consequently, it is frequently the case that adverse environment tips the balance inexorably towards disease. In this respect, the extremes of environmental variation can dominate variation in multifactorial disease susceptibility, in much the same way as is true for allelic variation in monogenic disease. Both types of variation represent opposite ends of the aetiological spectrum (Ward 1980).

An essential feature of multifactorial disease is the multiplicity of factors, which combine to define disease risk. On the environmental side of the ledger, the factors that contribute towards such disease as coronary heart disease, or cancer, are many and varied. In addition, the composition of environmental risk ranges from factors which, singly, are all important in defining risk (e.g. cigarette smoking and lung cancer), to factors which, by themselves, exert only a minor influence on risk (e.g. alcohol intake and hypertension). In similar fashion, a multiplicity of variant alleles combines to define genetic risk. Just as is true for environmental correlates of risk, individual alleles vary in the degree to which they influence risk. However, unlike the case for environmental factors, there is a definite structure to the pattern of genetic influence on disease susceptibility. This regular relationship, termed the *genetic architecture* of disease (Sing and Boerwinkle 1987), has been defined by evolutionary imperatives. For every population, the genetic architecture of disease has been shaped by the evolutionary history of individual alleles within that population. This has considerable implication for how genetic differentiation influences the distribution of disease risk among ethnic groups.

The basic principle, illustrated in Figure 8.1, is due to an inverse relationship between allele frequency and the severity of allelic effect. Alleles with the greatest impact will occur infrequently within the population. Conversely, very common alleles will, by themselves, only cause minor perturbations in the distribution of disease risk. Although genetic architecture is fundamentally a continuum, it is conceptually useful to identify three components: rare Mendelian variants, 'major genes' and polygenes. Rare Mendelian variants, such as the functional variants at the LDL receptor gene, or the *BRCA1* gene, exert a primary and clinically significant effect on risk. For example, the excessive LDL cholesterol levels caused by functional mutations of the LDL receptor gene are relatively unaffected by genetic background, or by the immediate environment. Consequently, familial hypercholesterolaemia due to *LDLR* variants segregates as an autosomal dominant. Such functionally potent allelic variants are constrained by evolution to be few in number and rare in frequency. Hence, although important at the individual and family level, rare Mendelian variants contribute little to attributable risk at the population level.

At the other end of the architectural scale are the true polygenes, which are both common in frequency and ubiquitous in occurrence. While their collective impact on disease risk is large, accounting for upwards of 50 per cent of the additive genetic variance, their individual effects are minute. Hence, they are essentially undetectable for all practical purposes. However, in the aggregate, genetic variation in polygenes can contribute to variability in risk among ethnic groups, especially when genotype and environmental interactions are considered.

'Major genes' are both moderate in effect and in frequency. The impact of allelic segregation at individual 'major gene' loci is detectable (unlike the situation for polygenes). Also, individual alleles at 'major genes' are sufficiently common to exert a measurable impact on the population-attributable risk (unlike rare Mendelian variants). Accordingly, these genes represent the target towards which much of genetic epidemiology is directed. The effect of Mendelian segregation of the three common apolipoprotein E alleles, which can account for upwards of 5 per cent of total variation in cholesterol levels (Sing and Davignon 1985) represents an early and informative example of such genes. The fact that the same apolipoprotein E alleles also exert a significant effect on susceptibility to Alzheimer's disease serves notice that genetic architecture is multifaceted. Allelic variation at a single locus can influence distribution of risk for more than one disease.

In Figure 8.1, the number of alleles is indicated by rectangles in each column, and allele frequency by the height of each rectangle. Further, for illustration, allele frequencies have been rescaled for each category of genic effect. In reality, the frequencies of rare Mendelian variants are vanishingly small, while allele frequencies for 'major genes' and polygenes will tend to be polymorphic. In Figure 8.1, rare Mendelian variants are represented by five alleles with substantial effects, one more frequent than the others. Segregation of seventeen alleles defines the cumulative impact of the 'major genes', while thirty-three alleles contribute to the polygenic component. It will be noted that this is an abstraction since, in reality, the number of relevant alleles and their frequency varies by disease. Every disease has its own genetic architecture. It should also be stressed that the emphasis is on *alleles* rather than loci. Although many loci will be essentially diallelic, so that the locus effect is mainly defined by segregation of a single allele, other loci will have more than two segregating alleles. In the case of apolipoprotein E, LDL cholesterol levels in most populations are influenced by the segregation of three polymorphic alleles. In general, the insights obtained by molecular dissection of monogenic loci will undoubtedly apply to multifactorial disease. Genetic risk will be determined by a spectrum of molecular variants at each

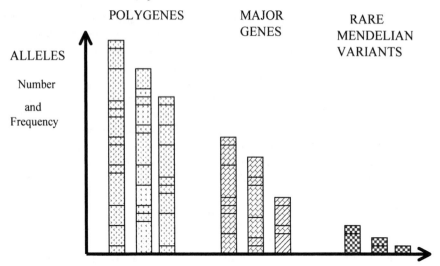

Figure 8.1 Genetic architecture of a complex disease. The magnitude of the contribution that individual alleles make towards risk of disease is represented on the horizontal axis, increasing from left to right. The vertical axis represents the number of alleles contributing to disease risk and their frequency. Within each column, the number of alleles is represented by the number of boxes, with allele frequency being represented by the height of individual boxes. Variation in shading is used to discriminate between the three categories of allelic risk (polygenes, 'major genes' and Mendelian variants). However, the discrete clustering of these categories along the horizontal axis is for illustrative purposes only. The theoretical distribution of risk is expected to be a smooth continuum, without breaks.

relevant locus, with every variant differing in terms of its population frequency and magnitude of effect.

The role of environmental factors, which can range from a modifying one to a dominant one, represents an added complexity. In the classical model, the joint contribution of genes and environment is usually represented by the equation: $P = G + E + G \times E$, with P representing the phenotype (in this case, risk of disease), G genetic factors, E environmental factors and $G \times E$ the interaction between genetic and environmental factors. This simple linear relationship indicates how variability in disease risk is collectively influenced by *genetic variation* within the population, plus *environmental variability* **and** the *interaction* between environmental and genetic factors. Hence, within a single population, the distribution of disease risk can be extremely complex. The conceptual complexity is increased when it is realised that environmental variation impacts on *each* component of the genetic architecture. Although somewhat tedious, it would be more insightful if disease risk were represented as a set of three of the above equations, one for each genetic category (polygenes, 'major genes' and Mendelian variants). The multiplicity of genotype–environmental interactions within each category also needs emphasis. Not only does each allele represented in Figure 8.1 have its own distribution within the population but *also* a unique set of environmental interactions.

The complex interactions between the multiple factors that contribute to risk of disease make identification of individual genetic risk factors a daunting task. The situation is even more difficult when ethnic groups are considered. As we have seen, the unique history of every ethnic group leads to considerable variability in the causal spectrum for monogenic disease. The aetiological complexity of multifactorial disease makes the distribution among ethnic groups infinitely more difficult to dissect. In large part, this is because ethnic groups are characterised not only by a unique constellation of alleles, but also by a unique set of environments. Hence, the aetiological underpinnings of multifactorial disease are likely to vary much more among ethnic groups than is commonly supposed.

In spite of these theoretical considerations, there is a common tendency to attribute ethnic differences in the risk of multifactorial disease to only a single, usually intrinsic, factor. This has the unfortunate effect of oversimplifying a complex multidimensional problem and reducing understanding. The attempts to explain the difference in hypertension risk between populations of African ancestry and those of European extraction are a case in point. For many years there has been a general, but unjustified, tendency to attribute the epidemiological differences in hypertension observed between United States Black people and United States White people to genetic factors. Differences in hypertension rates between United States Black people and White people were first noted in the 1930s. A quarter of a century later, the striking magnitude of the difference in risk was carefully documented by a, now classic, series of studies in the rural South (Comstock 1957, McDonough *et al.* 1964). These data made it abundantly clear that rates of hypertension were up to two to four times greater in United States Black people than in their White counterparts. A broad variety of environmental factors were implicated, some unique to the Black community, some not. However, the overriding consensus was that much of the excess risk of hypertension in the Black community was due to their genetic distinctiveness.

Despite some dissent, the invocation of genetic differences as the underlying cause of this major public health problem remains implicit in much of the epidemiological literature. This focus on genetic influence is so pervasive that it almost constitutes bias. Here, it is relevant to note that, since the first surveys in the United States, nearly 70 years ago, the risk ratio has undergone significant change. In the 1950s and 1960s, when national rates of hypertension in the United States were extremely high, the risk ratio (for women) was as high as 4.4. Thirty years later, when the national prevalence was appreciably lower, the risk ratio had diminished to 1.8. Looking ahead, it appears likely that the risk ratio may increase again, since while rates of hypertension will continue their decline within the White population, the decline may slow, or become reversed, in the Black community. Even though the magnitude of the risk differential between US Black people and White people has fluctuated considerably during the past 70 years, the emphasis on genetic causation has remained constant. This is unexpected since, as noted earlier (p. 89), substantial temporal changes in disease risk implicate extrinsic, rather than intrinsic, factors. Most recently, the emphasis on genetic determinism has acquired new trappings. This is in the form of a hypothesis that US Black people are uniquely susceptible to risk of hypertension because the ancestral slave population was subject to extreme selection for salt retention during the infamous 'middle passage' (Wilson and Grim 1991). Although dressed up in evolutionary principles, and undoubtedly proposed in good faith, this supposition has little credibility. Neither the genetic model, nor the historical evidence, holds up under careful scrutiny. However, even though this latest theory has fallen into disrepute, the tendency to attribute this particular ethnic difference in disease risk to genetic causation still remains.

Much of this inappropriate emphasis on genetic causation might never have occurred had more note been taken of data from Africa itself. Even before the first documented study of elevated risk of hypertension among US Black people, data existed indicating that Africans in Africa experienced little hypertension (Donnison 1929). At the time when extensive epidemiological studies were defining the differential risk of high blood pressure between US Black people and White people, a variety of studies within Africa were showing a different picture. The results of those later studies pointed to environment, not genetics, as the more pertinent factor. In rural Africa, blood pressure was low and hypertension rare, especially in the more traditional communities (Akinkugbe and Ojo 1969). Moreover, when migration to urban centres occurred rates of hypertension increased markedly, as shown by Scotch's (1963) classic analysis of Zulus. Thirty years later, the risk differential between urban Zulus and rural Zulus remained notable, with the transition from a rural to an urban lifestyle being marked by a decrease in physical activity and an increase in obesity. More recently, yet another analysis of a population that is making the transition between a traditional lifestyle to an urbanised way of life, the Luo, shows the same characteristic risk differential for hypertension (Poulter *et al.*, 1990).

If environment was so obviously the critical factor in determining differential rates of hypertension within Africa, why was it possible to maintain the belief that genetic difference was the predominant cause of the risk differential between US Black people and White people? The answer is unclear, though it is likely that the debate will continue unabated for some time to come. However, the recent publication of a critical piece of evidence places the weight of evidence even more squarely in the environmental camp. The data, summarised in Figure 8.2, derive from the first careful comparative analysis of blood pressure and hypertension rates among a series of populations of African ancestry, ranging from West Africa to the United States, via the Caribbean. Seven populations of West African origin were extensively surveyed, using the same methodology, with careful attention to ensure comparable evaluation of potential risk factors. The results showed a clear-cut trend in the prevalence of hypertension with the three West African populations exhibiting the lowest rates and the US population the highest. The three Caribbean populations had intermediate prevalence rates. These results eliminate any residual concern that previous intercontinental comparisons might have been confounded by lack of comparability between different independent surveys. Location, not genes, is the primary discriminator.

The details are even more revealing. First, and most obvious, overall rates of hypertension are clearly associated with overall rates of obesity [as measured by body mass index (BMI)]. Here, BMI is used as a surrogate for the degree to which the population has adopted a 'Westernised' lifestyle with, among other aspects, increased caloric intake and reduced physical activity. The West African populations with the lowest rates of hypertension are also the leanest. Conversely, the African American community of Maywood, a suburb of Chicago, has twice the overall rate of hypertension and a significant excess of obesity. Overall, it is clear that the substantial differences between geographic regions are attributable to the differences in lifestyle factors that manifest themselves as differences in BMI.

Second, and perhaps even more telling, is the distribution within West Africa. It is notable that the difference in hypertension rates between rural

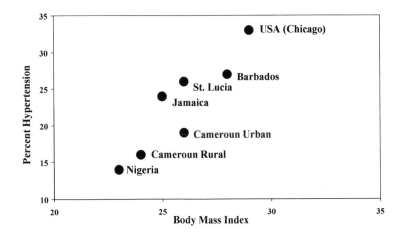

Figure 8.2   Hypertension in populations of West African origin. The distribution of prevalence of hypertension (vertical axis) among seven populations of West African origin, in terms of mean body mass index (BMI) for each population (horizontal axis). Both hypertension prevalence rates and mean BMI have been standardised by age and sex (after Cooper *et al.* 1997).

Nigeria (14.5 per cent) and urban Cameroon (19.1 per cent) is an appreciable fraction of the overall difference between West Africa (15.6 per cent) and the Caribbean (25.5 per cent). The rural–urban divide within West Africa represents a considerable change in the macro-social environment, as indicated in the difference in the distribution of BMI (22.2 versus 26.1). This results in a 20 per cent increase in hypertension from rural Nigeria to urban Cameroon. Within the Caribbean, the range in BMI values, from 25.7 (Jamaica) to 27.7 (Barbados), is much less, with a mean not much less than the value for the African American sample (28.9). This suggests a greater degree of similarity in lifestyle factors outside Africa than within Africa. Risk differentials for hypertension reflect this, with a 20 per cent increase in risk within Africa, which equals the 20 per cent increase from the Caribbean to the United States and exceeds the 20 per cent risk differential within the Caribbean. The importance of the macro-social environment is highlighted by the 63 per cent risk differential between West Africa and the Caribbean.

Taken together with the earlier studies, these results indicate that adverse environments, rather than deleterious genes, are the primary cause of the difference in hypertension rates *among* the populations of African ancestry. However, it also needs to be clarified that an absence of genetic causation to account for differences among ethnic groups does *not* mean an absence of ethnic-specific genes that give raise to ethnic-specific risk pathways. While this may seem paradoxical, the interpretation is clarified by considering the consequences of genetic differentiation for the genetic causation of complex disease.

Influence of genetic differentiation on genetic architecture of disease

Just as genetic differentiation results in a variable distribution of risk for monogenic disease among ethnic groups, the same is true for more complex multifactorial disease. The impact of population-specific variation in allele frequencies on the genetic architecture of disease is illustrated in Figure 8.3. As a consequence of their distinct evolutionary histories, both populations A and B have a different spectrum of alleles that contributes to disease risk. This is plotted on the 'species-specific' architecture illustrated in Figure 8.1. Alleles that are present in a population are represented by the shaded rectangles, while empty rectangles indicate alleles that are absent from one or other of the population. A number of consequences are immediately apparent. Most obvious is the fact that neither of the single populations contains all the relevant risk alleles. For example, instead of the five alleles of substantial effect that segregate as Mendelian variants, each population considered alone has only three (60 per cent of the total). The same is true for the 'major gene' and polygene categories, though to an increasingly lesser extent since the fraction of missing alleles declines in inverse proportion to allele frequency. More noteworthy, and more cogent for our argument, is the

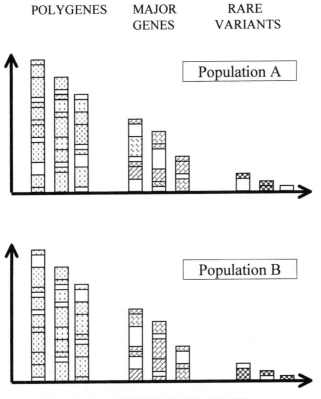

POLYGENES   MAJOR   RARE
             GENES   VARIANTS

Population A

Population B

ALLELIC CONTRIBUTION TO DISEASE RISK

Figure 8.3   Effect of genetic differentiation on the genetic architecture of disease risk. Representation of the genetic architecture of a complex disease in two populations, A and B, which are genetically distinct from each other. For each population, the genetic architecture of disease risk is depicted as in Figure 8.1. Risk alleles that are missing from either of the two populations (due to evolutionary factors such as genetic drift) are indicated by empty boxes.

even smaller proportion of alleles that are shared between the two populations. Since the probability that alleles are shared among populations is proportional to their evolutionary age (Thompson and Neel 1996), the rare (and evolutionary young) alleles of substantial effect will tend to be unique to individual populations while the more common polygenes will exhibit a much greater degree of sharing. As indicated in Figure 8.3, within each category of genic effect, there is a general tendency for the more frequent alleles to be shared among populations, while rarer alleles tend to be population specific in their distribution.

Figure 8.3 clearly indicates that the distribution of risk alleles will differ among populations. Hence, the distribution of genetic risk will differ among ethnic groups both in terms of which loci are involved and in the magnitude of effect associated with specific alleles. The main implication for the ethnic distribution of complex, multifactorial disease is that the differential distribution of allele frequencies for 'major genes' will dominate the ethnic-specific differences in genetic risk. Although differences in allelic variants that define Mendelian traits will be most marked, their overall rarity means they contribute little to differences in population risk. Conversely the majority of alleles at polygenic loci will have an ancient origin and will be widely dispersed among a broad variety of ethnically distinct populations. This leaves little opportunity for substantial differences among ethnic groups, and implies that the additive genetic background will be similar for most ethnic groups. In contrast, 'major gene' alleles, which individually contribute substantially to population-attributable risk, will tend to have an intermediate distribution of mutational ages and hence considerable variability in allelic frequency among ethnic groups (Figure 8.4).

When evaluating the distribution of disease risk among ethnic groups, it needs to be emphasised that not only will the set of relevant alleles vary, but so will the relevant environments. Moreover, the extent to which important environmental changes have occurred is also likely to differ by ethnic group. Thus, the intersection of genetic differentiation and environmental change can make an important contribution to ethnic differences in disease frequency. With genetic differentiation, the genotype by environmental interaction will necessarily vary by population. If the environment also varies among populations, which is usually the case, the interaction between genes and environments will be unique to each ethnic group. To the extent that ethnically distinct groups have a characteristic environmental milieu (which

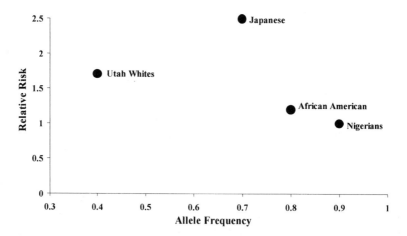

Figure 8.4   Relative risk of hypertension associated with the angiotensinogen *M235T* allele in ethnically distinct groups. Distribution of the population-specific relative risk of hypertension (vertical axis) associated with the *M235T* allele (methionine to threonine substitution at position 235), in terms of the population-specific allele frequency (horizontal axis).

is usually the case), the spectrum of genotype by environment interactions will likewise be increased across ethnic groups.

Conclusion

While exceedingly preliminary, the available genetic data emphasise that the variable risk of complex genetic disease among different ethnic groups cannot be attributed to a small number of independently acting discrete causes. Hypertension, like many other diseases of complex aetiology, varies appreciably in frequency among ethnic groups. When an ethnic group displays an elevated frequency, the public health consequences can be profound, as illustrated by the situation for African Americans in the United States. As a group, African Americans are readily characterised in terms of their excessive risk of hypertension and consequent morbidity and mortality. However, it is far less easy to discern the underlying reasons. It is clear that to fall back on 'ethnicity' as an explanation is at best a profession of woeful ignorance and at worst racist. Neither genetic background nor cultural milieu is sufficient to account for the risk of disease. Among populations of African ancestry, elevated frequency of a putative-risk allele does not predict a population-specific risk of disease. This appears true both in the low-risk environment of rural West Africa and the high-risk environment of urban United States. At the level of the individual, presence of the 235T variant exerts a physiological effect in all populations, but the pathophysiological implications are either negligible or irrelevant. Why populations of African ancestry should differ so markedly from Caucasian populations is an important challenge for epidemiology.

Ultimately, it has to be recognised that 'ethnicity' results from an irreducible mix of biological, social and cultural factors. Similarly, it is the equally complex interaction between genetic factors and environmental variables that leads to ethnic-specific disease profiles. Just as no single variable can provide an adequate identifier for 'ethnic affiliation', neither genes nor environment, considered in isolation, can provide an adequate causal explanation for the differences in disease frequency among ethnic groups. To attribute population differences in disease risk to underlying differences in the frequency of a 'susceptibility gene' is as meaningful as attributing differences in IQ to skin colour. It is almost as harmful. The tendency to seize on simple, but inadequate, explanations tends to forestall serious research into disease causation. It can also result in appropriately stigmatising the group. The way forward is to recognise that disease is the result of a complex interaction between genes and environments. This is particularly relevant for diseases that display marked differences in frequency, or severity, among ethnic groups. A corollary of this principle is that the profile of disease risk that may appear to indelibly characterise an ethnic group is, in fact, no more permanent than any single cultural attribute that appears to distinguish the group. Even if the genetic heritage of a group is slow to change over time, any change in the physical or macro-social environment can lead to the relatively rapid disappearance, or appearance, of disease. Witness the rise in the prevalence of diabetes in certain Amerindian and Micronesian populations in the space of less than two generations.

In conclusion, although ethnic associations with disease are often used as a descriptive label, this is really a confession of ignorance. Ethnic differences in disease risk result from a complex mix of genetic differentiation and ecological factors. To conclude that a specifiable percentage of the variance in disease risk can be attributable to ethnic factors explains nothing. Use of such labels merely identifies an association, which, if studied further, may ultimately lead to a deeper understanding of disease aetiology. Taken in isolation, the label is meaningless. Even worse, undue reliance on 'ethnicity' as a risk factor not only suppresses understanding but also increases the possibility that racist interpretations of disease risk will prevail.

Nonetheless, to disregard the ethnic variability in disease risk is equally misleading and can be just as deleterious. As this chapter indicates, ethnic variation in disease risk is a fundamental characteristic of our species. Fundamentally, it is a consequence of the distinct biological history and cultural history that, collectively, defines every ethnic group. To subscribe to the convenient fiction that the pathophysiology of complex disease, such as hypertension and diabetes, is invariant across ethnic boundaries represents a disservice to each ethnic group on two counts. In the first instance, it obstructs science by constraining our ability to develop a deeper and more comprehensive understanding of the full range of pathophysiology causing human disease. Ultimately, failure to comprehend the gamut of pathophysiology that leads to disease can only impede effective treatment. Second, and at a more immediate level, it inhibits our ability to develop appropriate and effective strategies for detecting and treating complex disease in ethnically diverse populations. In the final analysis, a reluctance to recognise the genetic (and socio-ecological) correlates of ethnic diversity in disease risk harms the very ethnic groups that the presumption of aetiological uniformity is designed to protect. Neither science, nor ethics would be well served by such a stance.

References

Akinkugbe, O.O. and Ojo, O.A. (1969) 'Arterial pressure in rural and urban populations in Nigeria', *British Medical Journal*, 2, 222–224.

Austerlitz, F. and Heyer, E. (1998) 'Social transmission of reproductive behaviour increases frequency of inherited disorders in a young-expanding population', *Proceedings of the National Academy of Sciences, USA*, 95, 15140–15144.

Bertranpetit, J. and Calafell, F. (1996) 'Genetic and geographical variability in cystic fibrosis; evolutionary considerations', *Variation in the Human Genome*, Ciba Foundation Symposium, 197, 97–118.

Comstock, G.W. (1957) 'An epidemiologic study of blood pressure levels in a biracial community in the southern United States', *American Journal of Hygiene*, 65, 271–315.

Cooper, R. and Rotimi, C. (1994) 'Hypertension in populations of West African origin: is there a genetic predisposition?', *Journal of Hypertension*, 12, 215–227.

Cooper, R., Rotimi, C., Ataman, S., McGee, D., Osotimehin, B., Kadiri, S., Muna, W., Kingue, S., Fraser, H., Forrester, T., Bennet, F. and Wilks, R. (1997) 'The prevalence of hypertension in seven populations of West African origin', *American Journal of Public Health*, 87, 160–168.

Devilee, P. (1999) '*BRCA1* and *BRCA2* testing: weighing the demand against the benefits', *American Journal of Human Genetics*, 64, 943–948.

Donnison, C.P. (1929) 'Blood pressure in the African native: its bearing on the aetiology of hyperplasia and arteriosclerosis', *Lancet*, I, 6–9.

Dragic, T., Litwin, V., Allaway, G.P., Martin, S.R., Huang, Y., Nagashima, K.A., Cayanan, C., Maddon, P.J., Koup, R.A., Moore, J.P. and Paxton, W.A. (1996) 'HIV-1 entry into CD4+ cells is mediated by the chemokine receptor CC-CKR-5', *Nature*, 381, 667–673.

Flint, J., Harding, R.M., Boyce, A.J. and Clegg, J.B. (1993) 'The population genetics of the haemoglobinopathies', *Clinical Haematology*, 6, 215–262.

Hartge, P., Struewing, J.P., Wacholder, S., Brody, L.C. and Tucker, M.A. (1999) 'The prevalence of common *BRCA1* and *BRCA2* mutations among Ashkenazi Jews', *American Journal of Human Genetics*, 64, 963–970.

Lewontin, R.C. (1972) 'The apportionment of human diversity', *Evolutionary Biology*, 6, 381–398.

Libert, F., Cochaux, P., Beckman, G., Samson, M., Askenova, M., Cao, A., Czeizel, A., Claustres, M., de la Rua, C., Ferrari, M., Ferec, C., Glover, G., Grinde, B., Guran, S., Kucinskas, V., Lavinha, J., Mercier, B., Ogur, G., Peltonen, L., Rosatelli, C., Schwartz, M., Pitsyn, V., Timar, L., Beckman, L., Parmentier, M. and Vassart, G. (1998) 'The Δccr5 mutation conferring protection against HIV-1 in Caucasian populations has a single and recent origin in Northeastern Europe', *Human Molecular Genetics*, 7, 399–406.

McDonough, J.R., Garrison, G.E. and Hames, C.G. (1964) 'Blood pressure and hypertensive disease among Negroes and whites', *Annals of Internal Medicine*, 6, 208–228.

Martinson, J.J., Chapman, N.H., Rees, D.C., Liu, Y.-T. and Clegg, J.B. (1997) 'Global distribution of the CCR-5 gene 32 basepair deletion', *Nature Genetics*, 16, 100–103.

Merryweather-Clarke, A.T., Pointon, J.J., Shearman, J.D. and Robson, K.J.H. (1997) 'Global prevalence of putative hemochromatosis mutations', *Journal of Medical Genetics*, 34, 275–278.

Neel, J.V. and Ward, R.H. (1970) 'Village and tribal genetic distances among American Indians, and the possible implications for human evolution', *Proceedings of the National Academy of Sciences, USA*, 65, 323–330.

Peltonen, L., Pekkarinen, P. and Aaltonen, J. (1995) 'Messages from an isolate: lessons from the Finnish gene pool', *Biological Chemistry*, 376, 697–704.

Pier, G.B., Grout, M., Zaidi, T., Meluleni, G., Mueschenborn, S.S., Banting, G. and Ratcliffe, R. (1998) '*Salmonella typhi* uses CFTR to enter intestinal epithelial cells', *Nature*, 393, 79–82.

Polednak, A.P. (1989) *Racial and Ethnic Differences in Disease*, Oxford: Oxford University Press.

Poulter, N.R., Khaw, K.T., Hopwood, B.E.C. *et al.* (1990) 'The Kenyan Luo migration study: observations on the initiation of a rise in blood dpressure', *British Medical Journal*, 300, 967–972.

Sajantila, A., Salme, A.-H., Savolainen, P., Bauer, K., Gierig, C. and Pääbo, S. (1996) 'Paternal and maternal DNA lineages reveal a bottleneck in the founding of the Finnish population', *Proceedings of the National Academy of Sciences, USA*, 93, 12035–12039.

Scotch, N.A. (1963) 'Sociocultural factors in the epidemiology of Zulu hypertension', (1963) *American Journal of Public Health*, 53, 1205–1213.

Scriver, C.R., Byck, S., Prevost, L., Hoang, L. and the PAH consortium (1996) 'The phenylalanine hydroxylase locus: a marker for the history of phenylketonuria and human genetic diversity', *Variation in the Human Genome*, Ciba Foundation Symposium, 197, 73–96.

Scriver, C.R. and Waters, P.J. (1999) 'Monogeneic traits are not simple: lessons from phenylketonuria', *Trends in Genetics*, 15, 267–272.

Shaper, A.G., Leonard, P.J., Jones, K.W. and Jones, M. (1969) 'Environmental effects of the body build, blood pressure and blood chemistries of nomadic warriors serving in the army in Kenya', *East African Medical Journal*, 46, 282–289.

Sing, C.F. and Boerwinkle, E. (1987) 'Genetic architecture of inter-individual variability in apolipoprotein, lipoprotein and lipid phenotypes', *Molecular Approaches to Human Polygenic Disease*, Ciba Foundation Symposium, 130, 99–121.

Sing, C.F. and Davignon, J. (1985) 'Role of the apolipoprotein E polymorphism in determining normal plasma lipid and lipoprotein variation', *American Journal of Human Genetics*, 37, 268–285.

Slatkin, M. and Rannala, B. (1997) 'The sampling distribution of disease-associated alleles', *Genetics*, 147, 1855–1861.

Stephens, J.C., Reich, D.E., Goldstein, D.B., Shin, H.S., Smith, M.W., Carrrington, M., Winkler, C., Huttley, G.A., Allikmets, R., Schriml, L., Gerrard, B., Malasky, M., Ramos, M.D., Morlot, S., Tzetis, M., Oddoux, C., di Giovine, F.S., Nasioulas, G., Chandler, D., Aseev, M., Hanson, M., Kalaydjieva, L., Glavac, D., Gasparini, P., Kanavakis, E., Claustres, M., Kambouris, M., Ostrer, H., Duff, G., Baranov, V., Sibul, H., Metspalu, A., Goldman, D., Martin, N., Duffy, D., Schmidtke, Estivill, X., O'Brien, S.J. and Dean, M. (1998) 'Dating the origin of the CCR5-Δ32 AIDS resistance allele by the coalescence of haplotypes', *American Journal of Human Genetics*, 62, 1507–1515.

Thompson, E.A. and Neel, J.V. (1996) 'Private polymorphisms: How many? How old? How useful for genetic taxonomies', *Molecular Phylogenetics and Evolution*, 5, 220–231.

Thompson, E.A. and Neel, J.V. (1997) 'Allelic disequilibrium and allele frequency distribution as a function of social and demographic history', *American Journal of Human Genetics*, 60, 197–204.

Tonin, P.N., Mes-Masson, A.-M., Futreal, P.A., Morgan, K., Mahon, M., Foulke, W.D., Cole, D.E.C., Provencher, D., Ghadirian, P. and Narod, S.A. (1998) 'Founder *BRCA1* and *BRCA2* mutations in French Canadian breast and ovarian cancer families', *American Journal of Human Genetics*, 63, 1341–1351.

Ward, R.H. (1980) 'Genetic epidemiology: promise or compromise?', *Social Biology*, 27, 87–100.

Ward, R.H., Frazier, B.L., Dew-Jaeger, K. and Pääbo, S. (1991) 'Extensive mitochondrial diversity within a single Amerindian tribe', *Proceedings of the National Academy of Sciences, USA*, 88, 8720–8724.

Weiss, K.M., Ferrell, R.E. and Hanis, C.L. (1984) 'A New World syndrome of metabolic diseases with a genetic and evolutionary basis', *Yearbook of Physical Anthropology*, 27, 153–178.

Wilson, T.W. and Grim, C.E. (1991) 'Biohistory of slavery and blood pressure differences in blacks today: a hypothesis', *Hypertension* 17 (Suppl.): I-22–I-28.

9 Approaches to investigating the genetic basis of ethnic differences in disease risk

Paul McKeigue

Introduction

Epidemiologists have two main approaches to distinguishing genetic and environmental explanations of ethnic differences in disease risk: studies of migrants and studies of the relationship of disease risk to proportionate admixture in populations of mixed descent. These epidemiological criteria indicate that most ethnic variation in disease risk is attributable to environment rather than to genes. For hypertension in West Africans compared with other groups, and for non-insulin-dependent diabetes in many non-European groups compared with Europeans, the epidemiological evidence points strongly to genetic explanations for the ethnic difference in disease risk. This is of practical importance, because, where suitable admixed populations exist, it is theoretically possible to map the genes that underlie these ethnic differences in disease risk by a novel approach that exploits admixture between human populations in a manner analogous to linkage analysis of an experimental cross. By conditioning on parental ancestry, and combining information from all markers on a chromosome in a multipoint analysis, it is possible in principle to extract all the information about linkage that is generated by admixture. Marker sets suitable for genome searches could be assembled by screening microsatellites, screening single-nucleotide polymorphisms or using subtractive hybridisation to discover restriction site polymorphisms that are informative for ancestry. To combine the marker data in a multipoint analysis and test for linkage, the posterior distribution of ancestry at each locus could be generated by Gibbs sampling and a score test constructed by averaging over this posterior distribution. This admixture mapping approach has far greater power than the allele-sharing linkage study designs that are now widely used to study the genetics of complex traits in humans. Suitable admixed populations exist in the Americas, Australia, southern Africa and circumpolar regions. There are obvious applications to studying the genetics of hypertension, diabetes, cancer and autoimmune disease.

Ethnic differences in disease risk that are likely to have a genetic basis

Epidemiological criteria for distinguishing between genetic and environmental explanations

Epidemiologists have developed standard criteria for distinguishing between genetic and environmental explanations of variation in disease risk between populations. The classic approach to this question is to study migrants: if an ethnic difference in disease risk has an environmental explanation, this difference is expected to 'wear off' within a few generations after migration (Reid 1971). For instance, the incidence of colorectal cancer is far lower in Japan than in the United States, but in Japanese Americans two generations after migration the risk of colorectal cancer approximates the risk in American White people (Haenszel and Kurihara 1968). If, on the other hand, an ethnic difference in disease risk has a genetic explanation, we would expect to observe such a difference consistently in all countries where a given migrant group has settled. We would also expect this ethnic difference to persist in populations where migrants have been settled overseas for many generations. An example of an ethnic difference in disease risk that meets these criteria is the high prevalence of non-insulin-dependent diabetes in South Asians (Indians, Pakistanis and Bangladeshis) compared with most other ethnic groups. Since the early years of the twentieth century, reports of a high prevalence of diabetes in migrant populations of Indian descent have come from many countries including Vietnam (Montel 1913), Singapore (Cheah *et al.* 1979), South Africa (Omar *et al.* 1985), Trinidad (Beckles *et al.* 1986), Fiji (Zimmet *et al* 1983) and England (McKeigue *et al.* 1991). Diabetes prevalence is as high in those Indian migrant populations that have been settled overseas since the mid-nineteenth century as in first-generation migrants from south Asia to England, or in urban populations in south Asia itself (Ramachandran *et al.* 1988, Ramachandran *et al.* 1992). These observations point to genetic explanations for the ethnic difference in disease risk (McKeigue *et al.* 1989). We have shown that the high risk of diabetes in South Asians occurs as part of a distinct phenotype including central obesity, insulin resistance and lipid disturbances (McKeigue *et al.* 1991). The expression of this diabetic phenotype is of course dependent on interaction with environmental factors, most importantly those that cause obesity. In low-income rural South Asian populations where most people are lean, the prevalence of diabetes is low (Ramachandran *et al.* 1992).

The most compelling evidence that some ethnic differences in disease risk have a genetic basis comes from studies in admixed populations (Chakraborty *et al.* 1986, Chakraborty and Weiss 1986). If the ethnic difference in disease risk has a genetic basis, we can predict that within an admixed population there will be a linear relationship between disease risk and proportionate admixture (M) from the high-risk population (estimated for each individual by typing marker polymorphisms) (Hanis *et al.* 1986). The risk ratio for disease associated with unit increase in M (estimated by a logistic regression analysis) within the admixed population will be the same as the observed risk ratio between the two 'founding populations' from which the admixed group is derived. As with any other epidemiological association, it is necessary to control for confounders in testing for association of proportionate admixture with disease risk. If adjusting for possible confounders such as socio-economic status does not reduce the risk ratio associated with unit increase in M, or reduces this risk ratio only slightly, it is unlikely that residual confounding can account for the remaining association.

Example: excess risk of hypertension in West Africans

One example of an ethnic difference in disease risk that meets these epidemiological criteria for a genetic explanation is the excess risk of hypertensive disease in West Africans compared with other groups. In people of West African descent settled in Europe and the Americas, prevalence of hypertension is two to five times higher than in Europeans (Boyle 1970, Chaturvedi *et al.* 1993). In England we have shown that average blood pressures are as high in those who have migrated directly from West Africa as in Afro-Caribbean migrants, even though these two groups have not shared a common environment for more than 200 years (Chaturvedi *et al.* 1993). In African American and Afro-Caribbean people, hypertension is inversely associated with genetic markers of European admixture (MacLean *et al.* 1974, Darlu *et al.* 1990). The slope of the regression of diastolic blood pressure on proportionate admixture in African Americans was estimated to be 14 mmHg per unit increase of admixture (MacLean *et al* 1974): approximately the same as the difference in means observed when African Americans without admixture were compared with European Americans (Boyle 1970). Adjustment for covariates including obesity and socio-economic status reduced the correlation between blood pressure and admixture only from 0.18 to 0.17, making it unlikely that residual confounding can account for the adjusted association (MacLean *et al.* 1974).

It is relevant also that clinical and epidemiological studies have identified a distinct phenotype of hypertension in people of West African descent. In comparison with hypertensive Europeans, hypertensive West Africans have elevated renal vascular resistance (Frohlich *et al.* 1984), low kallikrein excretion (Levy *et al.* 1977), raised urinary albumin excretion (Summerson *et al.* 1995), increased sensitivity of blood pressure to sodium (Luft *et al.* 1991), volume expansion (Lilley *et al.* 1976), low plasma renin (Sever *et al.* 1978) and poor response of blood pressure to angiotensin-converting enzyme inhibitors (Weinberger 1985). The risk of hypertensive end-stage renal failure and the rate at which renal function declines in treated hypertensive patients are far higher in people of West African descent than in Europeans (McClellan *et al.* 1988, Tierney *et al.* 1990, Peterson *et al.* 1997), even when differences in blood pressure are taken into account. The consistency with which this distinct hypertensive phenotype has been observed in African American and Afro-Caribbean populations of diverse West African origin suggests that these populations share a specific physiological disturbance predisposing to hypertension and renal damage [possibly a primary defect in a renal vasodilator mechanism (Warren and O'Connor 1980)].

Other examples

Some of the most striking ethnic differences in disease risk are seen with non-insulin-dependent diabetes mellitus (NIDDM). In some Native American, Pacific Islander and Native Australian populations, prevalence of diabetes before age 55 is more than 10 times higher than in Europeans (Wise *et al.* 1976). These risk ratios are reduced only slightly by controlling for obesity. As with hypertension in West Africans, diabetes in these high-risk populations is inversely associated with genetic markers of European admixture (Serjeantson *et al.* 1983, Chakraborty *et al.* 1986, Knowler *et al.* 1988). In some of these high-risk populations distinct phenotypes of diabetes can be identified: thus in West Africans diabetes is accompanied by favourable plasma lipid profile and low risk of coronary heart disease (Keil *et al.* 1995, Wild and McKeigue 1997), in contrast to the unfavourable plasma lipid profile and high risk of coronary heart disease in South Asians (McKeigue *et al.* 1991).

Some ethnic differences in disease risk for which epidemiological evidence points to genetic explanations are summarised in Table 9.1 (Zimmet 1992, Prineas and Gillum 1985, Qualheim *et al.* 1991, Mitchell *et al.* 1993, Hodge and Zimmet 1994, McKeigue *et al.* 1989, 1991, O'Dea *et al.* 1993, Miller *et al.* 1989, Hopkinson *et al.* 1994, Merrill and Brawley 1997, Congdon *et al.* 1992). It should be emphasised that this list excludes many other ethnic differences in disease risk for which epidemiological evidence supports environmental explanations. For example, migrant studies indicate that environmental factors account for the low risk of coronary heart disease in Japanese people compared with people of European descent (Worth *et al.* 1975). However, the high risk of coronary heart disease in people of South Asian descent around the world compared with other groups, persisting many generations after migration and unexplained by established coronary risk factors, is likely to have a genetic explanation (McKeigue *et al.* 1989).

For hypertension and diabetes the evidence that ethnic differences in risk have a genetic basis is compelling, as outlined above. For most of the other diseases listed one of the key lines of evidence – an epidemiological study showing that in an admixed population the disease is associated with proportionate admixture from the high-risk population – is lacking because such a study has not been done. A possible explanation for the negative results of some studies is that until recently it has not been technically feasible to estimate individual admixture accurately. At least forty marker loci must be typed to estimate individual admixture accurately. The form of the

Table 9.1 Ethnic differences in disease risk that are likely to have a genetic basis

Disease	High-risk groups	Low-risk groups	*Typical risk ratios between high-risk and low-risk groups*
Non-insulin-dependent diabetes mellitus	Pacific Islanders, Native Americans, Native Australians, South Asians (Zimmet 1992)	Europeans	5 to 12
Hypertension	West Africans (Prineas and Gillum 1985)	Europeans	2 to 5
Hypertensive renal disease	West Africans (Qualheim *et al.* 1991)	Europeans	6 to 20
Generalised obesity	Native Americans (Mitchell *et al.* 1993), Pacific Islanders, West African women (Hodge and Zimmet 1994)	Europeans	1–2 SD (continuous scale)
Central adiposity	South Asians (McKeigue *et al.* 1991), Native Australians (O'Dea *et al.* 1993)	Europeans	1 SD (continuous scale)
Coronary heart disease	South Asians (McKeigue *et al.* 1989)	West Africans (Miller *et al.* 1989)	2 to 3
Systemic lupus erythematosus	West Africans (Hopkinson *et al.* 1994)	Europeans	10
Prostate cancer	West Africans (Merrill and Brawley 1997)	Europeans	2 to 3
Angle-closure glaucoma	Inuit (Congdon *et al.* 1992)	Europeans	5 to 10

relationship between disease risk and admixture may yield insight into the underlying genetic model (Chakraborty and Weiss 1986). For instance, for an autoimmune disease such as systemic lupus erythematosus one could postulate a model in which heterozygosity at one or more loci influencing immune function is associated with increased risk. This would give an inverse U-shaped relationship between disease risk and proportionate admixture.

How many loci are likely to account for ethnic differences in disease risk?

If ethnic variation in risk of some diseases has a genetic basis, the possibilities for identifying the genes themselves depend upon whether the ethnic difference in risk results from small effects at many loci or from large effects at a few major loci. The studies reviewed above suggest that excess disease risk in one ethnic group compared with others is often associated with a distinctive phenotype, and with disturbance in a specific physiological pathway that is likely to be under the control of relatively few genes. This is consistent with arguments based on population genetics. If the trait on which there has been differential selection pressure is not the same as the trait under study, the loci that account for variation between sub-populations in the trait under study will in general be a subset of the loci that generate variation in the trait under study within sub-populations. Even if an ethnic difference in susceptibility results from drift rather than differential selection pressure, the same argument would apply.

For example, the high rates of non-insulin-dependent diabetes in many non-European populations have been attributed to differential selection for the ability to survive famine (Neel 1962). The pathogenesis of NIDDM involves disturbances in several physiological pathways, including beta-cell function, insulin-mediated glucose uptake, hepatic glucose production and body fat stores. It is likely, therefore, that only a subset of the genes that influences the risk of diabetes within populations also influences (in the same direction) the ability to survive famine.

This theoretical argument has experimental support. For instance the spontaneously hypertensive rat (SHR) strain, differs from its normotensive control (WKY) strain not only in blood pressure but in related traits such as insulin resistance and fatty acid metabolism (Aitman *et al.* 1997). As the SHR strain was selected for raised blood pressure, we would expect that all loci that generated variation in blood pressure within the ancestral population from which the SHR strain was derived would contribute to the SHR–WKY difference in blood pressure. The SHR–WKY difference between strains in a related trait such as insulin resistance, in contrast, would be accounted for by only those loci where the same alleles cause both raised blood pressure and insulin resistance. Experimental crosses have shown that multiple loci contribute to the SHR–WKY difference in blood pressure, whereas the difference in insulin resistance can be mapped to two major loci and the defect in fatty acid metabolism to only one of these two loci (Aitman *et al.* 1997).

Exploiting admixture to map genes that underlie ethnic differences in disease risk

Current attempts to map genes influencing complex traits such as hypertension or NIDDM are based on two main approaches: allele-sharing studies based on families with multiple affected members, or association studies of polymorphisms in candidate genes (Risch and Merikangas 1996). Both approaches have limitations. Allele-sharing studies lack adequate statistical power to detect genes of modest effect with realistic sample sizes (Risch and Merikangas 1996). Association studies have far greater statistical power than allele-sharing studies but depend upon knowing which gene to look at. A far more powerful method for mapping genes for complex traits is available to experimental geneticists, who detect linkage by typing crosses between inbred strains that differ in the trait under study. This experimental design has greater statistical power than allele-sharing designs in human families for fundamental statistical reasons: linkage analysis of an experimental cross compares means, whereas allele-sharing designs compare variances (Lander and Schork 1994).

The human counterpart of an experimental cross is admixture between two ethnic groups that have different risks of disease for genetic reasons. European maritime expansion since the fifteenth century has led to admixture of Europeans with other groups including Native Americans, West Africans, Pacific Islanders and Native Australians. In some cases people of mixed descent have formed endogamous populations isolated by geographic and social barriers from the founding populations: an example is the Anglo-Indian population of India.

Several writers have suggested that the linkage disequilibrium generated by admixture could be exploited to map genes underlying ethnic differences in disease risk (Chakraborty and Weiss 1988, Risch 1992, Briscoe *et al.* 1994, Stephens *et al.* 1994). Between any locus where genetic variation contributes to an ethnic difference in disease risk, and any loci where allele frequencies are different in the two ancestral ethnic groups, admixture will generate allelic disequilibrium. The statistical basis of this approach was first explored by Chakraborty and Weiss (1988), and subsequently by Stephens and colleagues, who named it 'mapping by admixture linkage disequilibrium' (Briscoe *et al.* 1994, Stephens *et al.* 1994). These groups examined the power to map a trait locus at which two alleles are expressed in a co-dominant manner – in other words a locus where the three possible genotypes are easily distinguished by the phenotypes they produce. They showed that such a trait locus could be detected in conventional allelic association studies with modest sample sizes, using markers spaced at 10 cM or less. This model is obviously not applicable to mapping genes for complex traits; in any case, a locus where two alleles are expressed in a co-dominant manner could easily be mapped by conventional linkage analysis. Under any realistic genetic model for a complex trait, power to detect the allelic association generated by admixture is low unless the information content for ancestry of the markers is very high (Kaplan *et al.* 1998).

Neither group was able to deal satisfactorily with one of the key methodological problems: the disequilibrium between alleles at unlinked loci that results from between-individual variation in proportionate admixture.

Chakraborty and Weiss (1988) suggested that statistical tests based on the history of admixture could help to establish whether association with marker alleles was attributable to linkage. This is not feasible in most admixed populations, where accurate individual histories of admixture do not extend further back than two generations. Stephens *et al.* (1994) suggested instead that individuals whose ancestry included admixture within the last two generations would be excluded from the analysis. This however would fail to eliminate disequilibrium between alleles at unlinked loci in populations such as Mexican Americans, where between-individual variation in proportionate admixture persists because of socio-economic stratification (Gardner *et al.* 1984).

To overcome these methodological limitations, we have developed an approach that has little in common with linkage disequilibrium mapping by allelic association, and is more directly analogous to linkage analysis of an experimental cross between inbred strains (McKeigue 1997, McKeigue 1998). For this reason 'admixture mapping' is a more appropriate term than 'mapping by admixture linkage disequilibrium'. Figure 9.1 below shows, for a pair of chromosomes in an F_2 sibship of mixed European–African descent, how crossing two ancestral strains generates variation in states of ancestry in the F_2 and subsequent generations. Chromosomal segments of European and African descent are represented respectively by broken lines and continuous lines.

In the second (F_2) and subsequent generations of mixed descent, ancestry on chromosomes varies between two states according to a stochastic process, so that at any given locus there may be 0, 1 or 2 alleles of African ancestry. The autocorrelation of ancestry along the chromosome conveys information about linkage. If only a few loci account for a difference in trait values between the two ancestral strains, this autocorrelation in the F_2 and subsequent generations will generate association of the trait with ancestry at marker loci that are linked to these trait loci.

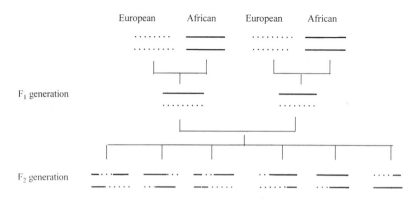
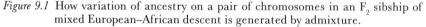

Figure 9.1 How variation of ancestry on a pair of chromosomes in an F_2 sibship of mixed European–African descent is generated by admixture.

The basis of admixture mapping is that instead of testing for allelic association, we combine information from marker genotypes to infer the states of ancestry at each locus on each chromosome of mixed descent. We then test for association of the trait with ancestry at the locus under study. By directly modelling the autocorrelation of states of *ancestry* at linked loci on chromosomes inherited from parents of mixed descent, rather than the association (disequilibrium) between *alleles* at these loci that is secondary to the autocorrelation of ancestry, we can extract all the information about linkage that is generated by admixture, as long as ancestry can be accurately assigned at each locus.

We can thus search the genome for loci where genetic variation accounts for ethnic differences in a trait. To map genes for hypertension in West Africans, for instance, hypertensive individuals who are descended from mixed West African–European unions at least two generations before are ascertained. A set of marker polymorphisms that have average information content for ancestry, defined as a function of allele frequencies (McKeigue 1998), of at least 30 per cent is chosen to span the genome at an average spacing of 2–5 cM. Affected individuals and their parents (sibs or offspring if parents are not available) are typed at these marker loci. Using a multipoint method the ancestry at each locus in each affected individual is classified as 0, 1 or 2 alleles African by descent. The statistical analysis tests for loci where in affected individuals the proportion of alleles that have African ancestry is higher than expected from the admixture (defined as the proportion of the genome that is of African ancestry) of both parents.

In generalising to recently admixed human populations the methods that have been developed for linkage analysis of an experimental cross, two problems arise: how to eliminate disequilibrium between the ancestry of alleles at unlinked loci, and how to assign ancestry of the alleles at each locus when markers that are fully informative for ancestry are not available? The methods that we have developed to overcome these two problems are described below.

Eliminating association between the ancestry of alleles at unlinked loci

Whereas in an experimental cross the ancestry of individuals can be controlled in the design, in recently admixed human populations admixture from the high-risk population varies between individuals: we cannot usually draw a sample consisting entirely of F_2 crosses, for instance. This variation in proportionate admixture from the high-risk population gives rise to association of the disease with alleles that have ancestry from the high-risk population at all loci on the genome, not just at loci that are linked to the disease under study. For instance, NIDDM in Pima Native Americans is inversely associated with the *[3;5,13,14]* haplotype at the *GM* locus (Knowler *et al.* 1988). This association arises not because the *GM* locus is linked to

NIDDM, but because the *[3;5,13,14]* haplotype is commoner in Europeans than in Native Americans and the presence of this haplotype in Pimas is inversely related to the proportion of Native American admixture (Knowler *et al.* 1988).

To eliminate this association between the ancestry of alleles at unlinked loci, it is sufficient to condition on parental admixture (defined as the proportion of the genome that has ancestry from the high-risk population) (McKeigue 1998). In epidemiological language, variation in parental admixture is a confounder of the association of disease with ancestry at the locus under study, and we can control for this confounding by using the entire parental genome as a matched control for the alleles at the locus under study.

Using a multipoint method to combine information from markers to assign ancestry at each locus

Experimental crosses are generally conducted with inbred strains, so that to assign ancestry at all points on the genome in an intercross it is sufficient to type markers at loci where different alleles have become fixed in each of the two parental strains. As human ethnic groups are not inbred strains, marker loci such as FY (Duffy blood group) at which different alleles have become fixed in each of the two founding populations are rare. Thus the information conveyed by typing a single marker will not usually be sufficient to assign the ancestry of each allele at the marker locus to one of the two founding populations. This problem can be overcome by using a multipoint statistical method to combine information from all markers to estimate ancestry at each locus. For clarity, the description of methods below is based on the example of a population of mixed European–West African descent, although the same principles apply to any pair of founding populations.

Although a multipoint analysis requires advanced statistical methods, the underlying principle is simple. We first choose a set of marker polymorphisms that have large differences in allele frequencies between European and Africans, spacing these markers at much higher density than the transitions of ancestry that occur on the chromosomes of individuals of mixed descent. If we type these markers in an individual and in that individual's first-degree relatives, we can assign haplotypes and reconstruct the sequence of marker alleles on each chromosome. Over any short interval, a haplotype in an individual of mixed descent will consist mainly of alleles that are commoner in one of the two founding populations than in the other. By combining information from these marker alleles, we can reduce the uncertainty with which ancestry at each locus is assigned as 0, 1 or 2 alleles African by descent.

To implement a multipoint analysis in practice, we can use a hybrid of frequentist and Bayesian approaches developed for 'missing data' problems (Little and Rubin 1987). For each locus, the *observed data* are marker phenotypes of affected individuals and their first-degree relatives. The *missing data* are the inheritance at the locus for each meiosis in the pedigree (whether the maternally derived or the paternally derived allele was transmitted), and the ancestry (European or African) of the two alleles at the locus in each founder in the pedigree. To test for linkage, we generate the posterior distribution of the missing data given the observed data and obtain a score test statistic and its variance (the observed information) by averaging over this posterior distribution. The critical part of the statistical analysis is to generate the posterior distribution of the missing data given the observed data. It is not feasible to obtain this distribution analytically, but if an appropriate statistical model can be specified and enough computing power is available it is possible to generate this distribution by Gibbs sampling, a Monte Carlo method in which subvectors of the missing data are updated one at a time with values from their posterior distributions (Thompson 1994, Gelman and Rubin 1996).

Statistical power and required sample size for admixture mapping studies

For a given value of the population risk ratio accounted for by the locus, the sample size required to detect linkage is not critically dependent on any other assumptions about the underlying genetic model (McKeigue 1998). Intercrosses (individuals who have both parents of mixed descent) contribute more information than backcrosses (individuals who have only one parent of mixed descent). Admixture mapping designs have far greater statistical power than conventional allele-sharing designs to detect genes of modest effect if these genes underlie ethnic differences in disease risk (McKeigue 1998).

The following comparisons are based on a multiplicative model ($f_2/f_1 = f_1/f_0 = \gamma$, where f_i is the penetrance of the genotype with i copies of the high-risk allele and γ is the genotypic risk ratio) and 90 per cent power to detect linkage at $P < 0.001$. For the admixture design we assume accurate assignment of ancestry of alleles at the disease locus, and for the affected sib-pair design we assume accurate assignment of identity-by-descent sharing at the disease locus. To detect a locus that accounts for a population risk ratio of 2, the admixture design requires only 322 equally admixed affected individuals, whatever the underlying allele frequencies or genotypic risk ratio. In contrast, the power of an affected sib-pair design depends critically on the underlying allele frequencies and genotypic risk ratio. With a genotypic risk ratio of 2, the required number of sib-pairs is between 2760 and infinity, depending on the underlying allele frequencies. As noted earlier, this statistical power advantage for admixture mapping compared with allele-sharing designs in human genetics is what we would expect by analogy with the equivalent design in experimental genetics.

To maximise the statistical power of an admixture mapping study, one should maximise the risk ratio between populations and minimise the number of loci likely to contribute to this risk ratio. In designing such studies, we can apply insights from epidemiology to refine the definition of the phenotype and to define the levels of environmental covariates that will maximise the population risk ratio. For instance, we have reviewed evidence that hypertension in West Africans has a distinct phenotype. If we define the phenotype of hypertension to include other features such as low plasma renin that are especially associated with African hypertension, the risk ratio for this phenotype in West Africans compared with Europeans will be higher than if the phenotype is defined simply as hypertension. As the risk ratio for hypertension in West Africans compared with Europeans is highest in lean individuals aged 30–59 years (Hypertension Detection and Follow-up Program Cooperative Group 1977), we can maximise the power of admixture mapping by restricting the collection of hypertensive probands to this weight category and age range.

Information about ancestry conveyed by a marker polymorphism

The ability to assign the ancestry of alleles at each locus depends upon choosing marker polymorphisms that are informative for ancestry and combining the information from marker genotypes in a multipoint analysis. The information about ancestry conveyed by a biallelic marker in an equally admixed population (McKeigue 1998) is equal to a statistic known as the *Wahlund variance* (Wahlund 1928) or *coefficient of gene differentiation* (Nei 1975) that we denote as f.

This is calculated as

$$f = \frac{\left(p_X - p_Y\right)^2}{\left[4\bar{p}\left(1 - \bar{p}\right)\right]} \quad \text{where} \quad \bar{p} = \tfrac{1}{2}\left(p_X + p_Y\right)$$

and p_X and p_Y are the *ancestry-specific allele frequencies* – the probability of allelic state 1 given that the ancestry of the allele is from population X, and the probability of allelic state given that the ancestry of the allele is from population Y. f represents the proportion by which heterozygosity at the locus is reduced as a result of division into two sub-populations of equal size that have different allele frequencies in relation to the heterozygosity of a total population formed by pooling these two populations. f lies between 0 (no information about ancestry) and 1 (different alleles fixed in the two sub-populations).

Relation of marker information content for ancestry to genetic distance

When genetic distance between human sub-populations is estimated from stable DNA polymorphisms, the most useful measure is the statistic F_{ST} (fixation index: sub-population total). F_{ST} for a single sub-population is defined as the average proportion by which heterozygosity is reduced in the sub-population compared with the ancestral total population from which it is derived (Wright 1951). Where (as is usually the case) we cannot measure allele frequencies in the ancestral total population, we can still estimate the mean F_{ST} value for two sub-populations, in relation to the ancestral total population, from allele frequencies in the sub-populations (Reynolds *et al.* 1983). If estimated from loci where there has been no mutation or selection since the two sub-populations separated, F_{ST} is a measure of genetic drift. The F_{ST} distance is defined as minus $\log_e(1 - F_{ST})$, which has expectation $t/2N$ where t is the number of generations since separation and N is the effective population size (harmonic mean over all generations and both sub-populations).

The mean f-value of stable polymorphisms is related to the F_{ST} distance between two sub-populations by the equation $f = F_{ST}/(2 - F_{ST})$. Thus for markers such as single-nucleotide polymorphisms (SNPs) and restriction site polymorphisms (RSPs), the mean f-value is slightly more than half the F_{ST} distance (since F_{ST} distances between human sub-populations are generally < 0.25). The distribution of f-values is however skewed to the right, as predicted from the neutral theory of evolution (Bowcock *et al.* 1991). Bowcock and colleagues have reported that the observed distribution of f-values of RSPs between human ethnic groups is even more skewed than the distribution predicted from the neutral theory, suggesting that the allele frequencies have diverged as a result of differential selection pressure as well as drift (Bowcock *et al.* 1991). Whatever the reasons for this highly skewed distribution of marker f-values, the practical implication for admixture mapping is that it is possible to identify markers that have f-values more than four times higher than the mean.

Using data from Cavalli-Sforza's group (Cavalli-Sforza *et al.* 1994), Table 9.2 shows F_{ST} distances for some pairs of human sub-populations between which admixture has occurred. Because the F_{ST} distance between Europeans and South Asians is only about one-third of the F_{ST} distance between Europeans and more genetically distant groups such as West Africans, it will be more difficult to assemble a marker set for admixture mapping in people of mixed European–South Asian descent than to assemble marker sets for admixture mapping in other populations.

Table 9.2 F_{ST} distances between ethnic groups that have undergone admixture (Cavalli-Sforza *et al.* 1994)

Pairs of sub-populations	F_{ST} distance
European–West African	0.15
European–Native Australian	0.15
European–Pacific Islander	0.13
European–Native American	0.11
European–South Asian	0.05

Number of markers required for a genome search

The *crossover rate* of ancestry (defined as minus half the gradient of the autocorrelation function at infinitesimal map distance) on chromosomes in the population under study determines the number of markers required for a genome search, the threshold P-value at which to declare significant linkage (Lander and Kruglyak 1995) and the mapping resolution of the study (Kruglyak and Lander 1995). The crossover rate is a function of the history of admixture (McKeigue 1997). The optimal strategy for admixture mapping is to conduct an initial genome search in a population where the ancestry crossover rate is low because admixture has occurred recently, and to proceed with fine mapping of the locus in a population where admixture has a longer history. To estimate the number of markers required for a genome search we have simulated multipoint analyses using a hidden Markov model (McKeigue 1998). Although these simulations are based on an ideal population in which the history of admixture is equivalent to an experimental cross producing non-overlapping generations F_2, F_3 ..., estimates of the required number of markers obtained in these simulations are likely to apply more generally. For these simulations we have specified a population where the ancestry crossover rate is 2 per morgan (equivalent to generation F_4), and 80 per cent of information about ancestry at each locus should be extracted by the multipoint analysis. The number of markers required for a genome search varies from about 600, if the markers have average f-value of 0.5, to about 1500, if the markers have average f-value of only 0.3.

Strategies for assembling marker sets

The information about ancestry extracted in a multipoint analysis depends only on the crossover rate, the marker spacing and the marker f-values. It does not matter whether the high f-values of the markers result from drift, mutation or disruptive selection. We can thus assemble a suitable marker set from microsatellites, RSPs, SNPs or any combination of these.

Screening single-nucleotide polymorphisms and restriction site polymorphisms

We have used published surveys of allele frequencies (Dean *et al.* 1994, Jorde *et al.* 1995, Poloni *et al.* 1995) to estimate the proportion of RSPs that have high f-values between Europeans and West Africans [or Bantu-speaking Africans, who are genetically close to West Africans (Cavalli-Sforza *et al.* 1994)]. When 105 RSPs were ranked by their f-values, the highest 5 per cent had mean f-value of 0.38 (Jorde *et al.* 1995, Poloni *et al.* 1995). As most RSPs are SNPs, we can predict that the proportion that have high f-values will be similar for SNPs and RSPs. Thus if we rely on SNPs to assemble a marker set for admixture mapping – 900 markers with average f-value of 0.40 – in populations of mixed European–West African descent, we can estimate that it will be necessary to screen a library of about 20,000 such polymorphisms. This estimate applies to any other pair of populations that are separated by F_{ST} distance of about 0.15. The assembly of libraries of SNPs, together with automated methods for typing them, is now under way on a large scale. This will make it feasible to assemble marker sets for admixture mapping.

Screening microsatellites

An alternative strategy for marker selection is to choose microsatellites that have high *f*-values when collapsed into biallelics (Dean *et al.* 1994, Shriver *et al.* 1997, Kaplan *et al.* 1998). Because mutation rates at microsatellite loci (about 10^{-3} per generation) are far higher than for SNPs (about 10^{-8} per generation), the distribution of *f*-values at microsatellite loci does not have a simple relationship to F_{ST} distance, even when selective neutrality applies (Shriver *et al.* 1995, Kimmel *et al.* 1996). Preliminary estimates suggest that the proportion of microsatellite loci that have high *f*-values is high: when microsatellite loci are ranked by their *f*-values between Europeans and West Africans, the highest 10 per cent have a mean *f*-value of about 0.5 (M. D. Shriver, personal communication). Screening 6,000 microsatellite loci would thus identify a set of 600 that have mean *f*-value of 0.5.

Using subtractive hybridisation to discover restriction site polymorphisms that are informative for ancestry

An alternative method of generating markers suitable for assigning ancestry would be to use representational difference analysis (Lisitsyn and Wigler 1993), a subtractive hybridisation technique that isolates base sequences that are present in one genome but absent in another genome or pooled sample of genomes. This could be used to discover RSPs where an allele that is common in one population is absent in the other. Although it would be necessary to map the polymorphisms before they could be used as markers, it is possible that as a means of identifying markers that are informative for ancestry, this would be more efficient than screening large numbers of known polymorphisms.

Conclusion

In principle, admixture mapping offers a powerful tool for investigating the genetic basis of ethnic differences in disease risk, overcoming some of the limitations of other approaches to studying the genetics of complex traits. Suitable populations are available in many countries, especially the United States. The assembly of marker sets for admixture mapping is feasible, although the optimal strategy will depend upon the balance between the initial cost of assembling the marker set and the subsequent cost of genotyping families. Diseases that may be amenable to study by this approach include diabetes, hypertension, obesity and systemic lupus erythematosus. Identification of the genes and the gene–environment interactions that underlie ethnic differences in susceptibility to these conditions would make fundamental contributions to our understanding of their aetiology.

References

Aitman, T.J., Gotoda, T., Evans, A.L., Imrie, H., Heath, K.E., Trembling, P.M., Truman, H., Wallace, C.A., Rahman, A., Dore, C., Flint, J., Kren, V. *et al.* (1997) 'Quantitative trait loci for cellular defects in glucose and fatty acid metabolism in hypertensive rats', *Nature Genetics*, 16, 197–201.

Beckles, G.L.A., Miller, G.J., Kirkwood, B.R., Alexis, S.D., Carson, D.C. and Byam, N.T.A. (1986) 'High total and cardiovascular disease mortality in adults of Indian descent in Trinidad, unexplained by major coronary risk factors', *Lancet*, 1, 1298–1301.

Bowcock, A.M., Kidd, J.R., Mountain, J.L., Hebert, J.M., Carotenuto, L., Kidd, K.K. and Cavalli-Sforza, L.L. (1991) 'Drift, admixture, and selection in human evolution: a study with DNA polymorphisms', *Proceedings of the National Academy of Sciences, USA*, 88, 839–843.

Boyle, E.J. (1970) 'Biological pattern in hypertension by race, sex, body weight, and skin color', *Journal of the American Medical Association*, 213, 1637–1643.

Briscoe, D., Stephens, J.C. and O'Brien, S.J. (1994) 'Linkage disequilibrium in admixed populations: applications in gene mapping', *Journal of Heredity*, 85, 59–63.

Cavalli-Sforza, L.L., Menozzi, P. and Piazza, A. (1994) *The History and Geography of Human Genes*, Princeton, NJ: Princeton University Press.

Chakraborty, R., Ferrell, R.E., Stern, M.P., Haffner, S.M., Hazuda, H.P. and Rosenthal, M. (1986) 'Relationship of prevalence of non-insulin-dependent diabetes mellitus to Amerindian admixture in the Mexican Americans of San Antonio, Texas', *Genetic Epidemiology*, 3, 435–454.

Chakraborty, R. and Weiss, K.M. (1986) 'Frequencies of complex diseases in hybrid populations', *American Journal of Physical Anthropology*, 70, 489–503.

Chakraborty, R. and Weiss, K.M. (1988) 'Admixture as a tool for finding linked genes and detecting that difference from allelic association between loci', *Proceedings of the National Academy of Sciences, USA*, 85, 9119–9123.

Chaturvedi, N., McKeigue, P.M. and Marmot, M.G. (1993) 'Resting and ambulatory blood pressure differences in Afro-Caribbeans and Europeans', *Hypertension*, 22, 90–96.

Cheah, J.S., Lui, K.F., Yeo, P.P.B. and Ahuja, M.M.S. (eds) (1979) 'Diabetes mellitus in Singapore: results of a country-wide population survey', in *Epidemiology of Diabetes in Developing Countries*, New Delhi: Interprint, p. 93–102.

Congdon, N., Wang, F. and Tielsch, J.M. (1992) 'Issues in the epidemiology and population-based screening of primary angle-closure glaucoma', *Survey of Ophthalmology*, 36, 411–423.

Darlu, P., Sagnier, P.P. and Bois, E. (1990) 'Genealogical and genetical African admixture estimations, blood pressure and hypertension in a Caribbean community', *Annals of Human Biology*, 17, 387–397.

Dean, M., Stephens, J.C., Winkler, C., Lomb, D.A., Ramsburg, M., Boaze, R., Stewart, C., Charbonneau, L., Goldman, D., Albaugh, B.J. *et al.* (1994) 'Polymorphic admixture typing in human ethnic populations', *American Journal of Human Genetics*, 55, 788–808.

Frohlich, E.D., Messerli, F.H., Dunn, F.G., Oigman, W., Ventura, H.O. and Sundgaard Riise, K. (1984) 'Greater renal vascular involvement in the black patient with essential hypertension. A comparison of systemic and renal hemodynamics in black and white patients', *Mineral and Electrolyte Metabolism*, 10, 173–177.

Gardner, L.I.J., Stern, M.P., Haffner, S.M., Gaskill, S.P., Hazuda, H.P., Relethford, J.H. and Eifler, C.W. (1984) 'Prevalence of diabetes in Mexican Americans. Relationship to percent of gene pool derived from native American sources', *Diabetes*, 33, 86–92.

Gelman, A., Rubin, D.B. (1996) 'Markov chain Monte Carlo methods in biostatistics', *Statistical Methods in Medical Research*, 5, 339–355.

Haenszel, W. and Kurihara, M. (1968) 'Studies of Japanese migrants. I. Mortality from cancer and other diseases among Japanese in the United States', *Journal of the National Cancer Institute*, 40, 43–68.

Hanis, C.L., Chakraborty, R., Ferrell, R.E. and Schull, W.J. (1986) 'Individual admixture estimates: disease associations and individual risk of diabetes and gallbladder disease among Mexican-Americans in Starr County, Texas', *American Journal of Physical Anthropology*, 70, 433–441.

Hodge, A.M. and Zimmet, P.Z. (1994) 'The epidemiology of obesity', *Baillere's Clinical Endocrinology and Metabolism*, 8, 577–599.

Hopkinson, N.D., Doherty, M. and Powell, R.J. (1994) 'Clinical features and race-specific incidence/prevalence rates of systemic lupus erythematosus in a geographically complete cohort of patients', *Annals of the Rheumatic Diseases*, 53, 675–680.

Hypertension Detection and Follow-up Program Cooperative Group (1977) 'Race, education, and prevalence of hypertension', *American Journal of Epidemiology*, 106, 351–361.

Jorde, L.B., Bamshad, M.J., Watkins, W.S., Zenger, R., Fraley, A.E., Krakowiak, P.A., Carpenter, K.D., Soodyall, H., Jenkins, T. and Rogers, A.R. (1995) 'Origins and affinities of modern humans: a comparison of mitochondrial and nuclear genetic data', *American Journal of Human Genetics*, 57, 523–538.

Kaplan, N.L., Martin, E.R., Morris, R.W. and Weir, B.S. (1998) 'Marker selection for the transmission/disequilibrium test in recently admixed populations', *American Journal of Human Genetics*, 62, 703–712.

Keil, J.E., Sutherland, S.E., Hames, C.G., Lackland, D.T., Gazes, P.C., Knapp, R.G. and Tyroler, H.A. (1995) 'Coronary disease mortality and risk factors in black and white men. Results from the combined Charleston, SC, and Evans County, Georgia, heart studies', *Archives of Internal Medicine*, 155, 1521–1527.

Kimmel, M., Chakraborty, R., Stivers, D.N. and Deka, R. (1996) 'Dynamics of repeat polymorphisms under a forward-backward mutation model: within-and between-population variability at microsatellite loci', *Genetics*, 143, 549–555.

Knowler, W.C., Williams, R.C., Pettitt, D.J. and Steinberg, A.G. (1988) 'Gm3;5,13,14 and type 2 diabetes mellitus: an association in American Indians with genetic admixture', *American Journal of Human Genetics*, 43, 520–526.

Kruglyak, L. and Lander, E.S. (1995) 'High-resolution genetic mapping of complex traits', *American Journal of Human Genetics*, 56, 1212–1223.

Lander, E. and Kruglyak, L. (1995) 'Genetic dissection of complex traits: guidelines for interpreting and reporting linkage results', *Nature Genetics*, 11, 241–247.

Lander, E.S. and Schork, N.J. (1994) 'Genetic dissection of complex traits', *Science*, 265, 2037–2048.

Levy, S.B., Lilley, J.J., Frigon, R.P. and Stone, R.A. (1977) 'Urinary kallikrein and plasma renin activity as determinants of renal blood flow: the influence of race and dietary sodium intake', *Journal of Clinical Investigation*, 60, 129–138.

Lilley, J.J., Hsu, L. and Stone, R.A. 'Racial disparity of plasma volume in hypertensive man', *Annals of Internal Medicine*, 84, 707–711.

Lisitsyn, N. and Wigler, M. (1993) 'Cloning the differences between two complex genomes', *Science*, 259, 946–951.

Little, R.J.A. and Rubin, D.B. (1987) *Statistical Analysis with Missing Data*, New York: Wiley.

Luft, F.C., Miller, J.Z., Grim, C.E., Fineberg, N.S., Christian, J.C., Daugherty, S.A. and Weinberger, M.H. (1991) 'Salt sensitivity and resistance of blood pressure. Age and race as factors in physiological responses', *Hypertension*, 17(Suppl. I), 102–108.

McClellan, W., Tuttle, E. and Issa, A. (1988) 'Racial differences in the incidence of hypertensive end-stage renal disease (ESRD) are not entirely explained by differences in the prevalence of hypertension', *American Journal of Kidney Diseases*, 12(4), 285–290.

McKeigue, P.M. (1997) 'Mapping genes underlying ethnic differences in disease risk by linkage disequilibrium in recently admixed populations', *American Journal of Human Genetics*, 60, 188–196.

McKeigue, P.M. (1998) 'Mapping genes that underlie ethnic differences in disease risk: methods for detecting linkage in admixed populations by conditioning on parental admixture', *American Journal of Human Genetics*, 63, 241–251.

McKeigue, P.M., Miller, G.J. and Marmot, M.G. (1989) 'Coronary heart disease in South Asians overseas: a review', *Journal of Clinical Epidemiology*, 42, 597–609.

McKeigue, P.M., Shah, B. and Marmot, M.G. (1991) 'Relation of central obesity and insulin resistance with high diabetes prevalence and cardiovascular risk in South Asians', *Lancet*, 337: 382–386.

MacLean, C.J., Adams, M.S., Leyshon, W.C., Workman, P.J., Reed, T.E., Gershowitz, H. and Weitkamp, L.R. (1974) 'Genetic studies on hybrid populations. III. Blood pressure in an American Black community', *American Journal of Human Genetics*, 26, 614–626.

Merrill, R.M. and Brawley, O.W. (1997) 'Prostate cancer incidence and mortality rates among white and black men', *Epidemiology*, 8, 126–131.

Miller, G.J., Beckles, G.L.A., Maude, G.H., Carson, D.C., Alexis, S.D., Price, S.G.L., and Byam, N.T.A. (1989) 'Ethnicity and other characteristics predictive of coronary heart disease in a developing country – principal results of the St James survey, Trinidad', *International Journal of Epidemiology*, 18, 808–817.

Mitchell, B.D., Williams Blangero, S., Chakraborty, R., Valdez, R., Hazuda, H.P., Haffner, S.M. and Stern, M.P. (1993) 'A comparison of three methods for assessing Amerindian admixture in Mexican Americans', *Ethnicity and Disease*, 3, 22–31.

Montel, M.L.R. (1913) Anonymous Comptes rendus des travaux du Troisieme Congres Biennial tenu a Saigon. Saigon: Far Eastern Association of Tropical Medicine, 1913; Une question sur le diabete. pp. 522–3.

Neel, J.V. (1962) 'Diabetes mellitus: a "thrifty" genotype rendered detrimental by "progress" ', *American Journal of Human Genetics*, 14, 353–362.

Nei, M. (1975) *Molecular Population Genetics and Evolution*, Amsterdam: North-Holland.

O'Dea, K., Patel, M., Kubisch, D., Hopper, J. and Traianedes, K. (1993) 'Obesity, diabetes, and hyperlipidemia in a central Australian aboriginal community with a long history of acculturation', *Diabetes Care*, 16, 1004–1010.

Omar, M.A.K., Seedat, M.A., Dyer, R.B., Rajput, M.C., Motala, A.A. and Joubert, S.M. (1985) 'The prevalence of diabetes mellitus in a large group of South African Indians', *South African Medical Journal*, 67, 924–926.

Peterson, J.C., Adler, S., Burkart, J.M., Greene, T., Hebert, L.A., Hunsicker, L.G., King, A.J., Klahr, S., Massry, S.G., Seifter, J.L., Kusek, J.W., Agodoa, L.Y. *et al.* (1997) 'Effects of blood pressure control on progressive renal disease in blacks and whites', *Hypertension*, 30, 428–435.

Poloni, E.S., Excoffier, L., Mountain, J.L., Langaney, A. and Cavalli-Sforza, L.L. (1995) 'Nuclear DNA polymorphism in a Mandenka population from Senegal: comparison with eight other human populations', *Annals of Human Genetics*, 59, 43–61.

Prineas, R.J., Gillum, R., Hall, W.D., Saunders, E. and Shulman, N.B. (1985) (eds) Hypertension in blacks: epidemiology, pathophysiology and treatment. Chicago: Year Book, 1985; 2, U.S. epidemiology of hypertension in blacks. p. 17–36.

Qualheim, R.E., Rostand, S.G., Kirk, K.A., Rutsky, E.A. and Luke, R.G. (1991) 'Changing patterns of end-stage renal disease due to hypertension', *American Journal of Kidney Diseases*', 18, 336–343.

Ramachandran, A., Jali, M.V., Mohan, V., Snehalatha, C. and Viswanathan, M. (1988) 'High prevalence of diabetes in an urban population in south India', *British Medical Journal*, 297, 587–590.

Ramachandran, A., Snehalatha, C., Dharmaraj, D. and Viswanathan M. (1992) 'Prevalence of glucose intolerance in Asian Indians – urban–rural difference and significance of upper-body adiposity', *Diabetes Care*, 15, 1348–1355.

Reid, D.D. (1971) 'The future of migrant studies', *Israel Journal of Medical Sciences*, 12, 1592–1596.

Reynolds, J., Weir, B.S. and Cockerham, C.C. (1983) 'Estimation of the co-ancestry coefficient: basis for a short-term genetic distance', *Genetics*, 105, 767–779.

Risch, N. (1992) 'Mapping genes for complex diseases using association studies with recently admixed populations', *American Journal of Human Genetics*, 51(Suppl.), 13 (abstract).

Risch, N. and Merikangas, K. (1996) 'The future of genetic studies of complex human diseases', *Science*, 273, 1516–1517.

Serjeantson, S.W., Owerbach, D., Zimmet, P., Nerup, J. and Thomas, K. (1983) 'Genetics of diabetes in Nauru: effects of foreign admixture, HLA antigens and the insulin-gene-linked polymorphism', *Diabetologia*, 25, 13–17.

Sever, P.S., Peart, W.S., Meade, T.W., Davies, I.B., Gordon, D. and Tunbridge, R.D. (1978) 'Are racial differences in essential hypertension due to different pathogenetic mechanisms?', *Clinical Science and Molecular Medicine*, 4(Suppl.), 383s–386s.

Shriver, M.D., Jin, L., Boerwinkle, E., Deka, R., Ferrell, R.E. and Chakraborty, R. (1995) 'A novel measure of genetic distance for highly polymorphic tandem repeat loci', *Molecular Biology and Evolution*, 12, 914–920.

Shriver, M.D., Smith, M.W., Jin, L., Marcini, A., Akey, J.M., Deka, R. and Ferrell, R.E. (1997) 'Ethnic-affiliation estimation by use of population-specific DNA markers', *American Journal of Human Genetics*, 60, 957–964.

Stephens, J.C., Briscoe, D. and O'Brien, S.J. (1994) 'Mapping by admixture linkage disequilibrium in human populations: limits and guidelines', *American Journal of Human Genetics*, 55, 809–824.

Summerson, J.H., Bell, R.A. and Konen, J.C. (1995) 'Racial differences in the prevalence of microalbuminuria in hypertension', *American Journal of Kidney Diseases*, 26, 577–579.

Thompson, E.A. (1994) 'Monte Carlo likelihood in genetic mapping', *Statistical Science*, 9, 355–366.

Tierney, W.M., Harris, L.E., Copley, J.B. and Luft, F.C. (1990) 'Effect of hypertension and type II diabetes on renal function in an urban population', *American Journal of Hypertension*, 3, 69–75.

Wahlund, S. (1928) 'Zusammensetzung von Populationen und Korrelation-serscheinungen vom Standpunkt der Vererbungslehre aus betrachtet', *Hereditas*, 11: 65–106.

Warren, S.E. and O'Connor, D.T. (1980) 'Does a renal vasodilator system mediate racial differences in essential hypertension?', *American Journal of Medicine*, 69, 425–429.

Weinberger, M.H. (1985) 'Blood pressure and metabolic responses to hydro-chlorothiazide, captopril, and the combination in black and white mild-to-moderate hypertensive patients', *Journal of Cardiovascular Pharmacology*, 7(Suppl. 1), S52–S55.

Wild, S. and McKeigue, P.M. (1997) 'Cross-sectional analysis of mortality by country of birth in England and Wales 1970–1992', *British Medical Journal*, 314, 708–710.

Wise, P.H., Edwards, F.M., Craig, R.J., Evans, B., Marchland, J.B., Sutherland, B. and Thomas, D.W. (1976) 'Diabetes and associated variables in the South Australian Aboriginal', *Australian and New Zealand Journal of Medicine*, 6, 191–196.

Worth, R.M., Kato, H., Rhoads, G.G., Kagan, A. and Syme, S.L. (1975) 'Epidemiologic studies of coronary heart disease and stroke in Japanese men living in Japan, Hawaii and California: mortality', *American Journal of Epidemiology*, 102, 481–490.

Wright, S. (1951) 'The genetical structure of populations', *Annals of Eugenics*, 15, 322–354.

Zimmet, P., Taylor, R., Ram, P., King, H., Sloman, G., Raper, L.R. and Hunt, D. (1983) 'Prevalence of diabetes and impaired glucose tolerance in the biracial (Melanesian and Indian) population of Fiji: a rural–urban comparison', *American Journal of Epidemiology*, 118, 673–688.

Zimmet, P.Z. (1992) Kelly West lecture 1991: challenges in diabetes epidemiology from West to the rest', *Diabetes Care*, 15, 232–252.

10 Diabetes, ancestral diets and dairy foods

An evolutionary perspective
on population differences in
susceptibility to diabetes

Anthony J. McMichael

Epidemiological profile of non-insulin-dependent diabetes mellitus

The incidence of non-insulin-dependent (i.e. type II) diabetes mellitus (NIDDM) is increasing markedly in adult urban populations around the world. In the early decades of the twenty-first century this disease is destined to become a major global public health problem: the approximately 3 per cent of adults currently affected will become an estimated 5 per cent by 2025 [World Health Organization (WHO) 1998a] as populations 'age' and urbanise, and as obesity becomes more prevalent (WHO 1998b).

Two striking epidemiological features of NIDDM are the wide variation in prevalence between populations, and, at the individual level, the strong positive correlation with relative body weight. The more than tenfold difference in NIDDM prevalence between Pima Indians (of Arizona, United States) and Polynesians at the high extreme, South Asian and West Africans in the middle range, and European populations at the low extreme, could reflect population differences in genetic susceptibility, in exposure to environmental factors, or both. The persistence of elevated rates of NIDDM in South Asian migrants several generations after migration to the United Kingdom suggests that genetic factors are important (McKeigue 1997a). On the other hand, the similar elevations in NIDDM prevalence rates in urbanised Indian, Chinese and African migrant populations in Mauritius testify to the importance of environmental (presumably lifestyle) factors (Zimmet and Alberti 1997). So, too, does the approximately fivefold difference in NIDDM prevalence between rural and urban populations in Tamil Nadu, southern India, living a mere 20 miles apart (McKeigue 1997a).

In adult individuals, body mass index (BMI) is very strongly correlated with impaired glucose tolerance (IGT) and with NIDDM, especially if the increased adiposity is centripetal ('abdominal'). Short-term studies of the covariation of weight and glucose tolerance confirm that this is a causal relationship (Sims *et al.* 1973, O'Dea 1991). More recently, evidence from cohort studies in Western populations has shown that the incidence of IGT and of NIDDM is raised in individuals of low birth weight (particularly those with low ponderal index: i.e. low weight/length ratio), especially if those individuals also become overweight in adulthood (McKeigue 1997b). This increased risk may reflect the long-term consequences of fetal metabolic adaptation ('programming') to antenatal nutritional insufficiency (Barker 1994).

The role of insulin in diabetes

NIDDM is a serious metabolic disorder that causes end-organ damage to the kidneys, heart, blood vessels and retina. The disease process is the result of 'insulin resistance' – a reduction in the body's sensitivity to insulin. This pancreatic hormone is central to the metabolic production, storage and mobilisation of the body's main fuels: glucose and free (non-esterified) fatty acids.

Insulin secretion into the blood is stimulated by the post-prandial absorption of simple sugars (from carbohydrate), fatty acids (from fat) or amino acids (from protein). In persons of average BMI, insulin reduces blood glucose levels by replenishing liver stores of glycogen and by increasing the deposition of glucose as glycogen in muscle. Insulin also stimulates the liver to convert fatty acids to low-density lipoprotein cholesterol and triglycerides, which are then released into the bloodstream and, under insulin action, stored in peripheral adipose tissue. Insulin, conversely, inhibits the mobilisation of glucose and fatty acids from these storage tissues. Meanwhile, in circumstances of low intake of carbohydrate foods (as with Inuit Eskimos – see Van der Merwe 1992) excess dietary amino acids can be converted by the liver to glucose (by 'gluconeogenesis') or, in other circumstances, to lipids.

These major actions of insulin are summarised in Figure 10.1. The figure indicates that, under normal conditions, the dominant effect of insulin is to enhance the peripheral deposition of glucose and lipid as energy stores. Insulin has various other metabolic effects not shown here (including influencing urinary sodium and nitrogen excretion, sympathetic nervous system tone and leptin sensitivity).

The mechanism of impairment of insulin action has not yet been determined. It may entail the down-regulation of either cell-surface insulin receptor activity or intracellular transport of glucose, or some other modulation (Clausen *et al.* 1995). Insulin sensitivity is also reduced by leptin, the hormone secreted by adipose tissue (Bray 1996). Hence, in obese persons, raised leptin levels achieve negative feedback by reducing insulin action and thus limiting the further deposition of energy in fat cells (which may help explain the increase in insulin resistance associated with obesity). However, this relationship was presumably not important in hunter–gatherer populations, in whom obesity was a rarity. Indeed, in the historically usual non-obese circumstance, leptin's main role was probably in the hormonal triggering of ovulation in adequately nourished women.

Possible evolutionary sources of differences in insulin sensitivity genotype between populations

'Thrifty genes' and selective insulin resistance

Four decades ago, in a world with a much lower prevalence of obesity than exists today, it looked as if only a few populations (Pima Indians, Nauruans and other Polynesians, and Australian Aborigines) were particularly susceptible to diabetes. Further, the two main types of diabetes mellitus – adult-onset (NIDDM) and child-onset (insulin-dependent diabetes (IDDM) distinguished by insufficient pancreatic production of insulin) – had not then been differentiated.

The eminent population geneticist, J. V. Neel, postulated in 1962 that NIDDM in susceptible populations was due to their 'thrifty genotype', acquired evolutionarily in response to the precarious feast or famine dietary circumstances that had long prevailed (Neel 1962). In such circumstances, he argued, natural selection would have favoured those individuals with a heightened insulin release – a 'quick insulin trigger' – who were best able to store any temporary excess of dietary energy. This thrifty genotype, argued Neel, has now become 'detrimental' in the unfamiliar, modern, circumstance of continuous dietary abundance. In that setting, metabolic thrift causes obesity and, consequently, an unremitting demand on the pancreas to secrete insulin. Pancreatic exhaustion, he argued, leads to insulin insufficiency and, hence, diabetes.

Neel (1962) initially envisaged that only a minority of the world's ancestral populations had been subjected to unusual feast and famine selection pressures. Critics argued, however, that all ancient populations must have been confronted by recurring famines, particularly the early agrarian populations (including early Europeans). Agricultural societies everywhere, precariously reliant on several staple crops, have been chronically prone to famines (Solbrig and Solbrig 1994). This led Neel to suggest that the thrifty gene may indeed have once been universally acquired, but subsequently it would have been selected against in circumstances of dietary sufficiency in well-established agrarian populations. In those beneficent circumstances, he argued, metabolic thrift would have caused obesity and diabetes in early life, thereby reducing reproductive success.

Subsequently, medical science recognised that NIDDM differed biologically from (predominantly child-onset) IDDM, and, importantly, that NIDDM mostly did not cause disease until after the third decade of life. Hence, it was unlikely that NIDDM had been selected against via impaired reproductive success. Accordingly, in 1982, Neel substantially revised his hypothesis. He now proposed that the predisposition of certain populations to NIDDM was due to genetically based insulin resistance, acquired in response to hunter–gatherer diets that were low in carbohydrate but high in fat and meat (Neel 1982). Indeed, he argued that a selective insulin resistance would have maximised the availability of glucose in blood as an immediate fuel while also maximising the synthesis of fats (as triglycerides and low-density lipoproteins) from dietary fatty acids and meat-protein amino acids, and their deposition in adipose tissue as an energy store (see also Figure 10.1). This idea of selective insulin resistance has been further elaborated and corroborated in the 1990s (O'Dea 1992). Selective resistance occurs in several species of arid-land rodents when rendered obese in experimental feeding studies (Shafrir 1991), and it is evident in human subjects with impaired glucose tolerance and with NIDDM. The selectivity of insulin resistance is shown in Figure 10.1: the normal influence of insulin on pathways 1, 3 and 5 is impaired, while other insulin actions are unimpaired.

Several other suggestions have been proposed as to why particular populations have experienced such high rates of NIDDM over recent decades. Both O'Dea (1992) and Cooper (1993) have suggested that it is primarily a cultural transitional problem, occurring as metabolically susceptible populations change from traditional to modern diets. During the transition, there is a persistent, unconstrained, preference for energy-dense 'survival foods', high in fat and sugar. The resultant obesity potentiates any underlying tendency to insulin resistance. O'Dea (1991) has shown in young adult Australian Aborigines living in non-traditional urban-fringe settings that impaired glucose tolerance recedes when traditional diets and physical activity are resumed. Other studies have also shown that changes in body weight affect insulin sensitivity (Sims *et al.* 1973). O'Dea (1992) also points out that a rise in dietary fatty acids and their oxidation products in the blood could, via negative metabolic feedback, cause an increase in insulin resistance. Nevertheless, these scenarios assume a pre-existing susceptibility within the population in transition, most probably that of a selective insulin resistance genotype (O'Dea 1992, Cooper 1993).

The proposition that the genetic basis of NIDDM risk is a reduced insulin sensitivity rather than a heightened capacity for energy storage is supported by observations in Pima Indians that *individual* differences in insulin secretion and insulin sensitivity are predictive of subsequent diabetes and act independently of obesity (Lillioja *et al.* 1993). Further, the fact that the strength of the obesity–diabetes link varies greatly between populations suggests that in those populations in which obesity carries a high risk of diabetes there must be some additional genetic predisposition (Clausen *et al.* 1995).

Why are European populations at lower risk of NIDDM than other populations?

The recent accrual of epidemiological evidence indicates that most, not just a minority, of the world's populations are prone to NIDDM in the wake of increasing obesity (Stern 1991). European and Europe-derived populations are the main exception. Is there a plausible evolutionary explanation for

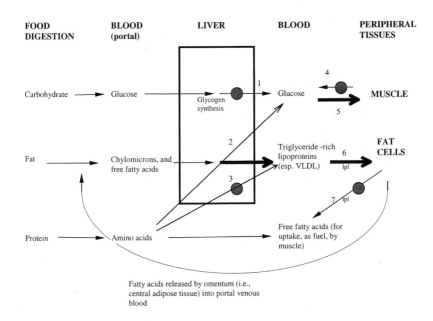

Figure 10.1 The principal actions of insulin in relation to the synthesis, deposition and mobilisation of the body's two main metabolic fuels, glucose and fatty acids. Pathways normally enhanced by insulin are shown as thick arrows, and those normally inhibited by insulin are shown with a filled circle impeding the arrow. (Selective insulin resistance affects pathways 1, 3, 5, thus allowing peripheral storage of lipids but raising the blood concentration of glucose.) lpl, lipoprotein lipase.

how the postulated background hunter–gatherer condition of selective insulin resistance could have been particularly selected against in the ancestors of today's low-risk European populations? Direct selection pressure against insulin-resistant individuals in well-fed early European agrarians, via the enhanced occurrence of diabetes (and fetal impairment) in pregnancy, is unlikely because early agrarian populations in Europe did not feast; they subsisted, often miserably.

Neel's (1982) reformulation of an insulin-resistant genotype rather than an insulin-driven metabolic thriftiness as the basis of NIDDM susceptibility changes the evolutionary scenarios that one must postulate. There is no longer a need to invoke periodic acute food shortages as the main selective pressure that acted on ancestral populations. Further, palaeo-anthropologists consider it unlikely that, during the great human dispersal around the world over the past 100,000 years, frontier hunter–gatherer groups knowingly risked starvation. After all, most frontier movement presumably occurred in order to increase food security. Nevertheless, famines must have been caused sporadically by climatic disasters, and marked changes in dietary profile often faced those who ventured furthest – of which the ancestors of Amerindians are a key example.

The proto-Amerindians, spreading from eastern Siberia across the temporarily exposed tundra of the Beringian land-bridge around 30–20,000 years ago and then confined in the Alaskan region by vast ice-sheets that did not retreat until around 12,000 years ago, would have eaten few plant foods. In modern times, the northern Inuit (Eskimos) obtain 90 per cent of their dietary energy from meat and fat (Van der Merwe 1992). The colonisation of the Pacific several thousand years ago by island-hopping seafarers originating from East Asia may have entailed heavy reliance on fish, chickens and pigs, both *en route* and after settlement on islands that often had limited cultivation potential (Diamond 1997). However, acute food shortages *en route* are considered to have been unlikely, because of the prudent safe-return-if-necessary strategy of 'latitude sailing' which precluded running out of rations (Allen and Cheer 1995). Hence, it is unlikely that the ancestors of the Amerindians and the Pacific Islanders (both known to have very high NIDDM rates today) experienced unusual feast or famine selection pressures during their migrations – although both populations may have experienced more recent acute famines (Brand-Miller and Colagiuri 1994).

The emerging view, then, is that it is the European populations who are metabolically 'deviant'. Other, non-European, populations remain genetically closer to the widespread ancestral human genotype that occurred in response to the dietary circumstances of the glaciated Pleistocene pre-agrarian world (Brand-Miller and Colagiuri 1994). To evaluate this idea we will examine the diet and the evolutionary history of early humans in more detail.

Early human evolution

The hominids, splitting off from the ancestral chimpanzee line around 5–6 million years ago, spent the first 98 per cent of their time in eastern and southern Africa (Stanley 1996). The early hominids (principally the Australopithecines, from around 4–2 million years ago) were predominantly vegetarian and probably had a moderate insulin sensitivity – albeit less than that of their forest-dwelling primate ancestors. In addition to the wild fruits, berries and seeds eaten by both apes and hominids, a large part of the Australopithecine diet comprised the fibrous roots and tubers from the open woodland and savannah, associated with the large grinding molars evident in Australopithecine fossil remains.

Earth entered a rapidly cooling and drying Pleistocene world, from around 2.5 million years ago (associated with a radical disruption of the oceanic circulation of heat, as the Panama isthmus closed the gap between North and South American continents). New survival pressures impinged acutely on the hominids, resulting in the emergence of the *Homo* genus in response to radical changes in habitat and food supplies (Stanley 1996). Vegetation receded in the eastern African cradle of humankind, grasslands spread, and grazing ungulate species increased in number and their herds increased in size. To survive, early humans had to rely more on meat, especially in the dry season. This radical change in early human diet was associated with rapid enlargement of the brain (Stanley 1996, Aiello 1997), both as cause and consequence, the former reflecting the brainpower needed for successful hunting, the latter reflecting the extra energy supplement required by the lactating woman to support a large-brained dependent infant. Increased use of stone tools and fire between 2 and 1 million years ago, along with archaeological evidence of a marked increase in systematic cut marks on fossilised animal bones and a shift in the isotopic (strontium and carbon) profile of human bones, all indicate a substantial supplementation of plant foods with animal foods (Van der Merwe 1992, Aiello 1997). Although contemporary hunter–gatherers live in a warmer, inter-glacial, world, they typically obtain around 20–40 per cent of daily food energy from meat. The proportion may have been higher during the prevailing glaciations of the Pleistocene world (Foley 1995).

This meat-enriched, reduced carbohydrate diet presumably prevailed among early humans through to very recent times, reflecting the unusually glaciated conditions that have occurred over the past 2 million years (Stanley 1996). Such a diet would have selectively favoured the maintenance of blood glucose levels as the day-to-day body fuel, while synthesising and depositing fats as longer-term energy stores. In that setting, selective insulin resistance would have conferred survival advantage – an advantage amplified by selection pressure on adult women to supply sufficient glucose to the developing fetus during pregnancy and to the neonate during lactation (Brand-Miller and Colagiuri 1994). Adequate glucose supply is essential for fetal and neonatal brain development (Barker 1994).

During the past 100,000 years, the modern human species, *Homo sapiens*, began dispersing out of north-east Africa to all continents (except Antarctica). During most of that time the colder and dryer environments of the most recent (Wurm) glaciation, from around 90–13,000 years ago, would have widely limited the availability of plant foods. This would have been particularly so for populations entering the tundras and frost-affected regions of Siberia, Europe, East Asia and, particularly, the temporarily exposed Beringian land-bridge and northern North America. Populations of easily hunted large prey animals existed in some of these environments. Indeed, the immigrant Amerindians and Australian Aborigines arrived in a landscape replete with 'naive' megafauna, thought to have provided a meat bonanza for several thousand years before extinction of those large mammals ensued (Diamond 1997). Modern humans would therefore have reached the beginnings of the agricultural era, from around 10,000 years before present (BP), in a relatively insulin-insensitive (i.e. insulin-resistant) state.

Soon after the end of the last glaciation, the ecology and diet of humans had begun to change radically. In particular, in response to the transformation of regional profiles of plant and animal species caused by a globally averaged 5°C warming over several thousand years, primitive forms of agriculture began to appear (Diamond 1997). In several locations and at different times, as human numbers outstripped supplies of wild foods, various regional populations became slowly but irrevocably committed to an agricultural economy. This entailed a major shift in dietary profile, with around 75 per cent of dietary energy now coming from starchy cereal grain carbohydrates and, for the great majority of peasant-agriculturalists, rather little energy coming from meat. Such agrarian diets had a substantially higher glycaemic index than that of hunter–gatherers (Thorburn *et al.* 1987, Brand-Miller and Colagiuri 1994). Given this unprecedented regional diversification of dietary nutrient profiles, Brand-Miller and Colagiuri (1994) have proposed that the extent to which the ancestral insulin insensitivity has been retained is inversely proportional to the duration of a particular population's exposure to agriculture. How do observations around the world match this simple bivariate prediction?

Agriculture as determinant of population metabolic genotype?

Archaeologists identify five or six main independent centres of agriculture (Solbrig and Solbrig 1994, Diamond 1997). The oldest was in the Middle East (the 'fertile crescent') beginning around 10,000 BP. This was the primary centre from which farming spread north west, throughout Europe, over the ensuing five millennia. Next, chronologically, were the Papua-New Guinea highlanders beginning garden-based horticulture around 9000 BP; then northern China (the Yang Shao people, cultivating millet) and South-East Asia (the original home of rice), separately, beginning around 8,000 BP. Then came Central America and Peru, each around 7,000 BP; the Indus Valley civilisation around 6,000 BP; and eastern Africa around 5,000 BP. The last two may not have been truly independent centres – archaeological and genetic evidence indicates the diffusion of domesticated plants, animals, and human agrarian genes from the older Middle Eastern centre (Diamond 1997).

Rice cultivation spread later to southern China, and then, around 4,000 BP, to Indonesia, Sri Lanka and southern India. Rice cultivation was introduced into Japan and the Philippines from the Asian mainland within the past 2–3,000 years. The colonisers of the Pacific originated from that East Asian Pacific coast several thousand years ago. They took various gardening and farming skills with them, along with yams, taro, breadfruit and chickens – which they supplemented with locally available coconuts, fish and turtles. Meanwhile, Eskimos, Australian Aborigines, and some of the northern Amerindians had essentially no contact with agriculture. The Pima Indians, descended from the Hokohaw, depended on foraging and hunting, supplemented with some agriculture during the past 2,000 years.

NIDDM rates in today's populations

In today's world, after allowing for differences in the prevalence of obesity, NIDDM rates are distinctly low in populations of European origin (Stern 1991). Among urbanising populations with increasing levels of obesity, NIDDM rates have become high in Amerindian groups in North America and Australian Aborigines, both of whom have had little or no exposure to large-scale agriculture. NIDDM rates have increased in the Japanese, who have been exposed to agriculture for much less time than European populations (Diamond 1997). The very high rates in Polynesian and Micronesian populations could reflect their relatively late exposure to a limited range of agriculture, but the picture is complicated by the unusually high prevalence of obesity in those island populations. In the United States, the NIDDM rates are much higher in African American than in Caucasian populations. The higher rates in populations of West African descent, now living in the United States and Caribbean, may reflect a relatively later and lesser reliance on agriculture than in the main Eurasian centres of agriculture.

The picture, however, is not clear-cut. Arab populations, for example, are at high risk of NIDDM (Al-Mahroos and McKeigue 1998), yet much of the Arab region has a history of long-term involvement in irrigated farming on the desert fringes (Solbrig and Solbrig 1994). Rates of NIDDM appear to be low in China, but other evidence indicates that rates in overseas Chinese populations, with higher levels of obesity, are substantially elevated (Zimmet and Alberti 1997). Nor is it correct to talk simplistically of the 'European' experience since there were no primary centres of agriculture within temperate Europe.

Spread of farming in Europe

Genetic and linguistic analyses indicate that, from around 9,000 years ago, the populous farming communities of the Fertile Crescent began diffusing north west across Europe, in a 'wave of advance', at approximately 1 kilometre per year (Diamond 1997). According to Cavalli-Sforza and colleagues (1994) there is a resultant gradient of 'farmers' genes' that runs diagonally across Europe from Turkey to Brittany, accounting for an estimated 28 per cent of all genetic variation between the sub-populations of Europe. As these farmers' genes numerically overwhelmed the smaller hunter–gatherer gene pools of ancient Europe, the agriculturalists' greater insulin sensitivity would have become prominent. However, Cavalli-Sforza's estimates for Europe have been contested; other genetic analyses suggest that there were earlier, more important, infusions of strains of genes into Europe when various non-farming human cultures entered from the eastern fringes (Richards *et al.* 1996). So, if farmers' genes were not the dominant influence in the European genetic evolution of *Homo sapiens* populations, and, further, if much of the evolutionary adaptation to farming occurred on-site during subsequent millennia, there is little basis for positing a markedly greater insulin-sensitising experience of European populations.

Perhaps there is something more than duration of 'exposure' that distinguishes the farming and dietary experience of early Europeans and therefore accounts for their distinctly low susceptibility to NIDDM today. Further, any such distinctive genetic divergence in susceptibility to NIDDM could only have occurred over just the last few thousand years. Is this plausible? The selection pressure would need to have been rather intense – similar to that of malaria, which appears to have evoked the evolution of various haemoglobinopathies and thalassaemias during several thousand years (perhaps also associated with agrarianism and settled living). Therefore, might some other factor in the European dietary experience have heightened the selection pressure to relax the low insulin sensitivity that had been acquired by humans during the meat-eating Pleistocene? A tantalising clue has recently been suggested (Allen and Cheer 1996).

The lactose tolerance connection

The Fertile Crescent farmers were not only the first to domesticate wild plants; they also made the radical breakthrough of domesticating goats, sheep and, later, cattle. This was a natural extension of pre-existing pastoralism in the Euphrates River Valley (Kretchmer 1993), and led to agrarian communities from around 7,000 BP consuming non-human milk and milk products (Sherratt 1981, Mallory 1989). The result today is that tolerance of lactose (milk sugar) is much more prevalent in European populations (and in the several African pastoralist groups that migrated from the Middle East across the then-verdant Sahara several thousand years ago) than in other non-European populations, most of whom have not traditionally consumed unfermented milk products. In Scandinavia, for example, nearly all persons are lactose tolerant, whereas in East Asian and Amerindian populations nearly all are lactose intolerant and milk products are not consumed. In some other cultures in predominantly lactose-intolerant populations, such as southern India, Tibet and much of Africa, dairy foods are consumed exclusively as fermented (i.e. lactose-depleted) milk products, such as yoghurt and buttermilk.

Human infants can digest the disaccharide lactose from breast milk and thus absorb its component simple sugars (glucose and galactose). In nature, this enzymatic capacity becomes redundant after weaning and, ever the energy conserver, natural selection has acted to switch off the lactase enzyme by mid-childhood (Kretchmer 1993). However, the introduction of dairy foods into the early Middle Eastern agrarian diet created a selection pressure for retention of lactase, to capture the considerable energy available directly from the lactose component of milk and, relatedly, to avert the intestinal discomfort of lactose intolerance and the resultant reluctance to consume milk. In situations of subsistence farming, such marginal gains in energy availability can be crucial to survival.

Lactose tolerance is inherited as a simple Mendelian dominant allele

(Kretchmer 1993). Population geneticists estimate that, if the gene for lactase retention had a selection coefficient of around 5–10 per cent (i.e. high, but quite plausible), then population adaptation with eventual predominance of lactose tolerance would have occurred within around 6,000 years (Cavalli-Sforza *et al.* 1994). The selection pressure relating to maximising energy uptake may have been amplified by the beneficial effect of lactose on calcium uptake. As farming populations spread into less sunny northern European climes, so the ultraviolet-powered production of vitamin D in skin declined and, with it therefore, the intestinal absorption of calcium. Lactose, like vitamin D, facilitates the absorption of calcium, which averts disabling, bone-deforming rickets (and which, via a misshapen pelvis, can directly impede reproductive success). This critical additional function of lactose probably explains the lactose tolerance gradient in European populations today, ranging from around 50 per cent in Italy to over 80 per cent in France and Germany, to over 95 per cent in Scandinavia (Kretchmer 1993). The lactase enzyme was, apparently, an agent of demic expansion in European history that facilitated nutritionally secure advances at the frontier.

This historical analysis indicates that the proto-European farmers had for long consumed an unusually glycaemic diet, high in simple carbohydrates from cereal grains and supplemented milk. This may have caused a very strong selection pressure for relaxation of the ancestral pre-agrarian insulin insensitivity. Not only is lactose moderately glycaemic in its own right, but whole milk with its protein content as secretagogue is a potent stimulus for insulin release (Allen and Cheer 1996). These early Europeans were therefore ingesting a diet unprecedentedly high in simple sugars – from stone-ground cereals, other cultivated plants and whole milk – while also experiencing heightened release of insulin. There would have been a dual benefit in enhancing the clearance of glucose from the blood and storing it as energy: first, more efficient capture of dietary energy, and, second, minimisation of the adverse consequences of hyperglycaemia (including the risk to the fetus from exacerbation of maternal glucose intolerance).

Such a thesis has recently been proposed by Allen and Cheer (1996), who have demonstrated a negative correlation ($r = -0.56$) between the prevalence rates of lactose tolerance and diabetes in over forty different populations around the world. European populations lie at one extreme of their scatter plot of data, with high prevalence of lactose tolerance and low rates of diabetes. This fortuitous coincidence of agrarian plant-based diets and consumption of unfermented dairy foods may thus underlie the relative non-susceptibility of European populations to NIDDM.

A good test of this hypothesis will be the future diabetes experience of Papua-New Guinea highlanders. They have been agrarians for almost as long as Europeans, eating a moderately glycaemic diet that includes taro, yams and bananas. But they have not had dairy foods. If the onset of urbanisation and increased obesity induces in them a susceptibility to diabetes similar to that already evident in their lowland compatriots, this would support the posited important extra role of lactose-containing dairy foods in rendering proto-Europeans less susceptible to diabetes. It would also be interesting to obtain data on NIDDM prevalence in other little-studied populations that are direct descendants of ancient hunter–gatherers, such as Lapps, Eskimos and Siberian native populations (Cavalli-Sforza *et al.* 1994). Similarly, in Europe, the Basques represent an enclave of ancient hunter–gatherer genes that were apparently not much diluted by the various genetic waves that have flowed across Europe over the past 20,000 years (Cavalli-Sforza *et al.* 1994).

The development of modern molecular genetic epidemiology will provide further insights into the nature and extent of genotypic differences between regional populations. As this information accrues, so the chance of making firmer inferences about the evolutionary influences upon variations in susceptibility to disease processes will increase.

Conclusion

Differences in population susceptibility to various disease processes may be better understood by exploration of their ancient, divergent, evolutionary paths. In relation to NIDDM, one of the world's great contemporary disease entities, European and Europe-derived populations may be at distinctly lower risk than most other populations because of characteristics of their ancestral diet. This diet is likely to have incurred selection pressures in favour of an increase in insulin sensitivity.

These insights into the interplay between environment, diet, human biology and disease occurrence are a salutary reminder of the intrinsically ecological dimension of human population health and disease. We have, with cultural development, hugely buffered our relationship with the natural world. However, we cannot finally discard the heritage of the long and more intimate relationship that prevailed over the many millennia of evolution of the modern human species.

It is important not to misinterpret such analyses as pointing to constitutional metabolic 'weaknesses' in particular populations. After all, various studies in populations known to be at particularly elevated risk of NIDDM, such as the Yanomama Indians of South America, several North American Indian groups and Australian Aborigines, have shown that, in the absence of obesity, the prevalence of glucose intolerance is low and that of frank diabetes is zero. Hence, despite the putative long-standing differences between populations in their insulin sensitivity genotype, non-obese populations living in energy balance with their local dietary environment do not display metabolic abnormalities.

Finally, there is a strong implication in this analysis for the importance of maintaining cultural diversity as we evolve towards a more globalised world; of ensuring that our ways of living retain the basic profile of dietary nutrients and net energy balance for which human biology has evolved. Any future increases in NIDDM incidence in human populations around the world will be a signal that our culture is distancing us unduly from the foundation conditions of healthy life.

References

Aiello, L. (1997) 'Brains and guts in human evolution: The Expensive Tissue Hypothesis', *Brazilian Journal of Genetics*, 20, 141–148.

Allen, J.S. and Cheer, S.M. (1995) '"Civilisation" and the thrifty genotype', *Asia-Pacific Journal of Clinical Nutrition*, 4, 341–342.

Allen, J.S. and Cheer, S.M. (1996) 'The non-thrifty genotype', *Current Anthropology*, 37, 831–842.

Al-Mahroos, F. and McKeigue, P.M. (1998) 'High prevalence of diabetes in Bahrainis', *Diabetes Care*, 21, 936–942.

Barker, D.J.P. (1994) *Mothers, Babies and Disease in Later Life*, London: BMJ Publishing.

Brand-Miller, J.C. and Colagiuri, S. (1994) 'The carnivore connection: dietary carbohydrate in the evolution of NIDDM', *Diabetologia*, 37, 1280–1286.

Bray, G. (1996) 'Leptin and leptinomania', *Lancet*, 348, 140–141.

Cavalli-Sforza, L., Menozzi, P. and Piazza, A. (1994) *History and Geography of Human Genes*, Princeton, NJ: Princeton University Press.

Clausen, J.O., Hansen, T., Bjorbaek, C., Echwald, S.M., Urhammer, S.A., Rasmussen, S., Anderson, C.B., Hansen, L., Almid, K. and Winther, K. (1995) 'Insulin resistance: interactions between obesity and a common variant of insulin receptor substrate-1', *Lancet*, 346, 397–402.

Cooper, R.S. (1993) 'Ethnicity and disease prevention', *American Journal of Human Biology*, 5, 387–398.

Diamond, J. (1997) *Guns, Germs and Steel. The Fate of Human Societies*, London: Jonathan Cape.

Foley, R. (1995) *Humans Before Humanity*, Oxford: Blackwell Publishers.

Kretchmer, N. (1993) 'Lactose intolerance and malabsorption', in Kiple, K.F. (ed.) *The Cambridge World History of Human Disease*, Cambridge: Cambridge University Press, pp. 813–817.

Lillioja, S., Mott, D.M. and Spraul, M. (1993) 'Insulin resistance and insulin secretory dysfunction as precursors of non-insulin dependent diabetes mellitus: prospective studies in Pima Indians', *New England Journal of Medicine*, 329, 1988–1992.

McKeigue, P. (1997a) 'Cardiovascular disease and diabetes in migrants: interaction between nutritional changes and genetic background', in Shetty, P. and McPherson, K. (eds) *Diet, Nutrition and Chronic Disease. Lessons from Contrasting Worlds*, Chichester: John Wiley, pp. 59–70.

McKeigue, P. (1997b) 'Diabetes and insulin action', in Kuh, D. and Ben-Shlomo, Y. (eds) *A Life Course Approach to Chronic Disease Epidemiology*, Oxford: Oxford University Press, pp. 78–100.

Mallory, J.P. (1989) *In Search of the Indo-Europeans*, London: Thames and Hudson.

Neel, J.V. (1962) 'Diabetes mellitus: a "thrifty" genotype rendered detrimental by "progress"', *American Journal of Human Genetics*, 14, 353–362.

Neel, J.V. (1982) 'The thrifty genotype revisited', in Kobberling, J. and Tattersall, R. (eds) *The Genetics of Diabetes Mellitus*, London: Academic Press, pp. 283–293.

O'Dea, K (1991) 'Westernisation, insulin resistance and diabetes in Australian Aborigines', *Medical Journal of Australia*, 155, 258–264.

O'Dea, K. (1992) 'Obesity and Diabetes in "The Land of Milk and Honey"', *Diabetes/Metabolism Reviews*, 8, 373–388.

Richards, M., Corte-Real, H., Forster, P., Macaulay, V., Wilkinson-Herbots, H., Demaine, A., Papiha, S., Hedges, R., Bandelt, H.J. and Sykes, B. (1996) 'Palaeolithic and Neolithic lineages in the European mitochondrial gene pool', *American Journal of Human Genetics*, 59, 185–203.

Shafrir, E. (1991) 'Animals with diabetes: progress in the understanding of diabetes through study of its pathogenesis in animal models', in Alberti, K.G.M.M. and Krall, L.P. (eds) *The Diabetes Annual/6*, Amsterdam: Elsevier, pp. 634–663.

Sherratt, A. (1981) 'Plough and pastoralism: aspects of the secondary products revolution', in Hodder, I., Isaac, G. and Hammond, N. (eds) *Pattern of the Past: Studies in Honour of David Clarke*, Cambridge: Cambridge University Press, pp. 124–143.

Sims, E., Danforth, E., Horton, E.S., Bray, G.A., Glennon, J.A. and Salans, L.B. (1973) 'Endocrine and metabolic effects of experimental obesity in man', *Recent Progress in Hormone Research*, 29, 457–496.

Solbrig, O.T. and Solbrig, D.J. (1994) *So Shall You Reap*, Washington, DC: Island Press.

Stanley, S. (1996) *Children of the Ice Age*, New York: Harmony.

Stern, M.P. (1991) 'Kelly West Lecture: Primary prevention of type II diabetes mellitus', *Diabetes Care*, 14, 399–410.

Thorburn, A.W., Brand, J.C. and Truswell, A.S. (1987) 'Slowly digested and absorbed carbohydrate in traditional bushfoods: a protective factor against diabetes?', *American Journal of Clinical Nutrition*, 45, 98–106.

Van der Merwe, R.J. (1992) 'Reconstructing prehistoric diet', in Jones, S., Martin, R. and Pilbeam, D. (eds) *The Cambridge Encyclopaedia of Human Evolution*, Cambridge: Cambridge University Press, pp. 369–372.

World Health Organization (1998a) *World Health Report 1998*, Geneva: WHO.

World Health Organization (1998b) *Obesity: Preventing and Managing the Global Epidemic. Report of a WHO Consultation on Obesity*, WHO/NUT/NCD/98.1 Geneva: WHO.

Zimmet, P. and Alberti, K. (1997) 'The changing face of macrovascular disease in non-insulin dependent diabetes mellitus: an epidemic in progress', *Lancet*, 350, Suppl 1, SI1–4.

11 Variations in health and disease

Race, ethnicity or 'nutrition transition'

Prakash Shetty

Introduction

Variations in biology arise as a result of advantageous 'mutation'. This phenomenon is essential for the survival of a species, since those mutations that are selected to persist either provide an advantage or are neutral or potentially neutral. 'Natural selection' brings about adaptation to the environment and 'genetic drift' contributes to variation on a small scale over a short period of time. Blyth in 1835 emphasised food as a forceful determinant of variation.

> Redundance or deficiency of nutriment affects chiefly the stature of animals. Those herbivorous quadrupeds which browse the scanty vegetation on mountains are invariably much smaller than their bretheren which crop the luxuriant produce of the plains; and although the cattle usually kept in these different situations are of diverse breeds; yet either of the breeds gradually removed to the other's pasture, would, in two generations, acquire many of the characters of the other, would increase or degenerate in size, according to the supply of nutritious food; though in either case, they would most probably soon give birth to true varieties adapted to the change.
>
> (Blyth 1835)

Blyth and Darwin both considered food a major environmental influence in evolution, but they were principally interested in morphological changes such as stature, configuration of teeth or change in size of specific organs; it is now well recognised that food and nutrition can potentially influence metabolism. McMichael (Chapter 10) has discussed what happens over a time frame of tens of thousands of years, over which environmental pressures and dietary influences, in particular, have contributed to the variations we see in disease patterns today. In this chapter, I shall confine myself to biological variations in health and disease risk among populations that appear as variations between groups of different race and ethnicity, which are largely the result of dietary and lifestyle changes that have occurred over a much shorter time frame – over months, years, decades and a few generations. In this chapter an attempt will be made to examine what appears as racial and ethnic variations in health and disease risk and to discuss them as genetic interactions with nutrition and as a manifestation of developmental and nutrition transition. These variations will be considered under three separate categories (Table 11.1): (1) No genetic variation and no effect due to nutritional change; (2) genetic variation but no effect due to nutritional change; and (3) genetic variation superimposed by effects of nutritional change.

No genetic variation: no effect of nutrition

In this section will be considered those physiological variables that appear to be comparable across the racial, ethnic or genetic divide and are not influenced even by wide variations in nutritional status of these population groups. One such physiological function is human lactation and the ability to synthesise adequate quantities of breast milk to meet the newborn infant's nutritional needs.

Human lactation

Lactation imposes a significant additional energy stress on women during their reproductive years. The general assumption therefore is that lactational performance denoted by the quantity of breast milk produced is likely to be determined by the nutritional status of the mother and her body's store of energy. Figure 11.1 shows that the volume of milk produced at peak lactation is remarkably similar in groups of women from a wide variety of racial, ethnic, cultural as well as nutritional backgrounds. It demonstrates that the volume of milk produced by the mother is not dependent on the woman's nutritional status represented by the body mass index (BMI). This scatter plot based on a meta-analysis of 1,726 measurements from over forty-one studies across

Table 11.1 Genetic and nutritional interactions

1.	No genetic variation: no effect of nutrition
	Lactation
2.	Genetic variation present: no effect due to nutrition
	Taste
	Bone mineral density
	Risk of osteoporosis
3.	Genetic variations and effect of nutrition transition seen:
	Sucrose–isomaltose malabsorption
	Obligatory nitrogen loss
	Risk of obesity and non-insulin-dependent diabetes
	Risk of cardiovascular disease

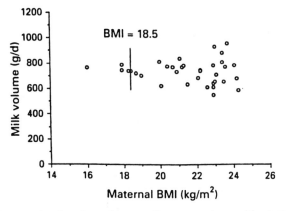

Figure 11.1 Scatter plot data from forty studies across the world relating breast milk
volume to the nutritional status of the mother based on maternal body
mass index (BMI) (Prentice *et al.* 1994).

the world (Prentice *et al.* 1994) shows that milk volume is constant across the
range of normal BMIs and is unaffected even when the BMI is low. It appears
that even small, presumably undernourished women, produce similar volumes
of milk during lactation as larger well-nourished mothers, indicating that
nutritional status does not compromise this vital physiological function. Of
the mother–infant dyad it is the infant's current size which is an important
determinant of milk volume. Human lactational performance thus depends
on factors such as the current size of the infant, with larger babies receiving
more milk and mothers with twins, even in poor developing societies, able to
breast feed twins by producing twice as much milk as that produced by similar
mothers with single infants (Prentice *et al.* 1986). Mothers across the world
of all racial and ethnic groups produce similar amounts of milk during peak
lactation. This is true in early lactation when no ethnic or racial differences
are demonstrable. However, during later lactation, say after 4–6 months, the
quantity of milk produced is largely dependent on cultural practices and the
mother's intention to wean the child (Prentice *et al.* 1986).

A variation in the quality of the breast milk is another factor in human
lactation that may be influenced by race, ethnicity and nutritional status.
The quality of the milk produced, e.g. the energy content of milk, is much
more difficult to assess because of complex diurnal, within feed and between
breast, changes in milk energy. It is virtually impossible to design a study to
obtain an integrated value for the energy in breast milk without affecting
the natural process of lactation. Since it is the fat content that may largely
influence the energy content and hence the quality of the breast milk,
comparisons of breast milk fat content may be helpful. However, a critical
review of the literature related to milk fat content shows that there are an
equal number of studies that show positive and negative associations with
nutritional status indicated by maternal BMI while yet others show no
association (Prentice *et al.* 1994). International or cross-ethnic comparisons
on the whole indicate that milk energy content is also apparently as robust

as the milk volume. Race, ethnicity or nutritional state does not appear to affect either the quality or the quantity of human lactation.

The energy stress of human lactation is among the lowest measured for any mammalian species, and perhaps it is related to the very slow growth rate of the human infant (Prentice and Whitehead 1987). The incremental energy needs of a breastfeeding mother of a single infant is only 25 per cent of her non-lactating requirement, whereas for a rat dam with a litter of eight pups or a ewe feeding two fast-growing lambs the incremental needs may be around 300 per cent. Humans also have proportionately larger fat stores than many other mammalian species, which provide for a greater flexibility in meeting the additional energy needs of pregnancy. Both inter- and intrapopulation comparisons show no detectable relationships between maternal BMI and milk output, thus supporting the view that nutritional status does not affect the milk volume output. It also establishes the fact that the physiological function of human lactation is biologically very robust and does not vary with either racial or ethnic group or their nutritional state. Human lactation is one biological process that shows no racial or ethnic variation and is not affected by nutritional changes or the nutritional status of the mother.

Genetic variation present: no effect of 'nutrition transition'

Taste preferences

The sense of taste fulfils two distinct functions: (1) it is crucial in determining the acceptability of food and (2) it plays a role in the activation of physiological responses related to digestive function. Two interacting factors are involved in the variation of responses to taste stimuli seen among population groups – genetics and dietary experience. The best example of genetic influences on taste is the inherited sensitivity to phenyl-thio-carbamides (PTCs) (Blakeslee 1932, Cavalli-Sforza and Bodmer 1971). Individuals able to taste PTC compounds probably have a dominant gene, whereas non-tasters are homozygous for the recessive allele and the proportion of tasters may vary between 60 per cent and almost 100 per cent in a population. It has also been suggested (Greene 1974) that selective pressures have maintained PTC taste polymorphism in different geographic regions. Many bitter-tasting goitrogenic compounds occur naturally in common vegetables. The ability to taste PTC would limit the ingestion of naturally occurring goitrogens, and in goitre-endemic areas PTC tasters would have an adaptive advantage where iodine intake is low. This effect is a long-term process like lactose tolerance.

Genetic and dietary influences may act alone or in concert to produce cultural and ethnic variations in taste responses. The pleasantness of simple taste substances like sodium chloride, quinine and citric acid may be influenced by dietary experiences. Studies conducted in India have shown that sour and bitter substances are perceived as being more pleasant by poor socio-economic labourers than by medical students in India or student volunteers in the United States (Moskowitz *et al.* 1975). It was suggested that this cross-cultural difference was due to more extensive dietary exposure to sour and bitter taste among the poor labourers, although the effects of poor nutritional status were not excluded.

Differences in response to sucrose, lactose and sodium chloride solutions have been reported between Black and White infants and children 9–15 years old in North America (Desor *et al.* 1975, Greene *et al.* 1975). Black children preferred more concentrated solutions of all three taste stimuli than did White Caucasian children. Evaluation of taste responses to sucrose solution in infants 2–3 days old and at 6 months of age was carried out by Beauchamp and Moran (1982, 1984). Their studies showed that newborn and 6-month-old infants prefer sucrose to water but also that differences are seen between Black and White infants; Black infants ingest more sucrose than White infants but not more water. The investigation was enlarged to question whether this difference was due to differential dietary experiences of these two groups of infants, since some of the mothers were habituated to feeding their infants sweetened water with sugar, karo syrup or honey as an adjunct to milk. The infants were divided into two groups – one consisted of those infants fed sweetened water by their mothers during the 1-week period between taste tests, while the other acted as a control with no exposure. The infants consumed more sucrose stimuli than water. However, infants fed sweetened water the previous week showed a significantly greater intake of sucrose stimuli than the unexposed control infants. It was also confirmed that there were differences in the consumption of sucrose solution between the two racial groups (Black and White infants), Black infants consuming significantly more sucrose solution. When the two racial groups were compared with regard to prior exposure to sucrose, it was found that the racial differences persisted and did not interact with the feeding effect. Both racial groups showed an increase following dietary exposure to the sweetened feed over a period of just 1 week. Several aspects of human taste sensation show racial differences between Black people and White people and also demonstrate that these differences respond in similar ways to nutritional change or other physiological change over the short term.

Bone mass and risk of osteoporosis

The mass of a bone is given by its volume and its apparent density, i.e. mass per unit external volume. Genes control about 60–75 per cent of the variance of peak bone mass (i.e. density) and a much smaller proportion of the variance in rate of bone loss. Genetic influences on bone mass are mediated by body size, bone size and muscle mass. The genetic potential for bone accumulation can be frustrated by insufficient calcium intake, disruption of the calendar of puberty and inadequate physical activity. Two lines of evidence support a genetic basis for racial (Black/White) differences in bone mass (Parfitt 1997). First, the differences in bone mass of magnitudes of the order of 10–40 per cent is incommensurate with known non-genetic factors. Second, the differences are already evident in the fetus and increase progressively during growth, especially during adolescence, and these differences in peak bone mass persist throughout life.

Several studies have shown that bone density is much higher in Black African Americans as opposed to comparable populations of White European Americans (Meier *et al.* 1992, Ettinger *et al.* 1997). Some consistent findings in Black African Americans are a lower 24-hour urinary excretion of calcium despite similar dietary calcium intakes, with the calcium excretion being inversely associated with (radial) bone density, and a higher 1,25-dihydroxy-vitamin D level, but a lower 25-hydroxyvitamin D level than age-matched White people (Bell *et al.* 1985). Bone biopsies in Black people have also shown a lower bone turnover (Weinstein and Bell 1988). There were no racial/ethnic differences in the biochemical markers of bone formation such as serum alkaline phosphatase and osteocalcin or of bone resorption such as urinary hydroxyproline and pyridinoline (Daniels *et al.* 1997). Levels of testosterone (total, free and bioavailable) were higher in Black people while dehydro-epiandrosterone levels were lower (Ettinger *et al.* 1997). There are however, significant differences in the mechanism of bone formation with a lower rate of mineralised matrix apposition within each remodelling unit and a longer total formation period in Black people than in White people. The differences appear to be the result of more frequent and/or longer inactive periods in the life span of bone formation units in Black people which may allow for a greater overall deposition of bone mineral and thus explain the higher bone mass and better quality of bone in Black people than in White people (Parisien *et al.* 1997).

Several recent studies have indicated that adjustment for a wide range of nutritional and lifestyle differences are unable to explain the differences in bone mineral density seen between the Black people and White people in North America (Ettinger *et al.* 1997) and in South Africa (Daniels *et al.* 1997). Recent studies also do not show differences in bone mineral content or density between Asian American and Caucasian American youth (Bhudikanok *et al.* 1996), since the differences seen were largely attributable to differences in weight, pubertal stage and weight-bearing activity. Racial differences in bone metabolism and in bone mineral density are clearly evident. However, it has not been possible to demonstrate that differences in diet or lifestyle can influence or alter this racial or ethnic difference in bone metabolism which is linked to variations in disease risk such as osteoporosis.

Genetic variations superimposed by 'nutrition transition'

Sucrase–isomaltase deficiency (sucrose–isomaltose malabsorption)

Sucrose–isomaltose malabsorption is quite unlike lactose malabsorption. The occurrence of lactase deficiency follows a geographic and ethnic pattern related to the origin and spread of agriculture and dairying over nearly 10,000 years (Kretchmer 1977). Congenital sucrase–isomaltase deficiency occurs much less frequently and in a sporadic distribution in most investigated populations. Unlike the average North American population with a very low prevalence [0.2 per cent frequency of heterozygotes in a large series of intestinal biopsies from White American subjects (Peterson and Herber 1967, Welsh *et al.* 1978)] the disease occurs much more frequently in Eskimos and Canadian Indians. In contrast to the 10,000- to 15,000-year history of lactose, sucrose is new to the human diet and is particularly new in the diet of the Eskimo, who until recently lived on a diet of fat and protein practically devoid of carbohydrates. Under these circumstances, the metabolic requirement for glucose was derived from gluconeogenic amino acids. The recent introduction of sucrose-containing foods into the Eskimo diet has been considered a possible cause of the persistent diarrhoea and gastroenteritis that occur with considerable frequency among Eskimo infants and children during the post-weaning period. Studies on adult Eskimos indicate that this ethnic group has a high frequency of sucrose–isomaltose malabsorption (Gudmand-Hoyer *et al.* 1984). The absence of sucrose in the traditional diet of Eskimos so far was responsible for sucrose activity of the intestinal mucosa as a negligible factor in natural selection. The recent introduction of sucrose into the Eskimo diet has posed nutritional–environmental stress and has created a potential health problem. This highlights the real dangers arising from the introduction of modern foods in the diet of groups in whom selection has caused a high frequency of rare phenotypes (Auricchio and Troncone 1989). Unfortunately, the same is true of a wide range of disease risks where the changes in dietary composition over a short period of time have exposed populations to increased disease risk.

Obesity and non-insulin-dependent diabetes mellitus

The relative contributions of genetic and environmental factors in the aetiology of obesity and non-insulin-dependent diabetes mellitus (NIDDM) remains controversial and unresolved. Twin and adoption studies as well as familial distribution point towards an important genetic contribution in the aetiology of both obesity (Bouchard 1994) and NIDDM (Newman *et al.* 1987). Research studies in twins, as well as adoption and family studies, have helped assess the extent obesity and body weight in an individual is attributable to genetic factors and heritability. The *level of heritability* is simply the fraction of the variation within a population in traits such as BMI that can be explained by genetic transmission. Two large comprehensive studies of twins, adoptees and nuclear families have yielded heritability estimates of about 25–40 per cent of the individual differences in BMI or body fat (Bouchard 1994, 1997). Several studies have shown that obese children frequently have obese parents. In about 30 per cent of cases, both parents of obese children are obese. However, it has also been documented that about 25–35 per cent of obese people belong to families with normal weight parents, although the risk of being obese is higher if the parents are obese (Bouchard 1997). The risk of becoming obese if one or both parents are obese is calculated by the *lambda coefficient*. This is defined as the ratio of the risk of being obese when a biological relative is obese compared with the risk in the population at large, i.e. the prevalence of obesity in the population. The risk of obesity so estimated is about two to three times higher for an individual with a family history of obesity, and it increases further with the severity of obesity.

However, the post-World War II increase in prevalence of both these conditions with improvement in living standards, relative affluence and easy availability of food all point towards important environmental contributions. These include mainly the impact of 'nutrition transition', which encompasses both the effects of dietary change as well as the consequences of changes in lifestyles and physical activity patterns.

Dietary changes and nutrition transition

The human diet has changed profoundly over the long and gradual process of evolution from hunter–gatherers in pre-agricultural societies constantly confronted with variable and uncertain food supplies to a greatly improved and relatively stable food supply following the first agricultural revolution. The better nutrition and health resulted in lower mortalities, although as the population increased and the pressure on food supplies grew, this led to under nutrition and an increase in mortality. The industrial revolution, the second agricultural revolution and the sanitary revolution in Europe over the last 200 or more years contributed to the development of modern industrialised societies with vastly improved health and longevity. The associated agricultural and technological activities contributed to the modern diet, which is far removed from the diets of hunter–gatherers and peasant agriculture phases of human cultural evolution. The differences we find today between the diets of peasant agriculturists and modern affluent societies are similar to those between the largely rural populations of developing countries and the people of developed industrialised societies. Even within developing countries, particularly those in rapid transition, there are wide differences in the dietary patterns of the rural populations compared with their urban counterparts and particularly among the urban affluent of developing societies. Thus, the pace of dietary change appears to have accelerated to varying degrees in different parts of the world, with countries in transition currently demonstrating dramatic alterations in dietary patterns. The modernisation of societies that follows economic development seems to result in a dietary pattern that is high in saturated fats, sugars and refined foods and low in dietary fibre content. The relationship between these dietary changes and obesity and NIDDM are probably causal.

Changes in physical activity patterns and lifestyles

Accompanying this change in food consumption patterns with modernisation, industrialisation and urbanisation is the change seen in physical activity patterns. During the process of economic development, the changes in dietary consumption patterns of populations have often been accompanied by a decline in levels of physical activity as a result of increasingly sedentary lifestyles. In the industrialised world, physical activity has declined as a result of the increasing mechanisation of life. Time in a day or week dedicated to paid work has declined in several countries since the early 1960s and is the result of shorter work shifts, shorter weeks and longer vacations. The decline in time dedicated to productive work has been accompanied by a reduction in energy spent at work as a result of increasing mechanisation of occupational work (Ferro-Luzzi and Martino 1996). Concurrent with this decrease in the energy expenditure as a result of occupational activities, increased urbanisation, universal use of motor cars, mechanisation of most manual jobs outside the occupational sphere and increasing leisure time have aggravated this trend. The increased leisure time is more often than not dedicated to sedentary activities, such as television viewing, thus altering the structure of leisure time and encroaching on time normally allocated to other activities including weekday sleep.

During the process of economic development, communities in developing societies often evolve from rural societies, where physical activity is needed for agricultural production, into urbanised, industrialised communities, where the demand for physical labour and activity declines. The process of economic development and rural to urban migration has thus reduced demand on physical activity such as that needed for agricultural production. The additional pursuit of leisure time activities, similar to that of the developed world, has thus contributed to the emergence of obesity as a significant problem even in developing countries, particularly those in rapid transition. In developing societies, which are industrialising and have economies in rapid transition sedentary lifestyles have accompanied periods when per capita intakes are also increasing. Thus, changes in dietary intake, food consumption patterns and physical activity levels and the consequent changes in body weight and body composition are contributing to the increased risk of obesity and its co-morbidities, which includes NIDDM.

Pima Indians: Arizona versus Mexico

The Pima Indians of Arizona have the highest prevalence of obesity (Knowler *et al.* 1991) and NIDDM (Knowler *et al.* 1990). This is a classic example of a community that has evolved from subsistence to Westernised diet and lifestyles over a short period of time. The increasing prevalence of obesity is paralleled by changes in the diet and in physical activity, i.e. a 'nutrition transition' over a short span of time. It is likely that in the presence of a possible genetic susceptibility, such as the 'thrifty genotype' (Neel 1978) characteristic of this ethnic community, changes in diet and lifestyle are a causal determinant of obesity and the predisposition to NIDDM. One way of testing this hypothesis is to compare the Pimas of Arizona with a closely related population living under markedly contrasting conditions. Observations made among Pima Indians in an underdeveloped mountainous region of north west Mexico seem to support this hypothesis (Ravussin *et al.* 1994). The Mexican community also of Pima ancestry (separated about 700–1,000 years ago) have a markedly contrasting diet and lifestyle. They consume a traditional diet characterised by less animal fat and more complex carbohydrates in their daily diet, and, being traditional agriculturists, they continue to adhere to lifestyles which are characterised by great energy expenditure, since they are physically very active with seasonal variations in activity levels. The Mexican Pimas have much lower levels of obesity and prevalence of NIDDM than the Arizona Pimas (Table 11.2).

Australian Aborigines

Similarly in Australia, the classic studies of O'Dea have documented a high prevalence of obesity and NIDDM among the Australian Aborigines which is associated with the degree of 'Westernisation' of the diet and lifestyles of these populations (O'Dea 1991, 1992). In a more recent study (O'Dea *et al.* 1993) it was demonstrated not only that the indigenous population of Australia had a much higher risk of NIDDM but also with a long period of acculturation of over 100 years the aborigine community in central Australia had lipid profiles closely resembling those in the rest of the Australian population. The rapidity with which these changes can occur has also been well demonstrated. Thirteen Tarhumara Indians living a traditional life in northern Mexico were fed a diet typical of affluent societies for 5 weeks

Table 11.2 Comparison of characteristics of Pima Indians living in Mexico with those resident in Arizona (from Ravussin *et al.* 1994)

	Women		*Men*	
	Mexico	*Arizona*	*Mexico*	*Arizona*
Age (years)	36	36	48	48
Weight (kg)	59.8	90.0	69.5	90.5
Height (cm)	154	159	167	171
BMI	25.1	35.5	24.8	30.8
BP (s/d; mmHg)	114/73	117/72	127/77	130/79
Cholesterol (mg/dl)	149	168	143	181
NIDDM prevalence	10.5	37.0	6.3	54.0

Notes
BMI, body mass index; BP, blood pressure; NIDDM, non-insulin dependent diabetes mellitus; s/d, systole/diastole.

(McMurphy 1991). On average they gained 3.8 kg, i.e. 7 per cent of initial body weight, and demonstrated dramatic increases in plasma lipids and lipoprotein levels. This study demonstrates how changes in diet over a much shorter period of time in susceptible populations can manifest with variations in disease risk.

A second approach to testing the hypothesis that environmental influences contribute considerably to the patterns in disease risk is to impose changes in the diet and lifestyles which are in effect a reversion to the traditional diet and lifestyles of a population, i.e. a reversal of the process we call 'nutrition transition'. O'Dea (1984) in her classic studies achieved this by taking a group of Aborigines living in an urban lifestyle to their traditional country of north west Australia to live as hunter–gatherers for 7 weeks. The reversion of the nutrition transition by reverting to traditional diet and lifestyles including activities resulted in dramatic changes in just 7 weeks. All subjects lost on average 8 kg in body weight and improved their carbohydrate metabolism greatly.

Risk of cardiovascular disease

South Asians

Studies of migrant populations have largely contributed to our understanding of ethnic variations in disease risk and have provided important insights into the causative contributions of both genetics and the environment as well as the various levels of interactions that exist between the two. Ethnic variations in disease risk particularly of NIDDM and cardiovascular disease in migrant populations are discussed in the chapter by Anand and Yusuf (Chapter 12) in considerable detail. However, I would like to make one important point which relates to the role of 'nutrition transition' in these variations. Ethnic variations in NIDDM and coronary heart disease (CHD) risk among South Asians in the United Kingdom forms another important component of our understanding of this interaction between genetic and environmental factors. Migration is an important ecological experiment. As a result of the alteration in the environment those who had apparently successfully adapted to a different environment now manifest patterns of disease risk which were hitherto concealed. Genetic susceptibilities are expressed in these new environments. This is best illustrated by a brief comparison of the dietary patterns of South Asians with that of the indigenous British populations of European origin.

Plasma cholesterol is one of the strongest predictors of CHD risk within populations. Despite cross-sectional and case–control studies showing an association between raised plasma cholesterol and CHD among South Asians which is just as strong as in Europeans (McKeigue and Marmot 1989, Hughes *et al.* 1990, McKeigue *et al.* 1993), in no South Asian community so far studied in the United Kingdom are average plasma cholesterol levels in middle age higher than the national average of about 6.0 mmol/l (McKeigue *et al.* 1988 and 1991). Plasma cholesterol levels are related to average saturated fat intake, and studies among South Asians in the United Kingdom summarised by McKeigue and Sevak (1994) show no remarkable differences in dietary intakes of total, saturated and polyunsaturated fat (PUFA) intakes. In fact PUFA intakes among South Asians is on average higher than that of the native British population, and yet South Asians have a higher prevalence of NIDDM and an increased risk of CHD.

Obviously the present dietary intake and lifestyles of South Asians are different from their pre-migration diets and lifestyles and in particular their levels of physical activity. International migration is not essential for the manifestation of this increased risk, which is considered as an ethnic variation or susceptibility to disease risk. Internal migration – from rural to urban areas – and the consequent changes in diet and lifestyle are capable of precipitating similar patterns of disease risk (Table 11.3). Such internal, i.e. rural to urban, migration manifests in precisely the same way within their country of origin, with increased risk of obesity, NIDDM and CHD risk. This emphasises the fact that diet and lifestyle changes, which constitute the basis of the 'nutrition transition', are powerful forces that account for much of what we believe to be ethnic variations in chronic disease risk. These environmental changes allow for the expression of genetic susceptibilities that did not until then have the appropriate milieu to express themselves. There is increasing evidence that genetic predisposition in the South Asian population is probably manifest in markers such as lipoprotein (a) levels (Bhatnagar *et al.* 1995, Enas and Mehta 1998) and in markers of thrombosis and increased coagulability (Anand and Yusuf, this volume). Recent studies comparing Mexican Americans in San Antonio with Mexicans living in Mexico City further indicate that environmental factors can override even the genetic susceptibility in the expression of disease risk, in this case that of NIDDM (Stern *et al.* 1992).

Table 11.3 Urban–rural differences in chronic disease risk in developing societies

	Urban (%)	Rural (%)	Reference
NIDDM prevalence (Tamil Nadu)	8.2%	2.4%	Ramachandran (1998)
CHD prevalence (Delhi)	46.1%	5.9%	Chadha *et al.* (1990)
Cancer incidence (Delhi versus Barshi)	118.8	57.6	Gopalan (1997)

Notes
CHD, coronary heart disease; NIDDM, non-insulin-dependent diabetes mellitus;

Hypertension and the initiation of rise in blood pressure

The Intersalt Study is probably the most extensive standardised international epidemiological study that has looked at the relationship between salt and blood pressure. In this study (Intersalt Cooperative Research Group 1988), four remote populations – Yanomamo and Xingu Indians of Brazil, Papua New Guinea highlanders and villagers from rural Kenya – had average 24-hour urinary sodium excretion (as a proxy of sodium intake) markedly lower than the other forty-eight international centres. The highest sodium excretion and blood pressures from among these four low sodium intake populations were recorded in the Kenyan sample, which apparently was in transition between its traditional rural existence and a more Westernised way of life. As the men and women in rural Kenya with relatively low blood pressures migrated to Nairobi in search of employment their blood pressures showed a rise. This remarkable longitudinal follow-up study of Luo migrants (Poulter *et al.* 1990) was a natural experiment that demonstrated a change in blood pressure following migration from rural Kenya. The new urban environment affected the whole population distribution of blood pressure, which shifted to the right compared with the distribution observed among the non-migrant controls. Not only was the percentage of the population with hypertension greater among migrants but the percentage of those with low blood pressure was also less in the migrants than in the non-migrant control subjects. This study further implicates rural–urban migration and the accompanying 'nutrition transition' characterised by diet and lifestyle changes as being responsible for the development of hypertension. The Kenyan Luo migration study (Poulter *et al.* 1990) showed that changes in dietary sodium–potassium ratios and body weight increases, as well as possibly the stress associated with urbanisation, were all contributory to these manifestations.

Cancer risk

Migration studies also provide evidence of the important part played by environmental factors in the development of cancers among ethnic migrant groups. These environmental factors are again related largely to diet and lifestyle and hence encompass 'nutrition transition'. Parkin addresses this issue in Chapter 13. The risk of certain types of cancer in the same racial or ethnic group alters dramatically during migration from one geographic area to another, and, depending on the degree and rate of acculturation with the native population, ultimately mimics the pattern seen in the native population. The classic examples are the patterns of breast and stomach cancer seen in Japanese women following migration to Hawaii (Kolonel *et al.* 1980), patterns of stomach and colorectal cancers among Chinese men in several geographic locations (Parkin *et al.* 1992) and studies on the cancer patterns of migrants to Australia (McMichael and Giles 1988). These studies underline the role of 'nutrition transition' in the variations of cancer risk in relatively homogenous ethnic or racial groups.

Conclusion

Over the last century, the pace of dietary and lifestyle changes has accelerated to varying degrees in different regions of the world. Economic development and urbanisation has resulted in societies entering different stages of what has been called the 'nutrition transition'. Diets high in complex carbohydrates and fibre have given way to more varied diets with higher proportions of fats, saturated fats and sugars. Major shifts have occurred in the composition of our daily diet. Modern societies throughout the world are converging on a dietary pattern which is high in fat, and particularly high in saturated fat, sugar and refined foods, and low in dietary fibre and complex carbohydrates. Accompanying these changes are lifestyle changes such as a dramatic reduction in levels of physical activity and increases in smoking and alcohol intakes. We are thus, globally hurtling towards a monoculture of diet and lifestyle. These shifts in diet structure and lifestyle patterns that accompany economic development and modernisation are also paralleled by demographic shifts associated with higher life expectancy and reduced fertility rates. An associated epidemiological transition is also taking place as patterns of disease shift away from infectious and nutrient deficiency diseases towards higher rates of chronic diseases. These changes are reflected in better nutrition outcomes such as changes in body size, including stature, but also lead downstream to further increases in body size and body composition manifested as obesity as well as contributing to its co-morbidities with increases in degenerative disease risk. This 'nutrition transition' is the environmental change that precipitates and unmasks a genetic predisposition which under traditional environmental circumstances was favourable to the survival of the individual or community. Much of what we see today as ethnic variations, particularly among migrant minority groups, are also being seen within their own geographic location, when economic development occurs and initiates the process of 'nutrition transition'. Genetic variations do exist, but manifest themselves as variations in disease risk when the environment changes as it does during the 'nutrition transition'.

References

Auricchio, S. and Troncone, R. (1989) 'Nutrition, evolution and traditional diets in children', *Beitraege zur Infusionstherapie und Transfusionsmedizin*, 22, 1–9.

Beauchamp, G.K. and Moran, M. (1982) 'Dietary experience and sweet taste preference in human infants', *Appetite*, 3, 139–152.

Beauchamp, G.K. and Moran, M. (1984) 'Acceptance of sweet and salty tastes in 2-year-old children', *Appetite*, 5, 291–305.

Bell, N.H., Greene, A., Epstein, S., Oexmann, M.J., Shaw, S. and Shary, J. (1985) 'Evidence for alteration of the vitamin D–endocrine system in blacks', *Journal of Clinical Investigation*, 76, 470–473.

Bhatnagar, D., Anand, I.S., Durrington, P.N., Patel, D.J., Wander, G.S., Mackness, M.I., Creed, F., Tomenson, B., Chandrashekhar, Y. and Winterbotham, M. (1995)

'Coronary risk factors in people from the Indian subcontinent living in west London and their siblings in India', *Lancet*, 345, 405–409.

Bhudhikanok, G.S., Wang, M.C., Eckert, K., Matkin, C., Marcus, R. and Bachrach, L.K. (1996) 'Differences in bone mineral in young Asian and Caucasian Americans may reflect differences in bone size', *Journal of Bone Mineral Research*, 11, 1545–1556.

Blakeslee, A.F. (1932) 'Genetics of sensory thresholds: taste for phenyl thio carbamide', *Proceedings of the National Academy of Sciences, USA*, 18, 120–130.

Bouchard, C. (1994) 'Genetics of obesity: overview and research directions', in Bouchard, C. (ed.) *The Genetics of Obesity*, Boca Raton: CRC Press, pp. 223–233.

Bouchard, C. (1997) 'Genetics of human obesity: Recent results from linkage studies', *Journal of Nutrition*, 127, 1887S–1890S.

Cavalli-Sforza, L.L. and Bodmer, W.F. (1971) *The Genetics of Human Populations*, San Francisco: Freeman.

Chadha, S.L., Radhakrishnan, S., Ramachandran, K., Kaul, U. and Gopinath, N. (1990) 'Epidemiological study of coronary heart disease in an urban population of Delhi', *Indian Journal of Medical Research*, 92, 424–430.

Desor, J.A., Greene, L.S. and Maller, O. (1975) 'Preferences for sweet and salt in 9- to 15-year-old and adult humans', *Science*, 190, 686–687.

Enas, E.A. and Mehta, J.L. (1998) 'Lipoprotein (a): an important risk factor in coronary artery disease', *Journal of the American College of Cardiology*, 32, 1132–1134.

Ettinger, B., Sidney, S., Cummings, S.R., Libanati, C., Bikle, D.D., Tekawa, I.S., Tolan, K. and Steiger, P. (1997) 'Racial differences in bone density between young adult black and white subjects persist after adjustment for anthropometric, lifestyle, and biochemical differences', *Journal of Clinical Endocrinology & Metabolism*, 82, 429–434.

Ferro-Luzzi, A. and Martino, L. (1996) 'Obesity and physical activity', in Ciba Foundation Symposium 201, *The Origins and Consequences of Obesity*, Chichester: John Wiley & Sons, pp. 228–246.

Greene, L.S. (1974) 'Physical growth and development, neurological maturation, and behavioral functioning in two Ecuadorian Andean communities in which goiter is endemic. II. PTC taste sensitivity and neurological maturation', *American Journal of Physical Anthropology*, 41, 139–151.

Greene, L.S., Desor, J.A. and Maller, O. (1975) 'Heredity and experience: their relative importance in the development of taste preference in man', *Journal of Comparative Physiology & Psychology*, 89, 279–284.

Gopalan, C. (1997) 'Diet related non-communicable diseases in Asia' in Shetty, P. and McPherson, (eds) *Diet, Nutrition and Chronic Disease: Lessons from Contrasting Worlds*, Chichester: John Wiley & Sons, pp. 10–23.

Hughes, L.O., Wojciechowski, A.P. and Raftery, E.B. (1990) 'Relationship between plasma cholesterol and coronary artery disease in Asians', *Atherosclerosis*, 83, 15–20.

Intersalt Cooperative Research Group (1988) 'Intersalt: an international study of electrolyte excretion and blood pressure. Results for 24 hour urinary sodium and potassium excretion', *British Medical Journal*, 297, 319–328.

Knowler, W.C., Pettitt, D.J., Saad, M.F. and Bennett, P.H. (1990) 'Diabetes mellitus in the Pima Indians: incidence, risk factors and pathogenesis', *Diabetes Metabolism Reviews*, 6, 1–27.

Knowler, W.C., Pettitt, D.J., Saad, M.F., Charles, M.A., Nelson, R.G., Howard, B.V., Bogardus, C. and Bennett, P.H. (1991) 'Obesity in the Pima Indians: its magnitude and relationship with diabetes', *American Journal of Clinical Nutrition*, 53, 1543S–1551S.

Kolonel, L.N., Hinds, M.W. and Hankin, J.H. (1980) 'Cancer patterns among migrant and native born Japanese in Hawaii in relation to smoking, drinking and dietary habits', in Gelboin *et al.* (eds) *Genetic and Environmental factors in Experimental and Human Cancer*, Tokyo: Science Society Press, pp. 327–340.

Kretchmer, N. (1977) 'The geography and biology of lactose digestion and malabsorption', *Postgraduate Medical Journal*, 53, S65–72.

McKeigue, P.M. and Marmot, M.G. (1988) 'Mortality from coronary heart disease in Asian communities in London', *British Medical Journal*, 297, 903.

McKeigue, P.M. and Sevak, L. (1994) *Coronary Heart Disease in South Asian Communities: A Manual for Health Promotion*, London: Health Education Authority.

McKeigue, P.M., Laws, A., Chen, Y.D., Marmot, M.G. and Reaven, G.M. (1993) 'Relation of plasma triglyceride and apoB levels to insulin-mediated suppression of nonesterified fatty acids. Possible explanation for sex differences in lipoprotein pattern', *Arteriosclerosis & Thrombosis*, 13, 1187–1192.

McKeigue, P.M., Marmot, M.G., Syndercombe–Court, Y.D., Cottier, D.E., Rahman, S. and Riemersma, R.A. (1988) 'Diabetes, hyperinsulinaemia, and coronary risk factors in Bangladeshis in east London', *British Heart Journal*, 60, 390–396.

McKeigue, P.M., Shah, B. and Marmot, M.G. (1991) 'Relation of central obesity and insulin resistance with high diabetes prevalence and cardiovascular risk in South Asians', *Lancet*, 337, 382–386.

McMichael, A.J. and Giles, G.G. (1988) 'Cancer in migrants to Australia: extending the descriptive epidemiological data', *Cancer Research*, 48, 751–756.

Meier, D.E., Luckey, M.M., Wallenstein, S., Clemens, T.L., Orwoll, E.S. and Waslien, C.I. (1991) 'Calcium, vitamin D, and parathyroid hormone status in young white and black women: association with racial differences in bone mass', *Journal of Clinical Endocrinology & Metabolism*, 72, 703–710.

Meier, D.E., Luckey, M.M., Wallenstein, S., Lapinski, R.H. and Catherwood, B. (1992) 'Racial differences in pre- and post-menopausal bone homeostasis: association with bone density', *Journal of Bone Mineral Research*, 7, 1181–1190.

Mohan, V., Deepa, R., Haranath, S.P., Premalatha, G., Rema, M., Sastry, N.G. and Enas, E.A. (1998) 'Lipoprotein(a) is an independent risk factor for coronary artery disease in NIDDM patients in South India', *Diabetes-Care*, 21, 1819–1823.

Moskowitz, H.W., Kumaraiah, V., Sharma, K.N., Jacobs, H.L. and Sharma, S.D. (1975) 'Cross-cultural differences in simple taste preferences', *Science*, 190, 1217–1218.

Neel, J.V. (1978) 'Diabetes mellitus: a "thrifty genotype" rendered detrimental by "progress" ', *American Journal of Human Genetics*, 14, 353–362.

Newman, B., Selby, J.V., King, M.C., Skemenda, C., Fabsitz, R. and Friedman, G.D. (1987) 'Concordance for type 2 (non-insulin dependent) diabetes mellitus in male twins', *Diabetologia*, 30, 763–768.

O'Dea, K. (1984) 'Marked improvement in carbohydrate and lipid metabolism in diabetic Australian aborigines after temporary reversion to traditional lifestyle', *Diabetes*, 33, 596–603.

O'Dea, K. (1991) 'Westernisation, insulin resistance and diabetes in Australian aborigines', *Medical Journal of Australia*, 155, 258–264.

O'Dea, K. (1992) 'Diabetes in Australian aborigines: impact of western diet and lifestyle', *Journal of Internal Medicine*, 232, 103–117.

O'Dea, K., Patel, M., Kubisch, D., Hopper, J. and Traianedes, K. (1993) 'Obesity, diabetes, and hyperlipidemia in a central Australian aboriginal community with a long history of acculturation', *Diabetes Care*, 16, 1004–1010.

Parfitt, A.M. (1997) 'Genetic effects on bone mass and turnover – relevance to black or white differences', *Journal of the American College of Nutrition*, 16, 325–333.

Parkin, D.M., Muir, C.S., Whelan, S.L., Gao, Y.T., Ferlay, J. and Powell, J. (eds) (1992) *Cancer incidence in five continents*, Volume 6, Lyon, France: International Agency for Research on Cancer.

Parisien, M., Cosman, F., Morgan, D., Schnitzer, M., Liang, X., Nieves, J., Forese, L., Luckey, M., Meier, D., Shen, V., Lindsay, R. and Dempster, D.W. (1997) 'Histomorphometric assessment of bone mass, structure, and remodeling: a comparison between healthy black and white premenopausal women', *Journal of Bone Mineral Research*, 12, 948–957.

Poulter, N.R., Khaw, K.T., Hopwood, B.E., Mugambi, M., Peart, W.S., Rose, G. and Sever, P.S. (1990) 'The Kenyan Luo migration study: observations on the initiation of a rise in blood pressure', *British Medical Journal*, 300, 967–972.

Prentice, A.M. and Whitehead, R.G. (1987) 'The energetics of human reproduction', in Louden A.S.I. and Racey P.A. (eds) *Reproductive Energetics in Mammals*, Vol. 57, London: Symposia of the Zoological Society, pp. 275–304.

Prentice, A.M., Goldberg, G.R. and Prentice, A. (1994) 'Body mass index and lactation performance', *European Journal of Clinical Nutrition*, 48, S78–S89.

Prentice, A.M., Paul, A.A., Prentice, A., Black, A.E., Cole, T.J. and Whitehead, R.G. (1986) 'Cross-cultural differences in lactational performance', in Hamosh, M. and Goldman, A.S. (eds) *Human Lactation*, New York: Plenum Publishing Corporation, pp. 13–44.

Ramachandran, A. (1998) 'Epidemiology of non insulin dependent diabetes mellitus in India', in Shetty, P. and Gopalan, C. (eds) *Diet, Nutrition and Chronic Disease: An Asian Perspective*, London: Smith Gordon, pp. 38–41.

Ravussin, E., Valencia, M.E., Esparza, J., Bennett, P.H. and Schulz, L.O. (1994) 'Effects of a traditional lifestyle on obesity in Pima Indians', *Diabetes Care*, 17, 1067–1074.

Weinstein, R.S. and Bell, N.H. (1988) 'Diminished rates of bone formation in normal black adults', *New England Journal of Medicine*, 319, 1698–1701.

Welsh, J.D., Poley, J.R., Bhatia, M. and Stevenson, D.E. (1978) 'Intestinal disaccharidase activities in relation to age, race, and mucosal damage', *Gastroenterology*, 75, 847–855.

12 Ethnic variations and cardiovascular disease

Sonia Anand and Salim Yusuf

Introduction

The importance of the major risk factors for cardiovascular disease (CVD), such as elevated blood pressure, elevated cholesterol, cigarette smoking and diabetes, has been determined from epidemiological studies conducted primarily in populations of European origin (Lenfant 1994). However, relatively little attention has been focused on the importance of various risk factors among people of non-European ancestry, who constitute the majority of the world's population. Determining risk factors among various ethnic populations is important to provide us with clues regarding similarities and differences in disease causation and facilitates the development of specific prevention strategies appropriately tailored to distinct ethnic groups.

Worldwide patterns of disease and regional differences

Globally, the major non-communicable diseases are CVD, cancer and diabetes. In most developed countries CVD rates are declining due to CVD risk factor modification, and improved secondary prevention strategies. By contrast CVD rates are increasing in many developing countries. These increases are due to epidemiological transitions resulting from a decrease in deaths due to acute infectious diseases and an increase in chronic diseases. The World Heart Federation reports that CVD claims approximately 15 million lives in the world each year, with over 60 per cent of these deaths occurring in developing countries. By the year 2020, CVD will join infectious diseases as the leading cause of death and disability in these countries. The reasons for this transition include increasing life expectancy secondary to declines in childhood and adult deaths from infections, and an increase in the prevalence of CVD risk factors associated with industrialisation and urbanisation.

The burden of CVD varies substantially between geographic regions. Ethnic variations in disease rates are closely tied to geographic patterns of disease (Marmot 1995). An ethnic group refers to a population that shares common cultural characteristics, such as language, religion, diet, and has some biological similarity. Often the first clue that ethnic variations in disease burden exist comes from observed differences in rates and risk factors between countries. These differences have provided many of the initial hypotheses for the various associations between lifestyle factors and CVD. One of the first epidemiological studies to highlight the variation in coronary heart disease (CHD) rates between countries was the Seven Countries Study (Menotti *et al.* 1993). In this major longitudinal cohort study sixteen cohorts of men aged 49 to 59 years were examined and followed for CHD mortality and total mortality. Large differences in CHD mortality between countries were observed, with low CHD rates in Japan and the Mediterranean countries and high CHD rates in Finland and the United States. These differences were in a large part explained by differences in diet, serum cholesterol and blood pressure. The World Health Organization (WHO) MONICA project (monitoring of trends and determinants in cardiovascular disease) is a CVD surveillance project which includes 117 reporting units in forty centres from twenty-six countries (Bothig 1989). These data indicate a greater than fourteenfold difference in CHD mortality among men and more than an elevenfold difference in CHD mortality for women exist between countries (Figure 12.1).

The massive fluctuations in CVD mortality which have occurred over relatively short periods of time in selected countries demonstrate the powerful impact that socio-economic changes have on health. For example, the low rate of CVD in Japan is closely tied to the economic prosperity of that country. This is in contrast to the astounding increase in CVD that has occurred recently among eastern European countries almost in parallel with the economic decline and the political instability of this region. These changes have occurred too quickly to be ascribed purely to genetic changes, and they reinforce the fact that both genes and environmental factors must be

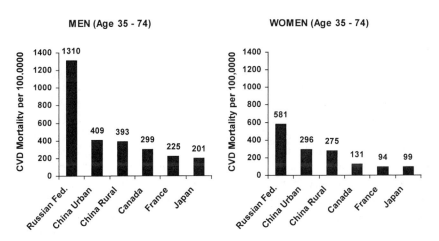

Figure 12.1 Cardiovascular disease (CVD) mortality in selected countries (American Heart Association 1999).

considered when trying to explain differences in CVD between regions and ethnic groups.

Ethnic variations in cardiovascular disease

People of European origin

People of European origin include those who originate from northern Europe, such as the Nordic countries and Germany, western Europe, including the United Kingdom and France, southern Europe, including Spain and Italy, and eastern Europe, which includes the Slavic countries.

Disease burden

Differences in the age-standardised mortality rates (ASMRs) vary widely between European populations. Data from the WHO indicate that the CVD mortality rate is sixfold higher among men and women in the Russian Federation than among people in France (Figure 12.1). In the 1990s, the ASMR for CHD among men in the Russian Federation was 737 per 100,000 compared with 94 per 100,000 among men in France (World Health Statistical Annual 1994). The cerebrovascular disease (CBVD) ASMR was 374 per 100,000 among men in the Russian Federation compared with 44 per 100,000 in France. Although the CVD mortality rates are much lower among women, large differences are seen among women between the different countries (Figure 12.1). Eastern European countries such as the Russian Federation, Hungary, and the Czech Republic have among the highest CVD rates in the world, which is in marked contrast to most economically stable European countries which have experienced declines in CVD mortality rates over the past 30 years.

Risk factors

CVD among European populations is mainly attributable to the major CVD risk factors, namely diets high in saturated fats, elevated serum cholesterol, elevated blood pressure, diabetes and smoking. The epidemic of CVD in the eastern European countries is related to high levels of smoking and excessive alcohol use along with diets high in saturated fat (Marmot 1995). However, CVD, like other epidemics, relates closely to social conditions, and its prevalence appears to be more strongly related to the social and cultural conditions of a society than to its genetic make-up. Research to explain why the Italian and French populations remain relatively 'protected' from CHD has yielded numerous hypotheses. It is likely that dietary differences account for an important component of the differences in disease rates. It is believed that the high consumption of oils high in mono-unsaturated fats, such as olive oil, and antioxidants is responsible for the low rates of CHD in Italy. In

France, the CHD mortality rate remains very low (Artaud-Wild *et al.* 1993). While this relative protection from CHD has been attributed by some to a high consumption of alcohol, in particular wine (Criqui and Ringel 1994), others believe the lower rate of CHD mortality may simply be due to a 'time-lag' between increases in consumption of animal fat and serum cholesterol concentrations (which have occurred only recently) and the expected increase in mortality (Law 1999).

Prevention

It is clear that major lifestyle change and vigilant treatment of conventional risk factors result in a decline in CVD rates. In Finland, an impressive 65 per cent reduction in CHD mortality and stroke was observed between 1972 and 1995. It is estimated that approximately 75 per cent of this decline in CHD mortality can be explained by a lowering of serum cholesterol by 14 per cent (0.93 mmol/l) in men and by 18 per cent (1.19 mmol/l) in women, reduction in diastolic blood pressure by 5 per cent (6.6 mmHg) in men and by 13 per cent (12.7 mmHg) in women and a significant reduction in smoking (by 18 per cent in men) (Vartiainen *et al.* 1994). In North America, a 30 per cent decline in CHD mortality occurred between 1980 and 1990. One-quarter of this decline is attributable to primary prevention efforts and about one-third is explained by secondary prevention efforts such as a reduction in serum cholesterol, diastolic blood pressure and smoking. In addition, about 40 per cent of this decline is attributed to improved medical and surgical management in patients with established coronary disease. More recently, in Poland during the 1990s, a rapid decrease (about 25 per cent) in CHD deaths in early middle age was observed. This decline is attributed in a large part to marked dietary changes, including an increased consumption of fruits and vegetables and a reduction in the consumption of animal fats (Zatonski *et al.* 1998).

Japanese

Disease burden

In parallel with a rise in economic prosperity, CVD rates in Japan have declined more markedly than those of Western countries, and the life expectancy in Japan is among the highest in the world. Mortality rates from CVD have traditionally been much lower in Japan than in Western countries (World Health Statistical Annual 1994). In Japan, the ASMR for CHD in men is 49 per 100,000, and in women is 18 per 100,000, which is one-quarter the rate of CHD in North America, and for CBVD it is 77 per 100,000 and 23 per 100,000 among men and women respectively (World Health Statistical Annual 1994). In addition, the pattern of CVD in Japanese men differs from that in Western populations, as in Japan men tend to experience relatively higher proportions of CBVD and less CHD (Iso *et al.* 1996).

Risk factors

A review of CVD risk factors in the Japanese population reveals that hypertension is the most important CVD risk factor, more so than cholesterol and cigarette smoking (Iso *et al.* 1996). Over the last 30 years blood pressure levels have declined in Japan as a result of improved diagnosis and treatment of hypertension. However, low serum cholesterol related to a diet low in saturated fat and cholesterol is also probably responsible for the low rates of CHD mortality observed in the Japanese. The prevalence of non-insulin-dependent diabetes mellitus (NIDDM) in Japanese men and women is higher than the rates in most Western countries. In the Hisayama prospective population-based study the prevalence of NIDDM was 13 per cent in men, and 9 per cent in women, and the relative risk of NIDDM for CVD was 3.0 (1.8–5.2) (Fujishima *et al.* 1996). Therefore, NIDDM appears to be an emerging and important risk factor for both stroke and CHD in the general Japanese population. However, during this period a two- to threefold increase in glucose intolerance and NIDDM, as well as obesity and hyper-cholesterolaemia (the mean cholesterol is only 10 per cent lower than in the United States in 1989), has been reported (Iso *et al.* 1996). The increase in diabetes, obesity and serum cholesterol is probably because of the 'Westernisation' of the Japanese lifestyle. It is possible that as cholesterol levels and glucose levels rise the impact of the high cigarette smoking may become manifest.

Prevention

With the increasing adoption of urban lifestyles in Japan, the rates of CHD risk factors could approach those of Americans. The differences in CHD rates between Japan and the United States demonstrate consistent relationships between diet, serum cholesterol and CHD. Recent studies have documented that the average serum cholesterol concentration among the Japanese has increased between 1980 and 1989. The age-adjusted total serum cholesterol levels increased from 4.84 to 5.22 mmol/l in men and from 4.91 to 5.24 mmol/l in women. This combined with the increased prevalence of cigarette smoking among Japanese men (59 per cent) suggests that Japan may soon experience a significant epidemic of CHD (Iso *et al.* 1996). Therefore, maintenance of a low-fat diet, avoidance of obesity through decreased energy intake and regular physical activity are likely to prevent the development of glucose intolerance. Avoidance of cigarette smoking is also critical. This change in the CVD risk factor profile has led to a changing pattern of CVD among the Japanese in Japan: a significant decrease in morbidity and mortality from CBVD but no increase in the risk of CHD. However, if the change in risk factors continues, CHD rates may show an increase in this population.

Chinese

Disease burden

Death rates from CVD (particularly CHD) have been increasing in China in recent decades (Woo and Donnan 1989). Although the CVD mortality rate in China is approximately the same as that in the United States, the CHD mortality rate is approximately 50 per cent lower than the rates observed in most Western countries, and the CBVD rate is significantly higher. In 1996, in urban China, the ASMR for CHD for men and women aged 35–74 was 100 per 100 000 in men and was 69 per100 000 in women (World Health Statistical Annual 1994). However, the ASMR for CBVD in men and women aged 35–74 was 251 per 100,000 in men and 170 per 100,000 in women (Thorvaldsen *et al.* 1995) (Figure 12.2). Comparison with five stroke registries from the West suggests that intracerebral haemorrhage occurs between two and three times more frequently in the Chinese than in White Caucasians (Hong *et al.* 1994). Only 6 to 12 per cent of strokes in White people are reported as intracerebral haemorrhages compared with 25 to 30 per cent of haemorrhagic strokes in the Chinese (Thorvaldsen *et al.* 1995).

Risk factors

A case–control study from Hong Kong of acute myocardial infarction (MI) sufferers indicates that conventional risk factors for CHD in the Chinese

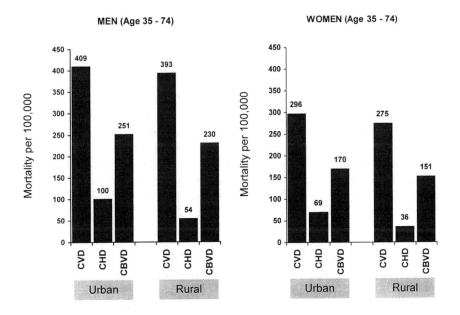

Figure 12.2 Coronary heart disease (CHD) and cerebrovascular disease (CBVD) mortality in urban and rural China (American Heart Association 1999).

remain important (Donnan *et al.* 1994). The odds ratio for AMI associated with cigarette smoking was 4.3 per cent, with hypertension 3.3 per cent and with diabetes 2.4 per cent. Although the mean serum cholesterol among the Chinese is low by Western standards, a prospective observational study of approximately 9,000 Chinese in urban Shanghai demonstrated that serum cholesterol was directly related (continuous relationship) to CHD mortality, even at these low levels (Chen *et al.* 1991). Cigarette smoking is highly prevalent among Chinese men as approximately 40–60 per cent of men smoke and there is evidence that these rates are increasing (Tao *et al.* 1989).

Geographic variations

Trends in morbidity and mortality from CVD within China indicate that the mortality rate attributable to CVD is higher in north China (Beijing) than in south China (Guangzhou) (People's Republic of China–United States Cardiovascular and Cardiopulmonary Epidemiology Research Group 1992). Furthermore, comparison of urban and rural areas in China indicate that CHD rates increase twofold in urban areas compared with rural areas, yet surprisingly the stroke rates do not differ by region (Figure 12.2). The prevalence of hypertension, mean serum cholesterol and mean body mass index (BMI) were all lower in the south than in the north, and lower in rural than in urban areas. However, the greatest differences in the prevalence of cigarette smoking exist between men and women (74 per cent versus 20 per cent) and this difference is observed in both urban and rural settings.

Migrant patterns

Data from Chinese migrants to Singapore and Mauritius provide evidence that the effects of exposure to urban environments lead to adverse risk factor profiles for CVD (Li *et al.* 1992, Hughes *et al.* 1990). In a comparative study of Chinese migrants to Mauritius the prevalence of CHD by electrocardiogram was six times greater (24 per cent versus 4 per cent) than in Beijing, China. The prevalence of diabetes and the mean serum cholesterol was also higher in Mauritius Chinese (5.5 mmol/l) than in Beijing Chinese (4.4 mmol/l), whereas the prevalence of hypertension and smoking was greater in Beijing (Li *et al.* 1992). Thus, although the prevalence of hypertension and smoking may decline with migration, the rates of obesity, late onset diabetes, elevated serum cholesterol and CHD tend to increase.

Prevention

Economic modernisation in China is resulting in an increased prevalence of conventional CVD risk factors over time in urban populations (Chonhua *et al.* 1993). This offers a major challenge for primary prevention among urban Chinese both in China and abroad, as the Chinese who have traditionally had a very low prevalence of CHD are not likely to remain protected from developing CHD with the change in lifestyles that follows migration or urbanisation. Important prevention strategies in this group include smoking cessation and maintenance of a 'traditional Chinese' diet (high vegetable, high tea, low fat consumption) to prevent the increase in BMI, diabetes, serum cholesterol and hypertension.

South Asians

The term South Asian refers to people who originate from the Indian subcontinent, i.e. Bangladesh, India, Pakistan and Sri Lanka.

Disease burden

Studies of South Asian migrants demonstrate that they suffer a higher mortality from CHD than other ethnic groups do. There are relatively few mortality studies from within India as there is no uniform completion of death certificates and no centralised death registry for CVD (Reddy 1993). However, the WHO and the World Bank data indicate that death attributable to CVD disease has increased in parallel with the expanding population in India, and it now accounts for a large proportion of the disability-adjusted life years (DALYs). Of all deaths in 1990, approximately 25 per cent were attributable to CVD, which is greater than the 9 per cent due to diarrhoeal diseases, the 12 per cent due to respiratory infections and the 5 per cent due to tuberculosis (Murray 1994). South Asian migrants to countries such as the United Kingdom, South Africa, Singapore and North America provide evidence that CHD mortality in South Asians is between 1.11 and 3.19 times higher than in other ethnic groups (Enas *et al.* 1992).

Temporal trends

In India the CHD rate is expected to rise in parallel with the increase in life expectancy due to an increase in per capita income and a decline in infant mortality. The average life expectancy increased from 47 years in 1960 to 58 years in 1990. This trend is expected to continue, with life expectancy at birth reaching 70 years by 2030, leading to large increases in CVD prevalence (Lowy *et al.* 1991). Although the CHD mortality rate of South Asians compared with other populations remains high, a decline in CHD rates has been observed in most South Asian migrants over the past 10 years. However, this decline has been less than that observed in the general population in many of these countries (Balarajan 1991, Sheth *et al.* 1999).

Risk factors

South Asians, despite having increased rates of CHD, do not display an excess of conventional CVD risk factors such as smoking, hypertension or elevated cholesterol (McKeigue *et al.* 1991, 1993). However, these factors remain strongly associated with the development of CHD in South Asians. Data from a case–control study (Pais *et al.* 1996) in Bangalore, India, in which 300 cases of acute myocardial infarction (MI) were compared with 300 age- and sex-matched controls, revealed an increasing risk of MI as the number of conventional risk factors increased. The odds ratio for MI associated with smoking was 3.6, for diabetes 2.6 and for hypertension 2.7. In this study serum cholesterol and lipid fractions did not differ between cases and controls, although the levels were similar to Western values. Cross-sectional studies of CHD risk factors in South Asians have identified that this group suffers a high prevalence of impaired glucose tolerance (IGT), central obesity, elevated triglycerides, and low high-density lipoprotein (HDL) cholesterol (McKeigue *et al.* 1991). The prevalence of IGT and NIDDM is four to five times higher in South Asian migrants than in Europeans by the age of 55 (20 per cent versus 4 per cent) (McKeigue *et al.* 1991, 1993). The prevalence of diabetes in South Asians in the UK was 10–19 per cent, in Trinidad 21 per cent, in Fiji 25 per cent, in south Africa 22 per cent, in Singapore 25 per cent and in Mauritius 20 per cent (McKeigue *et al.* 1991). In rural India the prevalence of diabetes is 3 per cent, and in urban India between 11 per cent and 30 per cent, which is similar to the rates reported among Indians living abroad (Ramachandran *et al.* 1992). In addition, there is increasing evidence that elevations in blood glucose are also risk factors for CHD, a condition that is also frequently observed to exist in South Asians. There is preliminary evidence that South Asians have elevated levels of lipoprotein (a) [Lp(a)] – a lipoprotein which is genetically mediated and associated with increased atherosclerosis and thrombogenesis (Anand 1998). However, the importance of Lp(a) in causing clinical events among South Asians is unclear.

Geographic variations

An urban–rural difference in CHD prevalence and risk factors is observed within India and abroad. Data from India demonstrate at least a twofold excess of CHD in urban compared with rural environments. A recent overview of prevalence surveys in India reported a ninefold increase in CHD in urban centres compared with a twofold increase in CHD rates among rural populations over two decades (Gupta and Gupta 1996). Associated with this increase in CHD rates in urban areas is an increase in the prevalence of lipid and glucose abnormalities. An increased prevalence of IGT and NIDDM, lower HDL cholesterol and higher triglycerides, increased abdominal obesity and BMI, and higher levels of hypertension is observed in the urban areas than in the rural areas. By contrast, the rates of tobacco smoking are higher within rural environments among both men and women.

Migration patterns

A recent study which compared the risk profiles of urban South Asians living in the UK with those of their siblings living in India revealed that the UK cohort had higher BMIs (27 versus 23), systolic BPs (144 mmHg versus 137 mmHg), total cholesterol (6.35 versus 5.0 mmol/l), lower HDL cholesterol (1.14 versus 1.27 mmol/l) and higher fasting glucose levels (5.4 versus 4.6 mmol/l) than their siblings (Bhatnagar *et al.* 1995). Therefore, adverse changes in CVD risk factors and CVD rates are observed when South Asians adopt an urban lifestyle, be it within their native countries or abroad following migration.

Hispanics

The term Hispanic includes Cuban Americans, Mexican Americans and Puerto Rican Americans. There are approximately 20 million Mexican Americans living in the United States, and they make up approximately 9 per cent of the United States population (American Heart Association 1999).

Disease burden

CVD is the leading cause of death among Hispanic men (26.9 per cent) and women (33.3 per cent) (American Heart Association 1999). The majority of information on CVD in Hispanics has been derived from studies in Mexican Americans. Although death certificate registries report that the ASMRs for major CVD among Mexican Americans are lower than those of African Americans and White people in the United States (Becker *et al.* 1988), recent data from the Corpus Christi Heart Project (CCHP), Texas, reported a greater incidence of MI in Mexican Americans than in non-Hispanic White people over a 4-year period (Goff *et al.* 1997). This population-based surveillance project conducted between 1988 and 1992 and comparing Mexican Americans with non-Hispanic White people reported age-adjusted incidence ratios of 1.52 (95 per cent CI 1.28–1.80) and 1.25 (95 per cent CI 1.10–1.42) among women and men respectively (Goff *et al.* 1997). The CCHP has reported a greater case fatality rate following MI among Mexican Americans than among non-Hispanic White people. Therefore, a lower CHD prevalence in Mexican Americans does not necessarily reflect a lower incidence of CHD. For CBVD, Hispanics under the age of 60 years have a significantly elevated CBVD death rate compared with non-Hispanic White people (men 32 versus 19 per 100,000, women 23 versus 18 per 100,000 respectively). However, in older age categories the CBVD rate in Hispanics is substantially lower than in White people (men 589 versus 765, women 535 versus 847 per 100,000) (Gillum 1995a). Therefore, overall the CBVD death rate over 45 years of age in Hispanics is lower than in White people (men 115 versus 147 per 100,000, women 110 versus 209 per 100,000) (Morgenstern *et al* 1997). Although a decline in CHD and CBVD mortality have occurred in

Mexican Americans over the past 20 years, this decline has been less than that which occurred among non-Hispanic White people (Stern and Gaskill 1987, Gillum 1995a).

Risk factors

The Hispanic Health and Nutrition Examination (HHANES) demonstrated that Hispanics suffer a high prevalence of conventional CVD risk factors such as hypertension (17 per cent prevalence), low HDL cholesterol < 0.90 mmol/l (15.2 per cent men, 5 per cent women), diabetes (24 per cent prevalence), physical inactivity (39 per cent) and obesity (29 per cent men, 39 per cent women) compared with non-Hispanic White people (American Heart Association 1999). The San Antonio Heart Study reported that Mexican Americans had 2.5 times the prevalence of NIDDM compared with the non-Hispanic White people as diagnosed by the oral glucose tolerance test (Haffner *et al.* 1992). Glucose intolerance appears to be the most influential risk factor for CHD among Mexican Americans (Goff *et al.* 1994). Furthermore, glucose intolerance also defines which Mexican Americans are more likely to suffer CHD events within their own population, as diabetic Mexican Americans are four times more likely to suffer an MI than their non-diabetic counterparts. They also observed that a socio-economic gradient within the Hispanic population existed, with diabetes being more prevalent in the lower socio-economic groups (Haffner *et al.* 1992). Furthermore, Mexican Americans have higher blood concentrations of triglycerides and lower HDL cholesterol levels than non-Hispanic White people (American Heart Association 1995).

Prevention

The burden of CHD among Hispanics is considerable, and prevention programmes addressing the high rates of obesity and the low levels of physical activity are needed to reduce the rate of glucose intolerance in this group. Promotion of these strategies is important given that Mexican Americans are less likely to receive treatment for diabetes, hypercholesterolaemia and hypertension than non-Hispanic White people (Goff *et al.* 1997). Therefore, it is critical that ethnically sensitive strategies to bring about both primary and secondary prevention in this growing group of Americans be developed.

Aboriginal or native populations

Owing to declining death rates from communicable diseases, increasing life expectancy and increasing adoption of 'Western' lifestyles (increased consumption of high-energy food and tobacco, reduced physical activity and increased stress as a result of the breakdown of traditional social structures), the rates of chronic degenerative diseases such as CVD, diabetes, cancer and mental illness are increasing among Aboriginal peoples. These trends parallel the epidemiological transition that is occurring in other developing populations throughout the world.

Disease burden

Although mortality rates for CVD among Aboriginal populations appear to be lower than people of European ancestry, CHD is the leading cause of death in North American Indian and Alaskan Natives (American Heart Association 1995). Although research in this ethnic group is limited, the Strong Heart Study (Howard *et al.* 1995), which was initiated in 1988, studied 4,549 American Natives aged 45–74 years from thirteen tribes in the southern United States. The prevalence estimates of definite MI in those aged 45–74 years was 2.8 per cent in men without diabetes, and 5.3 per cent in men with diabetes, 0.4 per cent in women without diabetes and 1.4 per cent in women with diabetes. Data from other United States studies indicate that Native Americans may have a lower prevalence of MI than White people (7.9 per cent), African Americans (6.1 per cent) and Hispanics (5.6 per cent) (Howard *et al.* 1995). There is little published information concerning the epidemiology of CBVD in native populations. In the United States the CBVD mortality rates under the age of 65 years is similar in Native Americans and White Americans, and substantially lower than rates in African Americans (Gillum 1995b). In Canada, CVD appears to account for the largest proportion of adult deaths among Aboriginal men and women. Although the CHD mortality rates among Aboriginal men and Canadian men are similar, the CHD mortality rate is 61 per cent higher among Aboriginal women. In addition, the stroke mortality rate is 44 per cent and 93 per cent higher among Aboriginal Canadian men and women respectively than the general Canadian population.

Temporal trends

As more Native Indians give up their traditional hunter–gatherer lifestyles and adopt 'urban' lifestyles the risk factors for CVD and CVD prevalence are expected to increase. Data from Canada in which the time periods 1979–83 and 1984–85 were compared revealed that a decline in CHD rates of 22 per cent occurred in Native men, whereas the rates of CHD increased by 5 per cent among Native women (Mao *et al.* 1992). The age-adjusted rates of CBVD mortality declined over the period from 1980 to 1990 in Native Americans by approximately 20 per cent, which is slightly lower than the 26 per cent decline observed in White Americans (Gillum 1995b).

Risk factors

The common CHD risk factors in Native men and women include diabetes, obesity, and low HDL cholesterol. The prevalence of cigarette smoking is increasing among Native Indians with wide variations seen between different tribes and reservations (Howard *et al.* 1995). The prevalence of diabetes in the Strong Heart Study was an astounding 48 per cent in the 45–64 year age group compared with approximately 5.5 per cent in the United States general population, and the prevalence of obesity was between 26 and 41 per cent, with an average BMI of 31 and a waist–hip ratio of 0.96 in men. Interestingly, the prevalence of hypertension and elevated serum cholesterol among Natives appears to be lower than in the general United States population. However, the prevalence of low HDL cholesterol is greater in this group as approximately 25 per cent of Native men have HDL cholesterol values less than 0.90 mmol/l.

Geographic variations

Studies in Aboriginal populations in North America have revealed that important regional and inter-tribal differences in CVD risk factors and disease rates exist (Howard *et al.* 1995, Gillum 1995b). The Strong Heart Study documented large inter-tribe differences in the prevalence of diabetes, IGT and cigarette smoking (Howard *et al.* 1995). Most of the current data on CVD rates and risk factors have come from studies of Native Americans living on reservations. There is relatively little information regarding these profiles among city-dwelling Native Americans.

Prevention

In order to devise preventive strategies for CVD in Native populations more research into the epidemiology of CVD and CVD risk factors must be performed. Specifically research into the epidemiology of CVD profiles of Native American Indians who do not live on reservations must be emphasised, as it is very likely that inner-city Natives may have different CVD risk factor profiles and disease rates than reservation populations. This information will be important in developing culturally sensitive risk factor modification and education programmes for Native populations.

Black people of African origin

The rates of CVD among Black people in Africa are relatively low compared with the rates in most Western countries. However, in urban centres in Africa, and among migrant Africans to the West Indies and the United States, the rates of CVD are similar or higher than the rates in most Western countries.

Africa

DISEASE BURDEN

CVD mortality data from countries in sub-Saharan Africa (SSA) are limited, as only 1.1 per cent of all deaths are registered with a central agency (Murray and Lopez 1997a). Data from other sources, such as sample registries, and small-scale population studies in 1990 indicate that the prevalence of acute MI in men and women of all ages was 3.4 per 100,000, and the mortality from acute MI in 1990 was 41 per 100,000 (Murray and Lopez 1997a). These rates are considerably lower than those of White people who live in Africa as well as the rates in most Western countries, which are on average five times higher (Murray and Lopez 1997a, b). Even so, in SSA, the proportional mortality rate from CHD accounts for 26 per cent of all deaths, and in the 60–70 year age group it accounts for over 80 per cent of all deaths (Murray and Lopez 1997a). Furthermore, the case fatality rate of CHD is higher in SSA than in Western countries, meaning that once an individual develops CHD in SSA, the probability of death is higher than in Western countries. This probably represents the limited access to acute and chronic treatment strategies in most parts of Africa.

RISK FACTORS

The prevalence of most conventional risk factors for CHD is lower among Black people than among other groups within Africa and the world, with the exception of hypertension and smoking among urban Black people (Seedat 1996, Berrios *et al.* 1997, Murray and Lopez 1997b). Data from the WHO Inter-Health Programme, a sub-study of the MONICA project, assessed the risk factor profile of men and women aged 35–64 years from the United Republic of Tanzania (Berrios *et al.* 1997). The prevalence of smoking was 37 per cent among men and 3.9 per cent among women; the mean BMI was 21 in men and 22 in women; the mean BP among men was 126/79 mmHg and 125/79 mmHg in women; the mean serum cholesterol was 4.1 mmol/l in men and 4.3 mmol/l in women. When compared with other developing and developed countries, the Tanzanian risk factor profile was more favourable, with the exception of smoking among men. Furthermore, the prevalence of multiple risk factors for CHD was low, as 65 per cent of the population has no identifiable risk factors, 30 per cent had a single risk factor and only 5 per cent had at least two risk factors compared with 50 per cent, 40 per cent, and 10 per cent respectively in the United States (Berrios *et al.* 1997).

GEOGRAPHIC VARIATIONS

In most urban and virtually all rural regions of SSA the prevalence of traditional CVD risk factors among Black people is low. However, with urbanisation an increase in conventional cardiovascular risk factors and CHD rates is expected (Akinkugbe 1985). In South Africa, the rapid migration of Black people to urban centres has led to increased poverty, obesity, hypertension, LDL cholesterol and a decrease in HDL cholesterol. Over time, given the increased migration of Black people to urban centres, this is likely to be the trend in most urban African centres.

PREVENTION

Prevention strategies such as reducing the availability of saturated fats and increasing the availability of mono-unsaturated fats, control of cigarette smoking by increasing the price of cigarettes, controlling the amount of salt consumption and promoting regular physical activity are required at the community level, especially among urban populations. Key primary and secondary prevention strategies among Black people include control of hypertension and tough anti-smoking campaigns.

West Indies

DISEASE BURDEN

In Trinidad, data obtained in 1989 reveal that the age-adjusted incidence of CHD in people of African origin was 7 per 1,000 person years at risk in men and 5 per 1000 person years at risk in women. The rate in men approximated men of European decent (6.45 per 1,000), whereas the rates among women were higher in Black people (5 versus 2.9 per 1,000). The rates in both sexes was substantially lower than that of men (16 per 1,000) and women (13 per 1,000) of South Asian origin in the same geographical region (Miller *et al.* 1989).

RISK FACTORS

The most prevalent and important risk factor among West Indian Black people is hypertension. In Trinidad, the St James survey showed that the prevalence of hypertension among African Black people was 33 per cent, diabetes 8.1 per cent and smoking 39 per cent (Miller *et al.* 1989). Furthermore, the mean HDL cholesterol (in mmol/l) in men was 1.03 and in women 1.30; the mean LDL cholesterol (mmol/l) was 4.04 in males and 4.11 in women. The most important predictors of CHD in this cohort were hypertension, high LDL cholesterol, low HDL cholesterol and diabetes mellitus.

United States of America

African Americans are the largest non-White population in the United States and represent approximately 12 per cent of the population.

DISEASE BURDEN

CVD is the leading cause of death among African Americans, and the incidence of both CHD and CBVD is higher in African Americans than in White Americans. Although the CHD mortality rate in African American men is slightly lower than White men (230 versus 246 per 100,000), it is higher among African American women than among White American women (165 versus 146 per 100,000) (American Heart Association 1995). Sudden cardiac death [defined by International Classification of Disease (ICD) codes 410–414] is also more common among African American men and women (Gillum 1989). In addition, the CBVD mortality rate is substantially higher among men (93 versus 63 per 100,000) and women (79 versus 59 per 100,000) than among their White counterparts (American Heart Association 1995). Although there has been a decline in mortality rates from CVD in both African Americans and White Americans over the past 30 years, these declines have been less marked in African Americans than those of European origin.

RISK FACTORS

Compared with White people, African Americans develop hypertension at an earlier age, and it is more severe (American Heart Association 1995) (Table 12.1). The reason for Black–White differences in the prevalence of hypertension is likely to involve a complex interaction between environmental responses to diet and stress, and a potential genetic–physiological difference such as differences in sodium–potassium excretion, perhaps linked to their origins in Africa and survival during migration to the United States. Serum cholesterol levels are not higher among African Americans than White Americans, and on average African Americans have higher HDL cholesterol levels than White people, despite the fact that African Americans suffer significantly more diabetes (American Heart Association 1995). The

Table 12.1 Conventional CVD risk factors among United States Black people and White people (American Heart Association 1999)

Risk factor	Black		White	
	Men	*Women*	*Men*	*Women*
Hypertension (%)	35.0	23.5	24.4	19.3
Smoking (%)	28.8	23.5	27.1	24.1
LDL cholesterol > 3.4 mmol/l (%)	43.8	41.5	49.3	42.9
HDL cholesterol < 0.8 mmol/l (%)	9.2	3.3	17.8	6.2
Diabetes (%)	7.3	9.1	5.2	4.5
BMI > 30 (%)	21.3	34.2	20.0	22.4
No leisure-time physical activity (%)	33.1	47.7	25.3	28.2

Notes
BMI, body mass index; LDL, low-density lipoprotein; HDL, high-density lipoprotein.

prevalence of cigarette smoking is greater among African American men (28.8 per cent versus 27.1 per cent) than among White men, and the rates are about the same in women (American Heart Association 1995). Obesity (defined as a BMI > 30) is an emerging problem among African Americans especially in women, and approximately 21 per cent of African American men and 34 per cent of women are obese compared with 20 per cent and 22 per cent of White American men and women respectively (American Heart Association 1995) (Table 12.1). Closely linked to the prevalence of obesity is a low prevalence of self-reported regular physical activity, and 33 per cent of men and 47 per cent of women are physically inactive compared with 25 per cent and 28 per cent of White American men and women respectively. Furthermore, the prevalence of diabetes in African Americans is higher than in White people, as African Americans aged 20–74 years have a NIDDM prevalence of 10 per cent compared with 5 per cent in White Americans (American Heart Association 1995). However, even after consideration of 'biomedical' differences in conventional risk factors, such as hypertension, diabetes, and obesity, other factors are likely to play a role in the slower decline in CVD rates observed among Black people. Differences in socio-economic status between African American and White people translate into decreased access to medical therapies and hospital services and results in the performance of fewer diagnostic tests and lower rates of coronary revascularisation procedures (Geronimus *et al.* 1996, Fang *et al.* 1996).

PREVENTION

As in other populations conventional CVD risk factors remain important; however, the dominant CVD risk factors among people of African origin is hypertension. Special efforts at detection, prevention and treatment of hypertension, both through lifestyle changes and through appropriate pharmacological therapy, are necessary. In the United States, the lower socio-economic status of Black people probably contributes to the higher disease burden. This Black–White differential in disease rates, risk factors and access to medical treatments necessitates that specific prevention strategies be initiated in this group. Such strategies include primary prevention programmes to prevent unhealthy lifestyle behaviours such as poor dietary practices and cigarette smoking. As these risk factors are closely tied to the low socio-economic status (SES), other factors besides conventional 'biomedical' risk factors need to be targeted. Health care providers must ensure equal access to health care services, especially among the lower SES Black populations (Schwartz 1999). However, in order to overcome the larger differential in SES between African Americans and White people, overall changes to social policy are required at the national level.

Importance of studies among migrant ethnic groups

Migrant groups living within a country are ideal populations to study variations in CVD rates and risk factors by ethnic group. Differences in disease rates observed in the same group living in different countries with different environmental exposures suggest that environmental influences are very powerful factors in the causation of CVD. Conversely, despite differences in the environments, similarities in disease rates within an ethnic group point to the existence of a predominant genetic propensity for risk of or for protection from CVD. Observational studies reveal that when members of a given ethnic group change to a new environment (by migration) their physical response to a given set of environmental factors usually differs from those who remain in their native lands. Early on in the period of migration, the pattern of disease risk of migrants may usually represent the patterns of their countries of origin. However, with time they may tend to mimic the population of their country of adoption. Comparing the mortality rates of long-settled migrants with the disease rates in their country of origin helps to establish the relative contribution of genetic and environmental influences on the variations in disease and mortality rates.

A study of multiple ethnic groups in the United States revealed that CVD mortality rates were highest among African Americans, followed by White people, and Hispanics (Frerichs *et al.* 1984). In contrast Japanese, Chinese, Koreans and Filipinos had a much lower CHD mortality risk. Another study conducted in California between 1985 and 1990 compared CHD and CBVD death rates in six ethnic groups. Once again, African American men and women in all age groups were found to have the highest CVD death rates. Hispanics, Chinese and Japanese had much lower CVD rates, although the CBVD deaths were proportionally a more important cause of death among

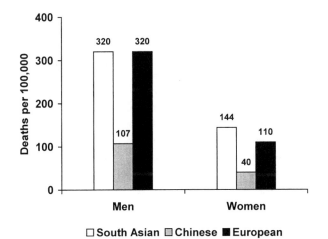

Figure 12.3 Variations in the rates of coronary heart disease (CHD) between ethnic groups in Canada (Sheth *et al.* 1999).

the Chinese and Japanese. Furthermore, a study which compared the rates of hospitalisation for CHD among Asian Americans with other Americans in Northern California revealed that the risk of hospitalisation for CHD was the lowest among the Chinese Americans (0.6) and the highest among the South Asians (3.7, $P < 0.001$) (Klatsky *et al.* 1994). Recent data from the UK reveals that although the CHD mortality rates were approximately 43 per cent higher among South Asian men and women than among the general UK population, among South Asians there has been a decline in CHD rates by 26 per cent in men and 18 per cent in women (Balarajan 1996). This is in keeping with a decline in CHD mortality in the UK as a whole over the past decade. In Canada, an analysis of the Canadian National Mortality Database of South Asians, Chinese and Canadians of European origin demonstrated that the ASMR per 100,000 for CHD in South Asian Canadians (men 320, women 144) was similar to European Canadians (men 320, women 110) but was much higher than the CHD mortality of Chinese Canadians (men 107, women 40) (Figure 12.3). Furthermore, a significant decline in CHD death rates from 1979–83 to 1989–93 was observed in all groups, with the greatest decline being apparent among South Asian men and women compared with European and Chinese Canadians respectively (men 22 per cent, 13 per cent, and 5.4 per cent, women 6 per cent, 4 per cent and 2 per cent) (Sheth *et al.* 2000).

Conclusion

CVD accounts for the largest percentage of deaths worldwide. To date, recognition and modification of the major CVD risk factors have led to declines in CVD in most Western countries, although these declines have lagged behind in most of the non-White population groups among them. Socio-economic development, urbanisation and increasing life expectancy have led to a progressive rise in the CVD rates in developing countries such as India and China. It is clear that conventional CVD risk factors such as elevated serum cholesterol, elevated blood pressure, cigarette smoking and glucose intolerance are the major risk factors for CHD and CBVD in most populations. However, other risk factors or protective factors (such as levels of endogenous fibrinolysis, dietary factors such as flavonoids and antioxidants) are likely to exist. Identification of these factors is important so that new approaches to the prevention of CVD in these populations may be developed. Research in ethnic populations who suffer adverse glucose and lipid changes upon adoption of urban lifestyles (i.e. Chinese, Hispanic, Aboriginal and South Asian) should be a priority as a greater proportion of these groups are adopting urban lifestyles, which is associated with observed increases in CVD rates. Furthermore, in developed countries, research into reasons for social and economic disparities and its impact on the distribution of CVD risk factors among ethnic groups must be continued to help develop specific interventions aimed at reducing the adoption of unhealthy lifestyle behaviours and to deal with barriers to access to health care services. Ultimately, all of this information will lead to the development of strategies for prevention which may be tailored to specific ethnic populations and generate important areas for future study.

References

Akinkugbe, O.O. (1985) 'World epidemiology of hypertension', in Hall. W.D., Saunders. E. and Shulman. N.B. (eds) *Hypertension in Blacks: Epidemiology, Pathophysiology, and Treatment*, St Louis: Year Book Publishers, pp. 13–16.

American Heart Association (1995) *Heart and Stroke Facts: 1996 Statistical Supplement*. Dallas, TX: American Heart Association.

American Heart Association (1999) *American Heart Association Statistical Facts*. Dallas, TX: American Heart Association.

Anand, S., Enas, E., Pogue, J., Haffner, S., Pearson, T. and Yusuf, S. (1998) 'Elevated lipoprotein (a) levels in South Asians in North America', *Metabolism*, 47, 182–184.

Artaud-Wild, S.M., Connor, S.L., Sexton, G. and Connor, W.E. (1993) ' Differences in coronary mortality can be explained by differences in cholesterol and saturated fat intakes in 40 countries but not in France and Finland. A paradox', *Circulation*, 88, 2771–2779.

Balarajan, R. (1991) 'Ethnic differences in mortality from ischemic heart disease and cerebrovascular disease in England and Wales', *British Medical Journal*, 302, 560–564.

Balarajan, R. (1996) 'Ethnicity and variations in mortality from coronary heart disease', *Health Trends*, 28, 45–51.

Becker, T., Wiggins, C. Key, C. and Samet, J. (1988) 'Ischemic heart disease mortality in Hispanic American Indians and non-Hispanic whites in New Mexico, 1958–1982', *Circulation*, 78, 302–309.

Berrios, X., Koponen, T., Huiguang, T., Khaltaev, N., Puska, P. and Nissinen, A. on behalf of the Inter-Health sites (1997) 'Distribution and prevalence of major risk factors of noncommunicable diseases in selected countries: the WHO Inter-Health Program', *Bulletin of the World Health Organization*, 75, 99–108.

Bhatnagar, D., Anand, I.S., Durrington, P.N., Patel, D. J., Wander, G.S., Mackness, M.I., Creed, F., Tomenson, B., Chandrashekar, Y. and Winterbottom, M. (1995) 'Coronary risk factors in people from the Indian subcontinent living in west London and their siblings in India', *Lancet*, 345, 405–409.

Bothig, S. (1989) 'WHO MONICA Project: objectives and design', *International Journal of Epidemiology*, 18 (Suppl. 1), S29–S37.

Chen, Z., Peto, R. MacMahon, S., Lu, J. and Li, W. (1991) 'Serum cholesterol concentration and coronary heart disease in population with low cholesterol concentrations [see comments]', *British Medical Journal*, 303, 276–282.

Chonhua, Y., Zhaosu, W. and Yingkai, W. (1993) 'The changing pattern of cardiovascular diseases in China', *World Health Statistics Quarterly* 46, 113–118.

Criqui, M.H. and Ringel, B.L. (1994) 'Does diet or alcohol explain the French Paradox?' *Lancet* 344, 1719–1723.

Donnan, S.P., Ho, S.C., Woo, J., Wong, S.L., Woo, K.S., Tse, C.Y., Chan, K.K., Kay, C.S., Cheung, K.O. and Mak, K.H. (1994) 'Risk factors for acute myocardial infarction in a southern Chinese population', *Annals of Epidemiology*, 4, 46–58.

Enas, E.A., Yusuf, S. and Mehta, J. (1992) 'Prevalence of coronary artery disease in Asian Indians', *American Journal of Cardiology*, 70, 945–949.

Fang, J., Madhavan, S. and Alderman, M.H. (1996) 'The association between birthplace and mortality from cardiovascular causes among black and white residents of New York City' *New England Journal of Medicine*, 335, 1545–1551.

Frerichs, R.R., Chapman, J.M. and Maes, E.F. (1984) 'Mortality due to all causes and to cardiovascular diseases among seven race-ethnic populations in Los Angeles County, 1980', *International Journal of Epidemiology*, 13, 291–298.

Fujishima, M., Kiyohara, Y., Kato, I., Ohmura, T., Iwamoto, H., Nakayama, K., Ohmori, S. and Yoshitake, T. (1996) 'Diabetes and cardiovascular disease in a prospective population survey in Japan: The Hisayama Study', *Diabetes*, 45 (Suppl. 3), S14–S16.

Geronimus, A.T., Bound, J., Waidmann, T.A., Hillemeier, M.M. and Burns, P.B. (1996) 'Excess mortality among blacks and whites in the United States', *New England Journal of Medicine*, 335, 1552–1558.

Gillum, R.F. (1989) 'Sudden coronary death in the United States: 1980–1985', *Circulation*, 79, 756–765.

Gillum, R.F. (1995a) 'Epidemiology of stroke in Hispanic Americans', *Stroke*, 26, 1707–1712.

Gillum, R.F. (1995b) 'The epidemiology of stroke in Native Americans', *Stroke*, 26, 514–521.

Goff, D.C., Ramsey, D., Labarthe, D.R. and Nichaman, M.Z. (1993) 'Acute myocardial infarction and coronary heart disease mortality among Mexican Americans and non-Hispanic whites in Texas, 1980 through 1989', *Ethnicity Disease*, 3, 64–69.

Goff, D.C., Jr, Ramsey, D.J., Labarthe, D.R. and Nichaman, M.Z. (1994) 'Greater case-fatality after myocardial infarction among Mexican Americans and women than among non-Hispanic whites and men. The Corpus Christi Heart Project', *American Journal of Epidemiology*, 139, 474–483.

Goff, D.C., Nichaman, M.Z., Chan, W., Ramsey, D.J., Labarthe, D.R. and Ortiz, C. (1997) 'Greater incidence of hospitalized myocardial infarction among Mexican-Americans than Hispanic Whites. The Corpus Christi Heart Project, 1988–1992', *Circulation*, 95, 1433–1440.

Gupta, R. and Gupta, V.P. (1996); Meta-analysis of coronary heart disease prevalence in India', *Indian Heart Journal*, 48, 241–245.

Haffner, S.M., Valdez, R.A., Hazuda, H.P., Mitchell, B.D., Morales, P.A. and Stern, M.P. (1992) 'Prospective analysis of the insulin-resistance syndrome (syndrome X)', *Diabetes*, 41, 715–722.

Hong, Y., Bots, M.L., Pan, X., Hofman, A., Grobbee, D.E. and Chen, H. (1994) 'Stroke incidence and mortality in rural and urban Shanghai from 1984 through 1991. Findings from a community-based registry', *Stroke*, 25, 1165–1169.

Howard, B.V., Lee, E.T., Cowan, L.D., Fabsitz, R.R., Howard, W.J., Oopik, A.J., Robbins, D.C., Savage, P.J., Yeh, J.L. and Welty, T.K. (1995) 'Coronary heart disease prevalence and its relation to risk factors in American Indians. The Strong Heart Study', *American Journal of Epidemiology*, 142, 254–268.

Hughes, K., Yeo, P.P., Lun, K.C., Thai, A.C., Sothy, S.P., Wang, K.W., Cheah, J.S., Phoon, W.O. and Lim, P. (1990) 'Cardiovascular diseases in Chinese, Malays, and Indians in Singapore. II. Differences in risk factor levels', *Journal of Epidemiology and Community Health*, 44, 29–35.

Iso, H., Komachi, Y., Shimamoto, T., Iida and M. (1996) *Trends for Cardiovascular Risk Factors and Disease in Japan: Implications for Primordial Prevention*, pp. 52–54.

Klatsky, A.L., Tekawa, I., Armstrong, M.A. and Sidney, S. (1994) 'The risk of hospitalization for ischemic heart disease among Asian Americans in northern California', *American Journal of Public Health*, 84, 1672–1675.

Law, M.R. (1999) 'Why heart disease mortality is low in France: the time-lag explanation', *British Medical Journal*, 318, 1471–1476.

Lenfant, C. (1994) 'Task force on research in epidemiology and prevention of cardiovascular diseases', *Circulation*, 90, 2609–2617.

Li, N., Tuomilehto, J., Dowse, G., Alberti, K.G., Zimmet, P., Min, Z., Chitson, P., Gareeboo, H., Chonghua, Y. and Fareed, D. (1992) 'Electrocardiographic abnormalities and associated factors in Chinese living in Beijing and in Mauritius. The Mauritius Non-Communicable Disease Study Group', *British Medical Journal*, 304, 1596–1601.

Lowy, A.G.J., Woods, K.L. and Botha, J.L. (1991) 'The effects of demographic shift on coronary heart disease mortality in a large migrant population at high risk', *Journal of Public Health Medicine*, 13, 276–280.

McKeigue, P.M., Shah, B. and Marmot, M.G. (1991) 'Relation of central obesity and insulin resistance with high diabetes prevalence and cardiovascular risk in south Asians', *Lancet*, 337, 382–386.

McKeigue, P.M., Ferrie, J.E., Pierpoint, T. and Marmot, M.G. (1993) 'Association of early-onset coronary heart disease in south Asian men with glucose intolerance and hyperinsulinemia', *Circulation*, 87, 152–161.

Mao, Y., Moloughney, B.W., Semenciw, R.M. and Morrison, H.I. (1992) 'Indian reserve and registered Indian mortality in Canada', *Canadian Journal of Public Health*, 83, 350–353.

Marmot, M. (1995) 'Coronary heart disease: rise and fall of a modern epidemic', in Marmot, M. and Elliot, P. (eds) *Coronary Heart Disease Epidemiology*, Oxford: Oxford University Press, pp. 3–19.

Menotti, A., Keys, A., Kromhout, D., Blackburn, H., Aravanis, C., Bloemberg, B., Buzina, R., Dontas, A., Fidanza, F., Giampaoli, S. *et al.* (1993) 'Inter-cohort differences in coronary heart disease mortality in the 25-year follow-up of the Seven Countries study', *European Journal of Epidemiology*, 9, 527–536.

Miller, G.J., Beckles, G.L., Maude, G.H., Carson, D.C., Alexis, S.D. and Price, S.G. (1989) 'Ethnicity and other characteristics predictive of coronary heart disease in a developing community: principal results of the St James Survey, Trinidad', *International Journal of Epidemiology*, 18, 808–817.

Morgenstern, L.B., Spears, W.D., Goff, D.C., Grotta, J.C. and Nichaman, M.Z. (1997) 'African Americans and women have the highest stroke mortality in Texas', *Stroke*, 28, 15–18.

Murray, C.J. (1994) 'Quantifying the burden of disease: the technical basis for disability-adjusted life years', *Bulletin of the World Health Organization*, 72, 429–445.

Murray, C.J. and Lopez, A.D. (1997a) 'Mortality by cause for eight regions of the world: Global Burden of Disease Study', *Lancet*, 349, 1269–1276.

Murray, C.J.L. and Lopez, A.D. (1997b) 'Alternative projections of mortality and disability by cause 1990–2020, Global Burden of Disease Study', *Lancet*, 349, 1498–1504.

Pais, P., Pogue, J., Gerstein, H., Zachariah, E., Savitha, D., Jayprakash, S., Nayak, P.R. and Yusuf, S. (1996) 'Risk factors for acute myocardial infarction in Indians: a case control study', *Lancet*, 348, 358–63.

People's Republic of China-United States Cardiovascular and Cardiopulmonary Epidemiology Research Group (1992) 'An epidemiological study of cardiovascular and cardiopulmonary disease risk factors in four populations in the People's Republic of China', *Circulation*, 85, 1083–1096.

Ramachandran, A., Dharmaraj, D., Snehalatha, C. and Viswanathan, M. (1992) 'Prevalence of glucose intolerance in Asian Indians', *Diabetes Care*, 15, 1348–1355.

Reddy, K.S. (1993) 'Cardiovascular diseases in India', *World Health Statistics Quarterly*, 46, 101–107.

Schwartz, L.M. (1999) 'Misunderstandings about the effects of race and sex on physicians' referrals for cardiac catheterization', *New England Journal of Medicine*, 341, 279–283.

Seedat, Y.K. (1996) 'Ethnicity, hypertension, coronary heat disease, and renal diseases in South Africa', *Ethnicity and Health*, 1, 349–357.

Sheth, T., Chagani, K., Nargundkar, M., Anand, S., Nair, C. and Yusuf, S. (2000) 'Ethnic differences in cause-specific mortality: south Asians, Chinese, whites in Canada', *Ethnicity and Health*, 234 (in press).

Sheth, T., Nair, C., Nargundkar, M., Anand, S. and Yusuf, S. (1999) 'Cardiovascular and cancer mortality among Canadians of European, south Asian and Chinese origin from 1979 to 1993, an analysis of 1.2 million deaths', *Canadian Medical Association Journal*, 161, 132–138.

Stern, M. and Gaskill, S. (1987) 'Secular decline in death rates due to ischemic heart disease in Mexican Americans and non-Hispanic whites, Texas 1970–1980', *Circulation*, 76, 1245–1250.

Tao, S.C., Huang, Z.D., Wu, X.G., Zhou, B.F., Xiao, Z.K., Hao, J.S., Li, Y.H., Cen, R.C. and Rao, X.X. (1989) 'CHD and its risk factors in the People's Republic of China', *International Journal of Epidemiology*, 18(3) (Suppl. 1), S159–S163.

Thorvaldsen, P., Asplund, K., Kuulasmaa, K., Rajakangas, A.M. and Schroll, M. (1995) 'Stroke incidence, case fatality, and mortality in the WHO MONICA project', World Health Organization monitoring trends and determinants in cardiovascular disease [published erratum appears in *Stroke* 1995, 26(8), 1504] *Stroke*, 26, 361–367.

Vartiainen, E., Puska, P., Pekkanen, J., Tuomilehto, J. and Jousilahti, P. (1994) 'Changes in risk factors explain changes in mortality from ischemic heart disease in Finland', *British Medical Journal*, 309, 23–27.

Woo, K.S. and Donnan, S.P. (1989) 'Epidemiology of coronary arterial disease in the Chinese [Review]', *International Journal of Cardiology*, 24, 83–93.

World Health Statistical Annual 1998, Geneva, World Health Organization.

Zatonski, W.A., McMichael, A.J., Powles, J.W. (1998) 'Ecological study of reasons for sharp decline in mortality from ischemic heart disease in Poland since 1991', *British Medical Journal*, 316, 1047–1051.

13 Ethnicity and the risk of cancer

D. Max Parkin

Introduction

Ever since international data on cancer incidence and mortality have been available, it has been clear that there are large differences in the risk of specific cancers in different populations. Muir (1996) cites the early observations of Hoffman (1915), drawing attention to the tenfold difference in mortality from cancer of the breast between Japanese and British women. If the primary variable of interest is ethnicity, or racial group, the differences observed within the same geographic locality are more meaningful since at least some of the environmental differences present in international comparisons are reduced or eliminated. There are plenty of examples of such studies from multi-ethnic populations in all parts of the world – for example the White and Black populations of Harare, Zimbabwe (Bassett *et al.* 1995), the Chinese, Indian and Malay populations of Singapore (Lee *et al.* 1988) and, above all, studies from the United States (Miller *et al.* 1996) (Figure 13.1).

The simple comparison of age-standardised incidence rates by cancer site may disguise some important differences between ethnic groups which vary by age group, or histological sub-type of cancer, pointing out the importance of different aetiological factors, known or unknown, related in some way to race or ethnicity. Thus, the Black–White difference in the incidence of breast cancer in the United States varies with age, with higher incidence in pre-menopausal Black women and higher incidence in White women after the menopause (Figure 13.2). The much higher incidence of oesophageal cancer in Black men than in White men in the United States is confined to squamous cell carcinoma; for adenocarcinoma the reverse is found.

What accounts for ethnic variation in risk?

Valid comparisons can only be made using valid data, and, although this seems a banal point to make, there are many instances of uncritical use of poor-quality data in comparative studies. Thus, in particular, international mortality statistics are of very variable quality, and care should be taken in their selection. Even within a single country, it is possible that differential

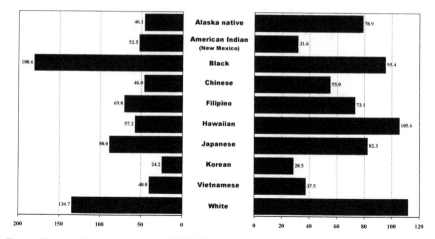

Figure 13.1 Incidence rates (per 100,000) of prostate (left) and breast(right) cancers, by race or ethnicity, in the United States [Surveillance, Epidemiology and End Results (SEER) program data, 1988–92, age-standardised to the United States population of 1970]. From Miller *et al.* (1996).

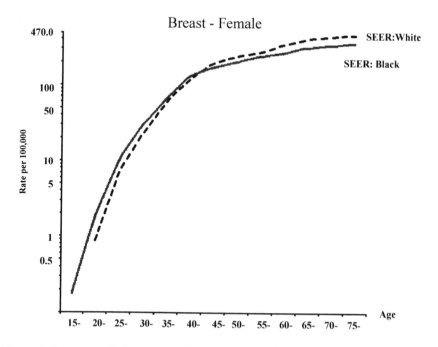

Figure 13.2 Age-specific incidence of breast cancer in the United States, SEER 1988–92, Black people versus White people (Parkin *et al.* 1997).

access to health care and diagnostic services by ethnic group *may* influence reporting rates of disease, though this is unlikely to be a major problem for cancer. A possible exception is in screening programmes. Screening may result in increases in reported incidence of disease, because of detection of latent cancers that would otherwise never have surfaced clinically. This is a particular problem with screening for cancer of the prostate (Brawley 1997) and for neuroblastoma (Bessho 1996), and it probably accounts too for part of the recorded increases in breast cancer incidence in some countries (Quinn and Allen 1995, Garne *et al.* 1997). Certainly, access to and acceptance of screening programmes has been shown to differ by ethnic group in several countries (Seow *et al.* 1997, Parker *et al.* 1998).

Differences in access to treatment certainly can affect outcome, so that survival rates from cancer are well known to vary by race or ethnicity (Baquet and Ringen 1986). Since mortality rates are determined by both incidence of disease and survival, this is a major consideration if mortality is being used, as it often is unconsciously, to provide information on cancer risk. From the data in Table 13.1, it is clear that differences of 50 per cent or more in mortality rates between the ethnic groups might easily occur as a consequence of survival differentials, rather than differences in incidence. From a public health point of view, statistics on numbers of deaths, person-years of life lost, etc., may be the relevant measure to use. There is also a considerable literature on the *reasons* for observed differences in survival between ethnic groups – do they represent variation in stage at presentation, tumour sub-types, host vulnerability, treatment received or response to it (Howard *et al.* 1992)? However, these do not concern us in this chapter, where the focus is on *differences in the risk of disease* by race or ethnicity, so we have chosen to concentrate upon statistics on cancer incidence.

Artefact aside, the principal question posed by observed inter-ethnic differences in risk is how much is due to variation in exposure (to 'carcinogens' or 'risk factors') and how much is the result of inherent differences in susceptibility to such exposures (and hence genetically determined).

Table 13.1 Five-year relative survival rate (%) by site and racial or ethnic group, United States Surveillance Epidemiology and End Results (SEER) Program, 1973–81 (Baquet and Ringen 1986)

Site	White	Black	Hispanic	Japanese	Chinese	Filipino	Hawaiian	Native Americans
Stomach	14	15	16	28	16	16	14	9
Colon	52	46	48	61	53	38	59	44
Rectum	49	37	44	55	44	45	42	24
Lung	12	11	11	14	15	12	16	5
Breast	75	63	72	85	78	72	78	53
Cervix	68	63	69	72	72	72	73	67
Bladder	74	50	70	72	74	49	48	37

From an epidemiological point of view, the variable 'ethnicity' or 'race' defines a constellation of genetic factors, which relate to susceptibility to a given cancer. Of course, there is considerable variation *within* a given ethnic or racial group (however this is defined), but there are often sufficiently large differences between them to yield distinctive patterns of risk. If 'ethnicity' is the variable of interest, the first consideration is to eliminate the effect of confounding variables, associated with the risk of disease and differentially distributed by ethnic group. As usual, such 'confounders' can be considered at several levels – so-called demographic variables such as social class (or occupation, educational level), place of residence, marital status, and so on, or more defined exposures such as tobacco, alcohol, diet, infection for which the demographic variables are themselves proxies.

In general, two approaches have been used to examine the relative contributions of ethnicity *per se* (genetic predisposition) and environmental exposures in determining risk.

1   *Descriptive studies*: These use pre-existing data sets in which the available variables include race or ethnic group, plus other rather non-specific indicators of exposure – for example, place of residence, socio-economic status, etc., as crude indicators of a whole host of environmental exposures.
2   *Analytical studies*: They involve individual data collection, by interview or biological materials (sometimes thereby attracting the name of 'molecular' epidemiology), or both, in multi-ethnic populations. The usual study designs (case–control, cohort) are used to estimate relative risk and prevalence of the different exposures, and to calculate the fraction of disease attributable to each 'exposure' – including 'ethnic group'.

Descriptive studies of ethnicity and cancer

A striking illustration of the likely influence of genetic factors on risk of cancer is provided by certain cancers of childhood. For several – for example Wilms' tumour and Ewing's sarcoma (Figure 13.3), there are very marked differences in incidence between ethnic groups for which no plausible environmental 'exposure' can be imagined. Any such exposure would have to be very carcinogenic (to act so early in life), very tissue specific, and be very unevenly distributed by ethnic group.

The most fruitful approach using routine data sources is through the study of migrants (Parkin and Khlat 1996). The rationale is quite simple. The risk of different cancers in a given migrant population is compared with that in the host population (similar environment, different genetics) and in the population living in place of origin (similar genetics, different environment). Ideally, such comparisons can take into account the age at migration, or the duration of residence in the two environments [original (origin), new (host)], as a crude means of quantifying 'exposure' to the new environment. They

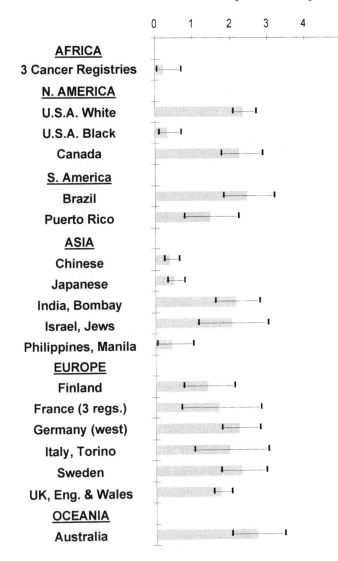

Figure 13.3 International variations in the incidence rates of Ewing's sarcoma in children (age-standardised incidence rates per million, and 95 per cent confidence intervals) (Stiller and Parkin 1996).

may also be able to compare the risk in the migrants with that in their offspring, who have lived in the new 'environment' throughout life. As noted earlier, all environmental exposures are subsumed by a single variable (place of residence). Many specific exposures are associated with this, not only via the external environment (air, soil, water), but also through socio-cultural factors (diet, fertility, smoking, etc.). Occasionally, there may be information on other indirectly associated variables (e.g. socio-economic status), which can be taken into account in estimating the ethnicity-associated component of risk.

Analytic studies of ethnicity and cancer

Estimation of the magnitude of the risk associated with different environmental exposures has been the staple fare of epidemiologists for more than 50 years. Methodological developments have allowed the refinement of the measurement of biomarkers of both exposure and outcome, which, despite the denomination of a multitude of new subspecialties, has not essentially altered the paradigms of methodology or deduction (McMichael 1994). Most research has focused on quantifying individual risk associated with exposure to environmental agents (the latter including behavioural variables – such as reproductive patterns). In general, there has been little interest in how much these may explain differences in risk between populations (Prentice and Sheppard 1989). Although 'ethnicity' is, and was, included as a variable in such analyses, in general there has been little interest in it as an explanatory variable *per se*. The importance of genetic susceptibility in modulating individual risk has become more obvious in recent years. This coincides with the development of new laboratory techniques. Until recently, genetic differences between populations were only recognisable through phenotypic markers such as blood group, the histocompatibility (HLA, human leucocyte antigen) system antigens, or the metabolism of marker substances. Now that direct genotyping has become possible, there is a rush of activity to identify genetic markers of risk with, again, the most effort focused upon individual differences within populations.

Genetic basis of cancer susceptibility

Genetically determined risk may be mediated by several mechanisms (Easton 1994, Ishibe and Kelsey 1997, Norppa 1997):

1   through germline mutations of genes which are normally concerned with the regulation of cell growth (oncogenes, tumour-suppressor genes);
2   variation in the genes (polymorphisms) which modulate the impact of environmental carcinogens
    – polymorphisms of carcinogen-metabolising enzymes
    – inherited differences in DNA adduct formation
    – variation in ability to repair DNA lesions induced by a carcinogen.

The risks associated with mutations to tumour-associated genes are very high. Genetic linkage studies among families with multiple cases of early-onset breast and/or ovarian cancer identified the gene *BRCA1*, located on chromosome 17q21 (Hall *et al.* 1990, Narod *et al.* 1991). In women carriers of this gene, the risk of breast cancer is increased thirty to fiftyfold in pre-menopausal women (Easton *et al.* 1995). However, the prevalence of the gene in the general population is low, so that the population-attributable fraction is small. For example, in the average White population, the prevalence of women carrying the gene (homozygotes or heterozygotes) is only around 1 in 800 (0.12 per cent) (Ford and Easton 1995), so that the population attributable fraction (PAF) calculated from the usual formula (Levin 1953)

$$\frac{P(r-1)}{1+P(r-1)}$$

is just 0.045 or 4.5 per cent.

On the other hand, most of the genetic polymorphisms in carcinogen-metabolising enzymes investigated to date confer only modest relative risks (often less than 2), but they are much more prevalent in the general population. For example, about 50 per cent of the population are glutathione-S-transferase-1 (*GSTM1*) deletion homozygotes (Rebbeck 1997); several studies have found that this genotype is associated with an increased risk of lung cancer, or of bladder cancer, although the relative risks are not high – around 1.5 on meta-analysis (d'Errico *et al.* 1996). The fraction of disease attributable to these polymorphisms could, therefore, be around 20 per cent.

How much of the risk *between* different ethnic groups might be accounted for by such genetic differences? This depends on the difference in the prevalence of susceptible genotypes in the different populations. The relative risk (RR) between two populations is given by:

$$RR = \frac{P_a(r-1)+1}{P_b(r-1)+1}$$

where P_a and P_b are the prevalences in the two populations, and r is the risk for those individuals with the susceptible genotype compared with those with the non-susceptible genotype (Gilliland 1997). The maximum relative risk between populations is therefore the ratio of the two prevalences; the actual risk depends on the values of P and r. Figure 13.4 illustrates a situation with a twofold difference in prevalence between populations – the relative risk between them increases with the value of r, but much more rapidly when the genetic susceptibility genotype is common.

Examples of ethnic differences in cancer risk

Malignant melanoma of the skin

This cancer shows very wide variations in cancer risk worldwide, from an

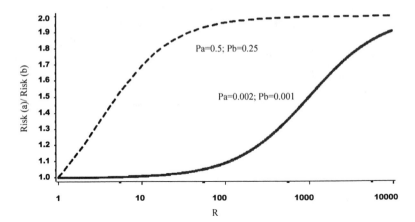

Figure 13.4 The relative risk between two populations (a and b) at different levels of
risk (R) associated with a particular genetic susceptibility, within each of
them. Upper curve: the prevalence of susceptibility genotype in population
a = 0.5 and in population b = 0.25. Lower curve: the prevalence of
susceptibility genotype in population a = 0.002 and in population b =
0.001.

age-standardised rate (in men) of over 30 per 100,000 in the predominantly
White population of New South Wales and Western Australia, to less than 1
per 100,000 in India, China and Japan (Parkin *et al.* 1997). It is well known
that exposure to solar ultraviolet (UV) radiation – particularly strong,
intermittent exposure resulting in sunburn – is a strong predictor of risk at
the individual level (Elwood and Jopson 1997). So, in studies of migrants
moving from regions with low to regions with high levels of ambient solar
irradiation (for example to Israel or Australia from different countries of
Europe) the incidence of melanoma increases. The increase is greatest in
individuals who migrate in childhood, rather than adults, because of the
greater cumulative exposure possible, and also, probably, because of the role
of UV radiation in inducing naevi in childhood (Khlat *et al.* 1992).

It is clear that UV exposure is not the whole explanation of international
differences, however, as shown by the striking variations in risk between
different ethnic groups within the same country – for example in the United
States or in Australia. The genetic basis for these differences is easily
recognised with such obvious phenotypic markers as cutaneous melanin. The
heavy pigmentation of the skin of populations of African descent is manifestly
protective against the induction of melanoma by UV light on the exposed
areas of skin; the incidence of acral lentiginous melanomas located on the
non-pigmented soles of the feet, or palms of the hand, is identical in the
Black and White populations of the United States (Stevens *et al.* 1990).
Melanin pigmentation is not the whole story, however. Populations of East
Asian origin – for example the Japanese – also have very low rates of

melanoma, despite relatively slight skin pigmentation, even when they move to sunny climates such as Australia (Grulich *et al.* 1995), California or Hawaii (Parkin *et al.* 1997), although, as for Black populations, the incidence of acral lentiginous melanoma (mainly on the soles of the feet) is much the same as in White populations (Elwood 1989). Dysplastic melanocytic naevi, which are frequently associated with malignant melanoma in White populations (up to one-third of cases), are very rare in Japan (Jimbow *et al.* 1989, Kuno *et al.* 1996); hence, differences in DNA repair mechanisms may also be involved.

Nasopharyngeal carcinoma

Nasopharyngeal carcinoma (NPC) is a rare malignancy in most parts of the world, but the incidence is relatively high in the southern provinces of China (Guangdong, Guanxi, Hunan and Fujian) (Li *et al.* 1979) and in Inuit (Eskimo) populations of Alaska and northern Canada (Nielsen *et al.* 1996). NPC occurs with moderately raised incidence in populations from South-East Asia: Vietnam, Philippines, Thailand and Malaysia (Parkin *et al.* 1997). An area of intermediate risk is also observed in north Africa (Shanmugaratnam 1982), although here the epidemiological features are a little different, with a peak of incidence occurring in adolescence and young adults. Within the high-risk areas of China, there are differences in rates between the several ethnic groups living there. The highest rates occur in the boat-dwelling Tankas living in central Guangdong, who have an incidence double that of land-dwelling Cantonese, who in turn have rates higher than those of the Hakka and Chiu-Chau dialect groups, living in eastern Guangdong (Li *et al.* 1985). The people of Fujian province are culturally similar to the Chiu-Chau people of Guangdong province, and so are their rates of NPC. In northern China, the incidence of NPC is not remarkable – in Tianjin the age-standardised rate in men is 1.6 per 100,000 (compared with 24.3 in Hong Kong), which is not much higher than in some European populations (Parkin *et al.* 1997).

Environmental risk factors for NPC have been extensively studied. The Epstein–Barr virus (EBV) is now generally accepted to be important in carcinogenesis at this site – the viral genome is present in all NPCs, and in monoclonal form, implying that its presence antedates the tumour; it is never found in normal epithelial cells in the nasopharynx (IARC 1997). However, infection with EBV is a ubiquitous human experience, so that it can by no means explain the striking geographic and ethnic patterns, and other agents must be involved. Among the environmental exposures, the most convincing are certain dietary items, particularly, in Asian populations, salted, preserved fish (Hildesheim and Levine 1993, IARC 1997), and, in North Africa, certain spices (Jeannel *et al.* 1990). It is far from clear whether these exposures can explain the geographic or ethnic patterns of NPC, but it does seem rather unlikely. The risk of NPC in Chinese living in the United States is high, and, although the risk of Chinese born in the United States is about half that of migrants born in China, it remains at least ten times higher than in the

White population of the United States (Buell 1974). Migrants to Israel from north Africa also have higher risks of NPC than the local population, and furthermore the offspring of such migrants retain their elevated risk comparison with individuals with locally born parents (Parkin and Iscovich 1997) (Figure 13.5). In Singapore, the different Chinese dialect groups preserve the ratio of risks observed in southern China, with the highest risk in Cantonese (double that in other dialect groups) and little change in incidence between the local born and the migrants from China (Lee *et al.* 1988). These observations suggest a genetic basis underlying some, if not most, of the geographic or ethnic differences in risk. Several studies within populations of southern Chinese origin have identified associations between HLA locus A and B antigens and NPC risk (Chan *et al.* 1983). It is not clear how much of the difference between populations could be attributed to HLA profiles, though Simons and colleagues (1976) did note that the frequency of the A2-B46 phenotype – associated with a relative risk of about 2 – was twice as common in Cantonese relative to the Chiu-Chau or Fujianese dialect groups, in parallel with the twofold difference in NPC incidence. In any case, the HLA phenotype may be only a marker for a more directly involved genetic mechanism. A linkage study based on affected sub-pairs among southern Chinese in China, Hong Kong, Singapore and Malaysia suggests that a gene

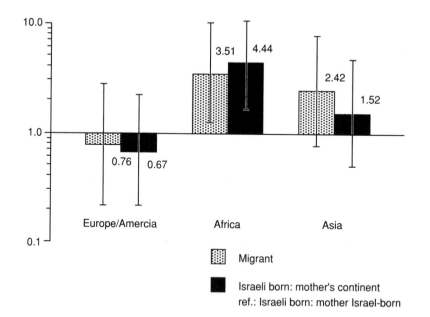

Figure 13.5 Nasopharynx cancer. Odds ratios (ORs) by birthplace, for migrants and Israeli-born cases with migrant mother. The reference category (baseline: OR = 1) is cases born in Israel with mother born in Israel (Parkin and Iscovich, 1997).

(or genes) closely linked to the HLA locus is associated with a twentyfold increased risk of NPC (Lu *et al.* 1990). Some cancers show deletions at specific regions of chromosome 9 (Lo *et al.* 1995). However, the genetic basis of susceptibility to NPC remains largely an enigma.

Breast cancer

For breast cancer, a clear inherited component has now been identified, with the cloning of two breast cancer susceptibility genes, *BRCA1* (chromosome 17q) and *BRCA2* (chromosome 13q). These two genes account for many of the familial cases of breast cancer. The effect of a germline mutation in one of the pair of alleles is to greatly increase the risk of developing breast cancer (Ford and Easton 1995).

The pattern of age-specific breast cancer risk in gene carriers is different from that of the general population, with, relatively, a much higher risk in young women (100-fold under age 30) than in older women (around tenfold at age 60) (Figure 13.6).

There are various estimates of the gene frequency in the population, but most place it, in Western populations, between 0.02 per cent and 0.1 per cent, probably around 0.06 per cent (Ford and Easton 1995). For a dominant gene, the carrier frequency is given by $q(2 - q)$, where q is the frequency of

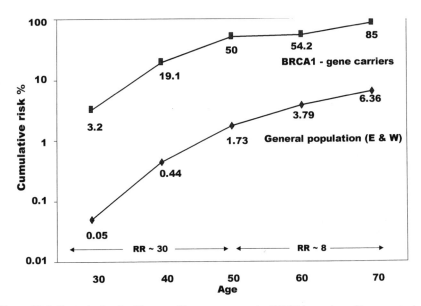

Figure 13.6 Cumulative incidence of breast cancer in *BRCA1* carriers (Easton *et al.* 1995) compared with the cumulative incidence in the general population of England and Wales in 1988–90 (Parkin *et al.* 1997).

the mutated gene. Thus, on average, around 0.12 per cent of the population will be carriers. It is therefore possible to estimate the proportion of breast cancers in the population which are due to *BRCA1* (Table 13.2).

Recently, it has been observed that *BRCA1* mutations are more common in women of Ashkenazi Jewish origin – around 1 per cent of this population are carriers (Goldgar and Reilly 1995). This is a population which is known to have a relatively high incidence of breast cancer – the cumulative incidence of breast cancer (0–69) in Israeli Jews of European origin is around 8.2 per cent compared with 5.2 per cent in Israeli Jews of African or Asian origin, 2.1 per cent in non-Jews living in Israel and between 4 per cent and 5 per cent in other populations from southern Europe (Spain, Slovenia, southern Italy) (Table 13.3).

Could these differences in incidence be due to variations in the prevalence of *BRCA1*? If the prevalence of *BRCA1* were ten times higher in Ashkenazi Jews than in the other populations in Table 13.3 (1 per cent versus 0.1 per cent), and the relative risk in the age range 20–69 was 50, then this could account for a difference as great as 1.5-fold (i.e. a relative risk in the

Table 13.2 Estimated percentage of breast cancer cases due to germline *BRCA1* mutations (Ford and Easton 1995)

Age (years)	Gene frequency (carrier frequency)		
	0.0002 (0.04%)	0.0006 (0.12%)	0.001 (0.2%)
20–29	2.6	7.5	11.9
30–39	1.7	5.1	8.2
40–49	0.7	2.2	3.6
50–59	0.5	1.4	2.4
60–69	0.3	0.8	1.3
20–69	0.6	1.7	2.8

Table 13.3 Breast cancer incidence in Mediterranean populations

	Cumulative incidence (0–69)%	Relative risk (95% CI)
Israel		
Jews born in Europe/America	8.2	1.0
Jews born in Africa/Asia	5.2	0.64 (0.61–0.67)
Non-Jews	2.1	0.27 (0.24–0.31)
Spain (nine cancer registries)	4.2	0.52 (0.51–0.53)
Slovenia	4.2	0.52 (0.50–0.54)
Southern Italy (Latina and Ragusa)	4.4	0.54 (0.50–0.58)

Source: Parkin *et al.* (1997).

comparison populations of 0.67). Thus, even in this particular circumstance, only part of the inter-population difference can be due to known genetic factors. This observation is not really surprising, since it is clear from studies of migrants to Israel that the observed incidence in groups of different origins (as defined by place of birth) can change markedly following migration, with Jews from North Africa, for example, having rates not greatly different from those in Jews of European origin, after 30 years or more residence in the new homeland (Steintz *et al.* 1989). The same effect is seen in Asian migrants to the United States: the marked increases in risk between generations (Ziegler *et al.* 1993) are in no way compatible with genetic variations as an explanation of the major part of the risk differentials between the United States and Asian countries (China, Japan, Philippines). In fact, for some observed differences in ethnicity, there is no need to call upon genetic difference by way of an explanation. From a case–control study in Atlanta and New Jersey of 1,241 young women (age 30–55) with breast cancer, Brinton and colleagues (1997) examined the relative risks due to reproductive variables (number of births, age at first birth, age at menarche) and lifestyle factors (body mass index, alcohol use, contraceptive use). With the relative risk and prevalence of these risk factors in White and Black women, the proportion of breast cancer cases that are attributable to them can be calculated. One can also estimate how much of the relative risk between the two populations can be explained – it was 1.21 – just about what is actually observed in Atlanta (1.20). This implies that, at equal levels of these variables, the rates would be the same.

Oral cancers

Day *et al.* (1993) used the data from a very large case–control study, with 1,065 subjects with oral cancer recruited in four centres, to determine how much of the observed differences in incidence rates between White people and Black people in the United States might be due to variations in exposures to carcinogens, rather than differential sensitivity to them. As with other investigators, they noted a strong effect of alcohol and tobacco smoking, which were multiplicative on risk. Population-attributable fractions for these two exposures were calculated, and, when the incidence rates in unexposed individuals were estimated, they were much the same in the four sex and ethnic groups, implying that these two exposures explain the difference in incidence. The odds ratios (ORs) for smoking were much the same in the two ethnic groups, but they were rather higher among Black people than among White people for alcohol drinking, though the differences were not statistically significant.

Cancer of the oesophagus

In a similar study, Brown and co-workers (1994) investigated the risk of squamous cell carcinoma of the oesophagus in men from three centres in the United States (124 White, 249 Black) in relation to smoking and alcohol status. It was noted already that incidence in Black people in the United States is much higher than in White people – the OR for the age group studied (30–79) is 6.9. The risk attributable to smoking and drinking was quite a bit higher for Black people than for White people (93 per cent versus 86 per cent), and this explains a large part of the difference in rates. However, there is still a small residual difference. Furthermore, the difference in population attributable ratios (PARs) is due to significantly higher relative risks for alcohol consumption for Black people than for White people rather than any difference in prevalence of exposure. In a further study (Brown *et al.* 1997), it was observed that the type of alcoholic beverage was not responsible for this difference. The higher relative risk in Black people could be due to other unexplored interactions with, for example, diet. Or it could be due to differences in genetic susceptibility to alcohol, through polymorphisms in genes controlling metabolic enzymes. CYP2E1 is a member of the cytochrome P450 family of enzymes that is inducible by ethanol and participates in the activation of nitrosamines. CYP2E1 shows some ethnic variation in the frequency of the major polymorphism of the encoding genes (Kato *et al.* 1992), and there is some evidence that there is an association between the c1/c2 and c2/c2 genotypes and the risk of oral carcinoma (Hung *et al.* 1997) and hepatocellular carcinoma (Yu, M.W. *et al.* 1995). However, Morita *et al.* (1997) and Hori and colleagues (1997) found no differences in the frequency of these genotypes in oesophageal cancer patients and normal subjects in Japan.

In contrast to the cytochrome P450 family, a striking association has been demonstrated between oesophageal carcinoma and polymorphisms in the genes controlling the alcohol-metabolising enzymes, alcohol dehydrogenase 2 (ADH2) and aldehyde dehydrogenase 2 (ALDH2). ADH2 is the enzyme responsible for metabolising alcohol to acetaldehyde, which is then metabolised further by ALDH2. The prevalence of the mutant alleles *ADH2*2* and *ALDH2*2* is much higher in Asian populations, and these alleles are rare in White populations or in those of African origin (Goedde *et al.* 1992). The *ALDH2*2* gene is dominant, so that heterozygotes have a reduced capacity to metabolise acetaldehyde, and this results in adverse reactions such as facial flushing and tachycardia. Up to 50 per cent of the general population in Japan, for example, are heterozygotes, and this tends to discourage excessive drinking. Nevertheless, Hori and colleagues (1997) found a strong association between the mutant gene and oesophageal cancer (OR = 4.4), and Yokoyama and co-workers (1996) observed an OR of 8 in alcoholics with oesophageal cancer and 12 in 'heavy drinkers'. Acetaldehyde is a known carcinogen in animals, and blood acetaldehyde levels following ethanol ingestion are greatly elevated in homozygotes (nineteenfold) and heterozygotes (sixfold) for *ALDH2*2* (Yamamoto *et al.* 1993).

These polymorphisms might explain the rather high rates of oesophageal cancer in Japan when compared with per capita intake of alcohol (Figure

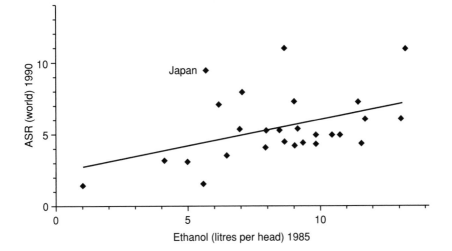

Figure 13.7 Comparison of age-standardised incidence rates of oesophageal cancer in men in 1990 (Parkin *et al.* 1997) with per capita consumption of ethanol in 1995 (IARC 1988) in twenty-eight national populations.

13.7) and the observation that the incidence among Japanese resident in the United States is higher than in the White population (Miller *et al.* 1996). We are not aware of any studies in multi-ethnic populations, containing a significant proportion of Asians, investigating the relative risks at different levels of alcohol consumption.

Bladder cancer

Bladder cancer was one of the first cancers for which variation in genetic susceptibility was suspected to play a role. Exposure to chemicals such as 2-naphthylamine and aminobiphenyls in occupational settings is a known hazard. Both require bioactivation in the body to form carcinogenic metabolites. The first step is N-hydroxylation (catalysed by the hepatic P450 enzyme CYP1A2), while a competing pathway is N-acetylation, catalysed by N-acetyl transferase 2 (NAT2) (Figure 13.8). The gene for NAT2 has two alleles – individuals homozygous for the 'slow' allele are slow acetylators and hence, theoretically, at higher risk of exposure to carcinogenic metabolites through the hydroxylation pathway. Although occupational exposures probably account for a small proportion of bladder cancers, this is not the case for the other major risk factor tobacco smoking, which with a relative risk of around 3 in men will account for 40–50 per cent of cases in Europe or the United States (Parkin *et al.* 1994). Tobacco smoke contains several carcinogenic arylamines, which are likely to be implicated in bladder carcinogenesis (IARC 1986).

Slow or fast acetylators can be identified by phenotype testing – the speed

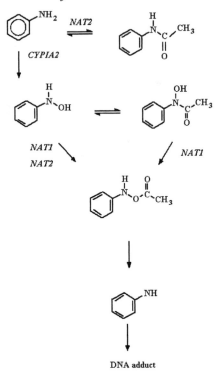

Figure 13.8 Pathways of aromatic amine metabolism.

of metabolism of marker drugs – isoniazid and caffeine have been the most used. A variety of studies suggest an OR for bladder cancer of around 1.5 in slow acetylators versus rapid acetylators (d'Errico *et al.* 1996). It is possible that different prevalences of this polymorphism might explain some of the difference in bladder cancer risk between ethnic groups. In Los Angeles (Yu *et al.* 1994) it was noted that the prevalence of tobacco smoking does not differ much between White people, Asians and Black people, though bladder cancer incidence certainly does. The prevalence of the slow acetylator phenotype follows the risk of bladder cancer (Table 13.4). Similarly, the levels of haemoglobin adducts of 3-amino-biphenyl (3-ABP) were higher in White than in Black people and Asians, at all levels of smoking. This difference is the consequence of the different prevalence of slow acetylators. The ratio of 3-ABP– haemoglobin (Hb) adducts in slow versus fast acetylators was 2.5, and for 4-ABP–Hb adducts 1.2 (not significant) after adjusting for smoking prevalence. Adjustment for prevalence of acetylator status made the ethnic differences in 3-ABP adducts non-significant. In a subsequent study (Yu, M.C. *et al.* 1995) the slow acetylation phenotype combined with the null genotype of the gene *GSTM1* (coding for glutathione-S-transferase, involved in conjugation of several reactive chemicals, including arylamines and

Table 13.4 Bladder cancer and acetylator phenotype in Los Angeles (from Yu *et al.* 1994)

	White	Black	Asian
Bladder cancer incidence[a]			
(cumulative rate, 0–74%)	1.81	1.06	0.76
Slow acetylator (%)	54	34	14
3-ABP–haemoglobin adducts (pg/g)	1.80	1.54	0.73
4-ABP–haemoglobin adducts (pg/g)	49.2	38.5	40.7

Note
a   From Parkin *et al.* (1997).

nitrosamines) resulted in higher levels of the 3- and 4-ABP–Hb adducts than did lower risk profiles (rapid acetylator and/or at least one functional *GSTM1* gene allele). The highest risk profile was seen in 27 per cent of White people, 15 per cent of Black people and 3 per cent of Asians.

Could it be, therefore, that NAT2 prevalence in different populations in part explains ethnic variation in the incidence of bladder cancer? The prevalences and risks in the Los Angeles study can, however, only explain a part of the observed differences [the corresponding attributable risks, with a RR of 1.5, are only 21 per cent (White), 14 per cent (Black) and 7 per cent (Asian)], so it is clearly not the sole explanation.

Conclusion

The triumph of epidemiology over the last 50 years in identifying the major environmental determinants of human cancer (infections, tobacco, diet, radiation, etc.) has inevitably led to an emphasis upon the role which exposure to them plays in determining individual differences in risk, as well as those between populations (Wynder and Gori 1977, Higginson and Muir 1979, Doll and Peto 1981). However, it has always been clear that, for many cancers, an important component of risk differentials between different races, or ethnic groups, is related to genetically determined susceptibility. Initially, some phenotypic correlates provided explanations (for example skin colour and susceptibility to skin tumours), but the recent rapid development of techniques of genotyping have greatly expanded the possibilities for investigation. So far, the direction of research has concentrated upon individual susceptibility to cancer, and the role that this may play in explaining inter-population differences has been of only secondary interest. However, it seems likely that some of the enigmas posed by international or inter-ethnic variations in risk – for example for some of the childhood cancers, for nasopharyngeal cancer, or even for such common cancers as lung (LeMarchand *et al.* 1992, Schwartz and Swanson 1997), stomach (Holcombe 1992) and cervix (Kjaer *et al.* 1988) – may stimulate research into possible underlying genetic mechanisms.

References

Baquet, C.R. and Ringen, K. (1986) *Cancer Among Blacks and Other Minorities: Statistical Profiles*, National Institute of Health Publication No. 86–2785. Bethesda, MD: National Cancer Institute.

Bassett, M.T., Levy, L.M., Chokunonga, E., Mauchaza, B., Ferlay, J. and Parkin, D.M. (1995) 'Cancer in the European population of Harare, Zimbabwe, in 1990–1992', *International Journal of Cancer*, 63, 24–28.

Bessho, F. (1996) 'Effects of mass screening on age-specific incidence of neuroblastoma', *International Journal of Cancer*, 67, 520–522.

Brawley, O.W. (1997) 'Prostate carcinoma incidence and patient mortality: the effects of screening and early detection', *Cancer*, 80, 1857–1863.

Brinton, L.A., Benichou, J., Gammon, M.D., Brogan, D.R., Coates, R. and Schoenberg, J.B. (1997) 'Ethnicity and variation in breast cancer incidence', *International Journal of Cancer*, 73, 349–355.

Brown, L.M., Hoover, R.N., Greenberg, R.S., Schoenberg, J.B., Schwartz, A.G., Swanson, G.M., Liff, J.M., Silverman, D.T., Hayes, R.B. and Pottern, L.M. (1994) 'Are racial differences in squamous-cell esophageal cancer explained by alcohol and tobacco use?', *Journal of the National Cancer Institute*, 86, 1340–1345.

Brown, L.M., Hoover, R., Gridley, G., Schoenberg, J.B., Greenberg, R.S., Silverman, D.T., Schwartz, A.G., Swanson, G.M., Liff, J.M. and Pottern, L.M. (1997) 'Drinking practices and risk of squamous-cell esophageal cancer among Black and White men in the United States', *Cancer Causes and Control*, 8, 605–609.

Buell, P. (1974) 'The effect of migration on the risk of nasopharyngeal cancer among Chinese', *Cancer Research*, 34, 1189–1191.

Chan, S.H., Day, N.E., Kunaratnam, N., Chia, K.B. and Simons, M.J. (1983) 'HLA and nasopharyngeal carcinoma in Chinese: a further study', *International Journal of Cancer*, 32, 171–176.

Day, G.L., Blot, W.J., Austin, D.F., Bernsteinl L., Greenberg, R.S., Preston-Martin, S., Schoenberg, J.B., Winn, D.M., McLaughlin, J.K. and Fraumeni J.F, Jr. (1993) 'Racial differences in risk of oral and pharyngeal cancer: alcohol, tobacco, and other determinants', *Journal of the National Cancer Institute*, 85, 465–473.

d'Errico, A., Taioli, E., Chen, X. and Vineis, P. (1996) 'Genetic metabolic polymorphisms and the risk of cancer: a review of the literature', *Biomarkers*, 1, 149–173.

Doll, R. and Peto, R. (1981) *The Causes of Cancer*, Oxford: Oxford University Press.

Easton, D.F. (1994) 'The inherited component of cancer', *British Medical Bulletin*, 50, 527–535.

Easton, D.F., Ford, D. and Bishop, D.T. (1995) 'Breast and ovarian cancer incidence in BRCA1-mutation carriers. Breast Cancer Linkage Consortium', *American Journal of Human Genetics*, 56, 265–271.

Elwood, J.M. (1989) 'Epidemiology and control of melanoma in white populations and in Japan', *Journal of Investigative Dermatology*, 92, 214S-221S.

Elwood, J.M. and Jopson, J. (1997) 'Melanoma and sun exposure: an overview of published studies', *International Journal of Cancer*, 73, 198–203.

Ford, D. and Easton, D.F. (1995) 'The genetics of breast and ovarian cancer', *British Journal of Cancer*, 72, 805–812.

Garne, J.P., Aspegren, K., Balldin, G. and Ranstam, J. (1997) 'Increasing incidence of and declining mortality from breast carcinoma; trends in Malmo, Sweden, 1961–1992', *Cancer*, 79, 69–74.

Gilliand, F.D. (1997) 'Ethnic differences in cancer incidence: a marker for inherited susceptibility?', *Environmental Health Perspective*, 105(S4), 897–900.

Goedde, H.W., Agarwal, D.P., Fritze, G., Meier, T.D., Singh, S., Beckmann, G., Bhatia, K., Chen, L.Z., Fang, B., Lisker, R., Paik, Y.K., Rothhammer, F., Saha, N., Segal, B., Srivastava, L.M. and Creizel, A. (1992) 'Distribution of ADH2 and ALDH2 genotypes in different populations', *Human Genetics*, 88, 344–346.

Goldgar, D.E. and Reilly, P.R. (1995) 'A common BRCA1 mutation in the Ashkenazim', *National Genetics*, 11, 113–114.

Grulich, A.E., McCredie, M. and Coates, M. (1995) 'Cancer incidence in Asian migrants to New South Wales, Australia', *British Journal of Cancer*, 71, 400–408.

Hall, J.M., Lee, M.K., Newman, B., Morrow, J.E., Anderson, L.A., Huey, B. and King, M.C. (1990) 'Linkage of early-onset familial breast cancer to chromosome 17q21', *Science*, 250, 1684–1689.

Higginson, J. and Muir, C.S. (1979) 'Environmental carcinogenesis: misconception and limitations to cancer control', *Journal of the National Cancer Institute*, 63, 1291–1298.

Hildesheim, A. and Levine, P.H. (1993) 'Etiology of nasopharyngeal carcinoma: a review', *Epidemiology Review*, 15, 466–485.

Hoffman F.L. (1915) *The Mortality from Cancer Throughout the World*, New Jersey: The Prudential Press.

Holcombe, C. (1992) '*Helicobacter pylori:* the African enigma', *Gut*, 33, 429–431.

Hori, H., Kawano, T., Endo, M. and Yuasa, Y. (1997) 'Genetic polymorphisms of tobacco- and alcohol-related metabolizing enzymes and human esophageal squamous cell carcinoma susceptibility', *Journal of Clinical Gastroenterology*, 25, 568–575.

Howard, J., Hankey, B.F., Greenberg, R.S., Austin, D.F., Correa, P., Chen, V.W. and Durako, S. (1992) 'A collaborative study of differences in the survival rates of black patients and white patients with cancer', *Cancer*, 69, 2349–2360.

Hung, H.C., Chuang, J., Chien, Y.C., Chern, H.D., Chiang, C.P., Kuo, Y.S., Hildesheim, A. and Chen, C.J. (1997) 'Genetic polymorphisms of CYP2E1, GSTM1, and GSTT1; environmental factors and risk of oral cancer', *Cancer Epidemiology, Biomarkers & Prevention*, 6, 901–905.

IARC (1986) *Monographs on the Evaluation of Carcinogenic Risks to Humans*, Vol. 38, *Tobacco Smoking*, Lyon: International Agency for Research on Cancer.

IARC (1988) *Monographs on the Evaluation of Carcinogenic Risks to Humans*, Vol. 44, *Alcohol Drinking*, Lyon: International Agency for Research on Cancer.

IARC (1997) *Monographs on the Evaluation of Carcinogenic Risks to Humans*, Vol. 70, *Epstein–Barr Virus and Kaposi's Sarcoma Herpesvirus/Human Herpesvirus 8*, Lyon: International Agency for Research on Cancer.

Ishibe, N. and Kelsey, K.T. (1997) 'Genetic susceptibility to environmental and occupational cancers', *Cancer Causes and Control*, 8, 504–513.

Jeannel, D., Hubert, A., deVathaire, F., Ellouz, R., Camoun, M., Ben Salem, M., Sancho-Garnier, H. and de Thé, G. (1990) 'Diet, living conditions and nasopharyngeal carcinoma in Tunisia: a case–control study', *International Journal of Cancer* 46, 421–425.

Jimbow, K., Horikoshi, T., Takahashi, H., Akutsu, Y. and Maeda, K. (1989) 'Fine structural and immunohistochemical properties of dysplastic melanocytic nevi: comparison with malignant melanoma', *Journal of Investigative Dermatology*, 92, 304S–309S.

Kato, S., Shields, P.G., Caporaso, N.E., Hoover, R.N., Jump, B.F., Sugimura, H., Weston, A. and Harris, C.C. (1992) 'Cytochrome P450II E1 genetic polymorphisms, racial variation and lung cancer risk', *Cancer Research*, 52, 6712–6714.

Khlat, M., Vail, A., Parkin, M. and Green, A. (1992) 'Mortality from melanoma in migrants to Australia: variation by age at arrival and duration of stay', *American Journal of Epidemiology*, 135, 1103–1113.

Kjaer, S.K., De Villiers, E.M., Haugaard, B.J., Christensen, R.B., Teisen, C., Moller, K.A., Poll, P., Jensen, H., Vestergaard, B.F. and Lynge, E. (1988) 'Human papillomavirus, herpes simplex virus and cervical cancer incidence in Greenland and Denmark. A population-based cross-sectional study', *International Journal of Cancer*, 41, 518–524.

Kuno, Y., Ishihara, K., Yamazaki, N. and Mukai, K. (1996) 'Clinical and pathological features of cutaneous malignant melanoma: a retrospective analysis of 124 Japanese patients', *Japan Journal of Clinical Oncology*, 26, 144–151.

Lee, H.P., Day, N.E. and Shanmugaratnam, K. (1988) *Trends in Cancer Incidence in Singapore 1968–1982*, Lyon, France: International Agency for Research on Cancer, pp. 1–161.

Le Marchand, L., Wilkens, L.R. and Kolonel, L.N. (1992) 'Ethnic differences in the lung cancer risk associated with smoking', *Cancer Epidemiology, Biomarkers and Prevention*, 1, 103–107.

Levin, M.L. (1953) 'The occurrence of lung cancer in man', *Unio Internationalis Contra Cancrum Acta*, 9, 531–541.

Li, C.C., Yu, M.C. and Henderson, B.E. (1985) 'Some epidemiologic observations of nasopharyngeal carcinoma in Guangdong, People's Republic of China', *National Cancer Institute Monographs*, 69, 49–52.

Li, J.Y., Liu, B., Li, G., Rong, S., Cao, D., Xu, Q., Liu, Z., Qiao, F., Gao, R., Rong, Z., Zhang, C., Zhou, Y., Dai, X., Xu, H., Ni, Z., Gu, X., Lu, Y., Wang, S., Gao, F., Cheng, Y., Liu, H., Wu, Y., You, X., Zhao, T., Xue, Z., Zhuang, Y., Zhang, D., Zhu, G., Fa, N., Hu, R. and Liu, Y. (1979) *Atlas of Cancer Mortality in the People's Republic of China*, Shanghai: China Map Press.

Lo, K.W., Huang, D.P. and Lau, K.M. (1995) 'p16 gene alterations in nasopharyngeal carcinoma', *Cancer Research*, 55, 2039–2043.

Lu, S.J., Day, N.E., Degos, L., Lepage, V., Wang, P.C., Chan, S.H., Simons, M., McKnight, B., Easton, D., Zeng, Y. and de-The, G. (1990) 'Linkage of a nasopharyngeal carcinoma susceptibility locus to the HLA region', *Nature*, 346, 470–471.

McMichael, A.J. (1994) ' "Molecular epidemiology": new pathway or new travelling companion?', *American Journal of Epidemiology*, 140, 1–11.

Miller, B.A., Kolonel, L.N., Bernstein, L., Young, J.L., Swanson, G.M., West, D., Key, C.R., Liff, J.M., Glover, C.S. and Alexander, G.A. (eds) (1996) *Racial/Ethnic Patterns of Cancer in the United States 1988–1992*, NIH Publication No. 96–4104, Bethesda, MD: National Cancer Institute.

Morita, S., Yano, M., Shiozaki, H., Tsujinaka, T., Ebisui, C., Morimoto, T., Kishibuti, M., Fujita, J., Ogawa, A., Taniguchi, M., Inoue, M., Tamura, S., Yamazaki, K., Kikkawa, N., Mizunoya, S. and Monden, M. (1997) 'CYP1A1, CYP2E1 and GSTM1 polymorphisms are not associated with susceptibility to squamous-cell carcinoma of the esophagus', *International Journal of Cancer*, 71, 192–195.

Muir, C.S. (1996) 'Epidemiology of cancer in ethnic groups', *British Journal of Cancer*, 29 (Suppl.), 12–16.

Narod, S.A., Feunteun, J., Lynch, H.T., Watson, P., Conway, T., Lynch, J. and Lenoir, G.M. (1991) 'Familial breast-ovarian cancer locus on chromosome 17q12–q23', *Lancet*, 338, 82–83.

Nielsen, N.H., Storm, H.H., Gaudette, L.A. and Lanier, A.P. (1996) 'Cancer in Circumpolar Inuit 1969–1988. A summary', *Acta Oncology*, 35, 621–8.

Norppa, H. (1997) 'Cytogenetic markers of susceptibility: influence of polymorphic carcinogen-metabolizing enzymes', *Environmental Health Perspective*, 105, 829–835.

Parker, S.L., Davis, K.J., Wingo, P.A., Ries, L.A. and Heath-CW, J. (1998) 'Cancer statistics by race and ethnicity', *CA Cancer Journal for Clinicians*, 48, 31–48.

Parkin, D.M. and Iscovich, J.A. (1997) 'The risk of cancer in migrants and their descendants in Israel: II carcinomas and germ cell tumours', *International Journal of Cancer*, 70, 654–660.

Parkin, D.M. and Khlat, M. (1996) 'Studies of cancer in migrants: rationale and methodology', *European Journal of Cancer*, 32A, 761–771.

Parkin, D.M., Pisani, P., Lopez, A.D. and Masuyer, E. (1994) 'At least one in seven cases of cancer is caused by smoking. Global estimates for 1985', *International Journal of Cancer*, 59, 494–504.

Parkin, D.M., Whelan S.L., Ferlay, J., Raymond, L and Young, J. (eds) (1997) *Cancer Incidence in Five Continents*, Vol. VII, IARC Scientific Publication No. 143, Lyon: International Agency for Research on Cancer.

Prentice, R.L. and Sheppard, L. (1989) 'Validity of international, time trend, and migrant studies of dietary factors and disease risk', *Preventative Medicine*, 18, 167–179.

Quinn, M. and Allen, E. (1995) 'Changes in incidence of and mortality from breast cancer in England and Wales since introduction of screening. United Kingdom Association of Cancer Registries', *British Medical Journal*, 311, 1391–1395.

Rebbeck, T.R. (1997) 'Molecular epidemiology of the human glutathione S-Transferase genotypes GSTM1 and GSTT1 in cancer susceptibility', *Cancer Epidemiology, Biomarkers and Prevention*, 6, 733–743.

Schwartz, A.G. and Swanson, G.M. (1997) 'Lung carcinoma in African Americans and whites. A population-based study in metropolitan Detroit, Michigan', *Cancer*, 79, 45–52.

Seow, A., Straughan, P.T., Ng, E.H., Emmanuel, S.C., Tan, C.H. and Lee, H.P. (1997) 'Factors determining acceptability of mammography in an Asian population: a study among women in Singapore', *Cancer Causes and Control*, 8, 771–779.

Shanmugaratnam, K. (1982) 'Nasopharynx', in Schottenfeld, D. and Fraumeni J.F. (eds) *Cancer Epidemiology and Prevention*, Philadelphia: Saunders.

Simons, M.J., Wee, G.B., Goh, E.H., Chan, S.H., Shanmugaratnam, K., Day, N.E. and deThé, G. (1976) 'Immunogenetic aspects of nasopharyngeal carcinoma, IV. Increased risk in Chinese of nasopharyngeal carcinoma associated with a Chinese-related HLA profile', *Journal of the National Cancer Institute*, 57, 977–980.

Steinitz, R., Parkin, D.M., Young, J.L., Bieber, C.A. and Katz, L., (eds) (1989) *Cancer Incidence in Jewish Migrants to Israel, 1961–1981*, IARC Scientific Publication No. 98, Lyon: International Agency for Research on Cancer.

Stevens, N.G., Liff, J.M. and Weiss, N.S. (1990) 'Plantar melanoma: is the incidence of melanoma of the sole of the foot really higher in blacks than whites?', *International Journal of Cancer*, 45, 691–693.

Stiller, C.A. and Parkin, D.M. (1996) 'Geographic and ethnic variations in the incidence of childhood cancer', *British Medical Bulletin*, 52, 682–703.

Wynder E.L. and Gori, G.B. (1977) 'Contribution of the environment to cancer incidence: an epidemiologic exercise', *Journal of the National Cancer Institute*, 58, 825–832.

Yamamoto, K., Ueno, Y., Mizoi, Y. and Tatsuno, Y. (1993) 'Genetic polymorphism of alcohol and aldehyde dehydrogenase and the effects on alcohol metabolism', *Arukoru Kenkyuto Yakubutsu Ison*, 28, 13–25.

Yokoyama, A., Muramatsu, T., Ohmori, T., Higuchi, S., Hayashida, M. and Ishii, H. (1996) 'Esophageal cancer and aldehyde dehydrogenase-2 genotypes in Japanese males', *Cancer Epidemiology, Biomarkers and Prevention*, 5, 99–102.

Yu, M.C., Skipper, P.L., Taghizadeh, K., Tannenbaum, S.R., Chan, K.K., Henderson, B.E. and Ross, R.K. (1994) 'Acetylator phenotype, aminobiphenyl-hemoglobin adduct levels, and bladder cancer risk in white, black, and Asian men in Los Angeles, California', *Journal of the National Cancer Institute*, 86, 712–716.

Yu, M.C., Ross, R.K., Chan, K.K., Henderson, B.E., Skipper, P.L., Tannenbaum, S.R. and Coetzee, G.A. (1995) 'Glutathione s-transferase M1 genotype affects aminobiphenyl-hemoglobin adduct levels in White, Black, and Asian smokers and nonsmokers', *Cancer Epidemiology, Biomarkers and Prevention*, 4, 861–864.

Yu, M.W., Gladek, Y.A., Chiamprasert, S., Santella, R.M., Liaw, Y.F. and Chen, C.J. (1995) 'Cytochrome P450 2E1 and glutathione S-transferase M1 polymorphisms and susceptibility to hepatocellular carcinoma', *Gastroenterology*, 109, 1266–1273.

Ziegler, R.G., Hoover, R.N., Pike, M.C., Hildesheim, A., Nomura, A.M., West, D.W., Wu-Williams, A.H., Kolonel, L.N., Horn-Ross, P.L., Rosenthal, J.F. and Hyer, M.B. (1993), *Journal of the National Cancer Institute*, 85, 1819–1827.

14 'Culture' in the field of race and mental health

Roland Littlewood

Consideration of the autonomy and ideological interests of particular human sciences is a matter for historical and cultural interpretation. In the absence of detailed accounts of everyday clinical practice, it is often difficult to assess the specific motivations for the practitioner of racist theories in psychiatry (Rackett 1992). The recent development of transcultural psychiatry in the United Kingdom may throw light on how individual practice relates to political contingencies, and how it develops a body of expert knowledge associated with 'culture' which becomes medical common sense.

Unlike the United States or Australia, Britain has never considered itself a nation of immigrants, yet considerable numbers of Europeans have settled here during the whole of the modern period. Cardiff, Liverpool and London have had substantial Black minorities since the eighteenth century. In the 1950s and 1960s, immigrants arrived from the Indian subcontinent and the British West Indies, and also from Eastern Europe, Hong Kong and West Africa. Although stimulated initially by government recruiting campaigns for unskilled labour, a series of increasingly restrictive immigration acts from the 1960s limited migration to dependent family members of those already established. The Irish Republic and the United Kingdom continue to have unrestricted movement between them, and more recently membership of the European Community encourages free migration between member states. The 1991 census lists the percentage population of England and Wales by self-reported ethnicity as White 94, Black Caribbean 1, African 0.4, Black other 0.4, South Asian 2.9, Chinese 1 (Balarajan and Raleigh 1992). Previous censuses had asked place of birth (or place of birth of the head of the household), which had the epidemiological advantage of particularising the countries of origin (and thus 'culture') in more detail, but the increasing numbers of children and grandchildren of migrants made any calculation of ethnicity from household origins more difficult. Given the popular British equation of 'immigrant' with 'Black', it is necessary to recall that the majority of migrants, in all but 1 year since the war, has been White, and that the largest single overseas-born minority community in Britain – perhaps 2 per cent of the population – is the Irish (Littlewood and Lipsedge 1982, revised 1997).

Although initially identified with certain individual psychiatrists' clinical and research interests, and the group they formed, transcultural psychiatry is now recognised as an 'interest' within the profession and as a 'section' within its representative body, the Royal College of Psychiatrists. It has been argued to be a response in the late 1970s to the comparatively large numbers of non-European psychiatric patients (Mercer 1986, Fernando 1988, Acharyya 1992, Littlewood 1992). However, the rates of illness among the Irish community have consistently been among the highest (Cochrane 1977, Littlewood and Lipsedge 1982, revised 1997), but little attention has been focused on them – just four academic papers (Brent Irish Mental Health Group 1986). 'Transcultural psychiatry' has come to be the psychiatry of people in Britain originating from the 'New Commonwealth' (over 200 academic papers and books), a category which excludes those from the predominantly White ex-Dominions (no papers published). It has become the euphemistic shorthand for Black mental health and treatment (Littlewood and Lipsedge 1982, revised 1997). As the term fell into disrepute among many of its practitioners, a variety of other terms have been proposed ranging from the bland 'ethnic issues' (Royal College of Psychiatrists 1989) to 'anti-racist psychiatry' (Fernando 1988, Littlewood and Lipsedge 1982, revised 1997). On the whole, the more 'race' is emphasised (in its current, political sense), the more psychiatrists are concerned with social and political analyses; if the terminology of 'transcultural' or 'immigrant' is used, the methodology tends to be purely medical.

Methodology was initially descriptive and epidemiological, emphasising the pattern and distribution of psychiatric illnesses familiar among English patients (e.g. Kiev 1963, Gordon 1965, Hemsi 1967). Interest was focused particularly on the differences in rates of psychiatric hospitalisation between different countries of origin. Two statistical findings which emerged in the 1970s continue to dominate the debate: higher rates of diagnosed schizophrenia and other psychoses among those of West Indian origin (Bagley 1971a and 1971b, Leff *et al.* 1976, Cochrane 1977) and higher rates of parasuicide and, more recently, eating disorders among South Asians (Cochrane 1977, Mumford and Whitehouse 1988, Littlewood 1995). Other striking findings such as the low rate of abnormal personality diagnosed in all ethnic minority groups and the relative infrequency of suicide, parasuicide and alcoholism among African Caribbeans or of schizophrenia among South Asians have elicited no interest at all (Littlewood and Lipsedge 1982, revised 1997). Perhaps surprisingly, given Britain's tradition of providing asylum for refugees, there have been relatively few psychiatric studies of their experiences (Kareem and Littlewood 1992).

The one case where we might claim that the psychiatric contribution to ideology has been fundamental – in theory, influence and personnel – was the 'social hygiene' movement of the late nineteenth and early twentieth centuries (Dowbiggin 1985, Gilman 1985). Through psychodynamic psychotherapy, its linear model of 'development' is still with us. Evolutionary social science regarded the social and moral evolution of human societies as part of the biological evolution of humankind; each individual, from fetus to adult, recapitulated the history of his/her race – in emotional, intellectual and moral development (Gould 1977); and, like the social organisation of non-Europeans, psychiatric illnesses could be placed on this single moral–biological trajectory, either as incompletely evolved primitive types or as degenerate forms (Wallace 1983, Dowbiggin 1985, Kuper 1988). It provided an element and powerful model in which virtually all biological, cultural and psychological patterns could be united along a single axis of progress and development. And it was evaluative – the further along the line, the better things were, more advanced, higher, more civilised – for morality was but the workings out of Nature. Kraepelin (1904, translated in 1975) explained the pattern of mental illness in non-Europeans as the consequence of their 'lower stage of intellectual development'.

The idiom of spatio-temporal development remains in such concepts as moral or intellectual retardation: the assumption is that psychopathy or mental handicap can be displayed (or even understood) as points along some single developmental trajectory, independent of personal meanings or historical context. Its most influential legacy remains that of psychoanalysis and thence other psychodynamic theories. Freud's debt to the Victorian evolutionary anthropologists is well known (Sulloway 1979, Wallace 1983) although he wrote little directly on 'racial' groups, but his predominantly female patients were seen, like non-Europeans, as just not so far along the evolutionary path (Mitchell 1974). Freud's non-Jewish colleagues were more prepared to discuss race (e.g. Lind 1914), and Jung, after a brief field trip to Kenya, equated cortical organisation with cultural history to warn Europeans that the African 'has probably a whole historical layer less', and thus 'living with barbaric races exerts a suggestive effect on the laboriously tamed instinct of the White race and tends to pull it down' (cited in Thomas and Sillen 1972). Jungian theories of the physical inheritance of racial archetypes still come perilously close to biological racism, and Jung's role in the Swiss and German debates on the 'Jewishness' of psychoanalysis seems ambiguous, to put it charitably (Cocks 1985). The association of biological difference with cultural difference always threatens to come close to racism. It is perhaps for that reason that most social scientists remain wary of sociobiology (Sahlins 1977); only with the development of population genetics has the correlation of genetic traits with culture again achieved some limited sort of respectability (e.g. Renfrew 1992).

Even psychoanalysts such as Roheim (1950) and Devereux (1980), who were far from prejudiced in their daily life, were prepared to argue for an equivalence between schizophrenia and non-European religions, and Bettelheim (1954) used childhood autism as the model of aboriginal culture. Whole societies, notably the adversaries of the Second World War, and later the Russians, were perceived by American and British analysts as in various stages of arrested psychological development, usually that of a childlike dependence on others (Benedict 1946, Adorno *et al.* 1950, Gorer and Rickman 1962). And the readings of their own societies offered by non-European psychoanalysts have frequently proposed something similar (Doi 1973, Obeyesekere 1990). Psychoanalytic anthropology has only recently moved away from taking non-European societies as exemplars of particular individual pathologies, an equation common in the nineteenth century (Rush's elision of black skin with leprosy, and Down's Mongolism – Szasz 1971), and later exemplified by Benedict (1935). The equation of the historical origins of cultural forms with their contemporary origin in individual patients makes psychoanalytical thinking continually vulnerable to pathologising societies, even though psychoanalysis has been generally influential in reframing the concept of race from a biological to a cultural understanding (Barkan 1992).

Freud's purely verbal and interpretive therapy and his lack of interest in psychotic patients or in genetic and biological explanations, together with the fact that he was Jewish, meant that only an attenuated form of psychoanalysis was taken up by the German hospital psychiatrists, the leading European theorists in the earlier part of this century (Cocks 1985). Even the last edition of the standard international text on psychiatric symptomatology, Jaspers' *General Psychopathology*, criticises Freud for 'cosmopolitanism', the standard Nazi/Stalinist code word for Jewish culture (Jaspers 1963). How 'Jewish' Freud's thinking actually was, has been the subject of recent debate (McGrath 1986, Gay 1987). By the 1940s, psychoanalytically orientated social scientists, aligned with American culture and personality theories or with the displaced Frankfurt School, were using psychodynamic concepts to deal with racism as a psychological phenomenon (e.g. Sterba 1947). No longer an explanation within scientific theories of development, racism itself became objectified as a pathological tendency (Willie *et al.* 1973), as a form of arrested development (Kovel 1970), or, indeed, as a mental illness which required therapy (*Psychiatry News* 1975). Psychometric tests identified racism as something carried by people using projection, concrete stereotypes and magical thinking (Adorno *et al.* 1950) – psychological patterns which not long before had been identified as characteristically Black (Kovel 1970). Now the Black and the racist were mirror images of the same psychopathological process. The historical and economic context of racism remained obscured. Xenophobia was identified as a morbid fear of the other, which, like any other phobia, could be categorised, assessed and treated.

Illness is a powerful political metaphor, and the abusive use of terms like 'mad' or 'retarded' is a common way of discrediting individuals or societies to whom we are opposed. Can we argue that the legacy of recapitulationist theory in psychoanalysis has any practical consequences for contemporary psychiatric practice? At a general level we can identify the (particularly North American) tendency to identify as psychological phenomena what, for other observers are educational, moral or political relations, together with recourse to an individualistic and therapeutic idiom for changing them (Rieff 1966, Gaines 1992).

More specifically, it might be argued that psychodynamic theories provide a justification for Western notions of power or development as medical matters, and hence as natural phenomena (Littlewood 1992). Their image of maturity is that of the individual who seeks personal autonomy against traditional social obligations, to free themselves of the meanings which cultures provide to construct personal experience (Lasch 1979). Psychoanalytical delineation of religion is that it is a neurosis, at best a compromise which will be unnecessary after full insight is attained. Psychoanalysis naturalises moral and political debate (Gorkin 1986) in a commodified world where evil no longer has any meaning, while at the same time it compels urgency – for sickness requires a surgeon. The idiom of 'maturity' and 'personal growth' argued by psychotherapists is that of self-sufficiency and self-knowing, rational, individuated and empowered. As with the Mental Health Movement, it offers as an image of health the idealised White male entrepreneur with psychology as itself a sufficient morality (Davis 1938, Kovel 1970, see Miller 1986). The process of therapy is that of contract in which the supplier (the analyst) remains as untouched by the procedure as possible, and indeed where any enduring personal engagement is recognised as unhealthy and counterproductive: not inappropriately termed 'counter-transference'. Yet consumer and producer have no absolute social role, for they change places: the analyst was once the analysand. It is probably in Latin America that psychodynamic psychoanalysis is now developing most rapidly; as if to articulate new values of exchange and experience when traditional obligations to authority and to family no longer have the same value.

We might wonder whether this idiom of individual psychological development as the index of social development will survive the recognition that the economic power of the countries of the Western Pacific Rim is predicated locally on rather different notions of psychological health. In therapeutic practice, the cultural and family obligations of small-scale societies are inevitably seen as regression (Deleuze and Guattari 1984, Kareem and Littlewood 1992). In the French Caribbean, the key to understanding local violence has been argued to be displaced Oedipal desires, originating in slavery but still generated anew in family life (André 1987) – although other French psychologists have argued that the Oedipal schema is itself European, and thus its application outside this context is inappropriate (Deleuze and Guattari 1984). Some psychoanalysts working with non-Western clients seem aware of this and are prepared to modify their notions of maturity (Kakar 1985). For theoreticians, however, any psychoanalytic reading of cultural forms seems to replicate Freud's *Totem and Taboo* (e.g. Obeyesekere 1990). The New Age therapeutic image of the *shaman* as the adjusted individual, in ecological balance with the environment, while reversing the racist evaluation, simply idealises the non-European as the child of unfettered Nature.

Although psychoanalysis was indebted to the evolutionary 'social hygiene' consensus, it was not itself employed in immediate justifications for genocide or the elimination of the mentally ill (Cocks 1985). Rapidly co-opted into an anti-racist position after the Second World War, it continues to see power and economics in terms of psychological development, to argue close parallels between psychopathology and non-European cultures, and offers a goal of psychological health and maturity which may be argued to be ethnocentric. There are close parallels with its understanding of gender (Mitchell 1974, Showalter 1985). The influence of psychoanalytic thinking on social work theory in Britain and America, and thence on public policy on social issues, has contributed an idiom of pathology to articulate Black–White relations, particularly in the pathologisation of the Black family as some discrete cultural entity, one which has been described as dysfunctional or even as 'a tangle of pathology' (Moynihan 1965); and this approach argues for individualistic 'therapeutic' coercion rather than for moral or political action.

We can identify three tendencies in British psychiatry: (1) a selective focus on Black rather than on White immigrants, irrespective of the actual rates of reported illness; (2) emphasis on increased rates rather than decreased rates, and thus on pathology rather than on successful coping strategies; (3) research carried out with hospitalised patients, and thus on psychotic illness rather than on unhappiness, adjustment problems, loss and coping (Cochrane and Stopes-Roe 1977, Fernando 1988).

In response to these three trends, transcultural psychiatry has developed as a fairly circumscribed sub-discipline. There have never been specialist qualifications and few training courses in it but the term appears in exam papers and syllabuses. For appointment to a post in an inner-city area, an expressed interest in 'transcultural psychiatry' is probably an asset; for it signifies some recognition of working with Black patients. By contrast, it has never been agreed whether the significant number of British psychiatrists who are of South Asian origin properly constitutes anything to do with transcultural psychiatry (Littlewood and Lipsedge 1982, revised 1997).

Explanations of the differential rates of illness among immigrant groups initially emphasised the experience of migration (Gordon 1965) and, later, the selective patterns of migration (the most vulnerable were those who chose to migrate) (Cochrane 1977), or considered that the 'culture' of the immigrant group was itself pathogenic in the new environments (Kiev 1963) (for critiques see Littlewood and Lipsedge 1982, revised 1997, Rack 1982). The debate has remained one conducted largely by psychiatrists and psychologists; the only social scientist involved in the 1960s argued for a Mertonian model of relative deprivation (Bagley 1971b, following Parker and Kleiner 1966), a suggestion which was not taken up. There was no interest in minorities' construction of selfhood, understanding of illness, patterns of psychological adjustment, recourse to mental health agencies or, indeed, their attitudes to professional medicine in general. One exception was a study of the range of the lexicon of affect (Leff 1973), which was later criticised as arguing for a less 'differentiated' Black psychology. Pathology is always a measure of difference, and medical understanding of culture was similarly one of cultural difference, employing easily accessible check lists of items such as religious affiliation, family pattern, employment and expectations in Britain, each of which could be argued to associate statistically with pathology one way or the other (e.g. Community Relations Commission 1976), although the papers usually simply reported epidemiological data rather than testing hypotheses. As Littlewood and Lipsedge (1982, revised 1997) and Mercer (1986) have argued, the approach of psychiatry is not only an emphasis on pathology but on the individual, in which questions of inter-group relations and economic power are reinterpreted through a focus on the individual as victim.

Although what we may term an 'epidemiological' approach still continues, a second and more critical set of ideas developed from the early 1980s after the death of a number of Black patients in psychiatric care (Mercer 1986). Some argued that the diagnoses given to people of non-European origin, particularly for schizophrenia, were frequently inappropriate or even wrong, biased by British psychiatric stereotypes about what constituted normality in different groups (Littlewood and Lipsedge 1978 and 1982, revised 1997), and that this could be demonstrated by using more rigorous research interviews with patients, and comparing the research diagnosis with the previous hospital diagnosis (Littlewood and Lipsedge 1982). Many West Indian patients who had been hospitalised with a diagnosis of schizophrenia were found to lack the symptoms of schizophrenia commonly regarded as of primary diagnostic significance in such studies as the World Health Organization's cross-national project on schizophrenia (itself modelled on British descriptive psychiatry). Similar debates have occurred in the United States (e.g. Kramer *et al.* 1975, Pope and Lipinski 1978, Adebimpe 1981, 1982). An earlier British study, which had showed that alcoholism was preferentially diagnosed among Irish people (Bagley and Binitie 1970), was cited to suggest that popular cultural stereotypes had carried over into medical practice. Increased salience was given to these issues by repeated findings that, independently of their diagnosis, non-White patients of quite diverse linguistic and cultural backgrounds were two to three times more likely to be hospitalised as involuntary patients under Britain's Mental Health Act than were similar groups of White people, whether these were native Britons or non-English-speaking European immigrants (Rwegellera 1980, Littlewood 1986, McGovern and Cope 1987a). This occurred independently of diagnosis. As in the United States (Sabshin *et al.* 1970, Cole and Pilisuk 1976, Geller 1988), there was some evidence of differences in medical treatment. Allowing for diagnosis and demographic differences, Black patients were more likely to be given physical treatment (Littlewood and Cross 1980, cf. McGovern and Cope 1991) and more likely to be given depot medications (Lloyd and Moodley 1992). It has become generally accepted that access to psychotherapy is easier for White people (Littlewood 1992).

The shift from cultural explanations – locating psychopathological differences within the characteristics of an individual's ethnicity – to explanations based on race (now viewed not as biology but as the social construction of ethnicity and its articulation with institutional interests and medical power) was accompanied by a shift from empirical, descriptive statistics to a more critical interpretative stance (Pillay *et al.* 1984). The medical approach was supported by studies which showed that the British-born children of West Indian immigrants were likely to have even higher rates of diagnosed schizophrenia than their migrant parents (McGovern and Cope 1987b, Harrison *et al.* 1988), and later that the incidence of schizophrenia in the African Caribbean population was increasing (Wessely *et al.* 1991). Perhaps not incidentally, these observations were made during the same period as Black unemployment soared [for the possible association between unemployment and schizophrenia in capitalist countries see Warner (1985)]. This was an unexpected finding; in most situations of international migration, if a migrating group have higher rates of psychiatric illness than the population they come to live among, their children born in the new country usually have levels of morbidity intermediate between the two. One of the British studies (Harrison *et al.* 1988) had used the internationally recognised WHO procedures for diagnosis – the 'first-rank symptoms' and a diagnostic decision tree – rather than the local hospital diagnosis. If one extrapolated from rates to lifetime risk, it appeared that Black Britons had a more than 10 per cent chance of becoming schizophrenic. Angry debate followed in the late 1980s among the psychiatric professionals in the Transcultural Psychiatry Society, some of whom left. The preference for statistical surveys was extensively criticised, but no convincing explanations were offered of the figures for British-born African Caribbeans, apart from a general conviction that psychiatrists were somehow still prejudiced, personally or theoretically (see Littlewood and Lipsedge 1982, revised 1997), and indeed the suggestion was made that studies of this sort should be abandoned (cf. Royal College of Psychiatrists 1989, Fernando 1991).

Mercer (1986: 116) has argued in a review that British transcultural psychiatry 'is neither a movement, an ideology nor the result of an institutional or policy initiative. Rather, it consists of a particular vocabulary, a specific set of terms of reference and a distinct grouping of a range of concerns'. He delineates a political spectrum of those involved from 'conservative' (Julian Leff), to 'centrist' (Philip Rack, John Cox), to 'left' (Maurice Lipsedge, Roland Littlewood) and 'radical' (Aggrey Burke). The almost complete absence of social scientists in the debates led to a reversal in explanation: the 'discourse on transcultural psychiatry' (Mercer 1986) was still couched in psychological terms, but now away from the Black patient to the White psychiatrist. The diagnostic differences were argued by many, to be not as 'real' ones, but reflections of racist bias on the part of psychiatrists. These were now urged to participate in Racism Awareness Training to change their attitudes. The minority press and some activist groups took up the issue of misdiagnosis, which was widely reported in a number of television documentaries. It became accepted by the media that British psychiatry was racist, even if few took the radical view that transcultural psychiatry was itself simply 'a crucial ... new operational method' of medicalising the existing oppression of the Black population (Black Health Workers and Patients Group 1983). In the best of these critiques, Mercer (1986) argued more rigorously, following David Armstrong, that the construction of ethnicity could be seen within the policies of the post-war British National Health Service which sought to enlist compliance through a focus on the patients' own social identity. These critiques were taken up by some social workers and community workers, but were greeted unfavourably by most doctors. By the 1970s, expressly racist views were only espoused publicly by fringe political groups, and the medical consensus was certainly one of equal opportunity and access to treatment. Psychiatrists in particular identified themselves as liberals (Littlewood and Lipsedge 1982, revised 1997). Anything recalling eugenic theories was medically and legally unacceptable (Childs 1993). Other doctors who had not been involved previously in the arguments now published studies which argued that any racial bias in treatment was rather an excessive caution which had actually led to the *underdiagnosis* of schizophrenia among Black people (Richardson and Hendrik-Gutt 1981, Dunn and Fahy 1990). Biological explanations – genetic or obstetric vulnerability, nutritional disadvantage – were not widely volunteered, presumably because of a feeling that any biological argument could not be separated from racist assumptions or even eugenic practice (Eagles 1991).

If psychosis was the object of interest for psychiatrists when looking at African Caribbeans, parasuicide and eating disorders were identified more commonly in South Asians and they were frequently explained by 'culture conflict' (Merrill and Owens 1986, Mumford and Whitehouse 1988, cf. Littlewood 1995). It was noted that this seemed to follow the popular stereotypes – West Indians as public and out of control, Asians as private and too controlled – a binary opposition which recalled the earlier perception of the Irish and the Jews (Billingsley 1970, Parmer 1981, Littlewood and Lipsedge 1982, revised 1997).

Transcultural psychiatry's shift from emphasising culture to emphasising racism was similar to that which has been described in the United States (Adebimpe 1984, Jones and Gray 1986), an attempt to situate the practice of psychiatry within a social field. Yet, the non-medical explanations which were offered remained simplistic, at times conspiratorial, but still individualistic rather than political. If patterns of 'psychopathology' were no longer located within the individual attitudes, experiences and actions of the designated patient, they were now to be found in those of the psychiatrist. The relativity of psychiatric categories seemed illustrated when a well-publicised study in Birmingham on the medical conception of the term 'cannabis psychosis' (diagnosed locally as ninety-five times more frequent among young Afro-Caribbean men than among a comparable group of White men) was accompanied by its virtual disappearance within 2 years (Littlewood 1988 and 1989).

To some it appeared that the new emphasis on the culture of psychiatry itself, however welcome, instead of examining the interaction between psychiatry and patient, left the latter as a mere cipher, a palimpsest on which psychiatric institutions simply inscribed their power. The possibility that 'real' psychopathology in Black people could in part be also understood as 'resistance' – an active, albeit unsuccessful, appropriation of the dominant symbolic system for personal ends – was dismissed as exoticism or romanticism (Burke 1984, Mercer 1986). The term 'culture' became discredited as apparently just a perceived attribute of individuals, rather than as the interactive matrix in which different forms of power, representation, ideology and social action clashed, compromised or coalesced (Littlewood and Lipsedge 1982, revised 1997). The 1990s have demonstrated some slight return to the idea of 'culture', largely because of objections that the critique of racism allowed little space to individual strategies of resistance, and criticisms that an emphasis on 'Black' groups conflated subtle differences of emphasis where they were not shared by all groups labelled as such.

Acknowledgement

This chapter uses some material of mine previously published in *Transcultural Psychiatry Research Review*, 30, 243–290.

References

Acharyya, S. (1992) 'The doctor's dilemma: the practice of cultural psychiatry in multicultural Britain', in Kareem, J. and Littlewood, R. (eds) *Intercultural Therapy*, Oxford: Blackwell Publishers, pp. 74–82.
Adebimpe, V.R. (1981) 'Overview: White norms and psychiatric diagnosis in black patients', *American Journal of Psychiatry*, 138, 279–285.
Adebimpe, V.R. (1982) 'Psychiatric symptoms in black patients', in Turner, S.M. and Jones, R.T. (eds) *Behaviour Therapy in Black Populations*, New York: Plenum.
Adebimpe, V.R. (1984) 'American blacks and psychiatry', *Transcultural Psychiatric Research Review*, 21, 83–111.
Adorno, T.W., Frenkel-Brunswick, E., Levinson, D.J. and Sanford, R.N. (1950) *The Authoritarian Personality*, New York: Harper.
André, J. (1987) *L'inceste Focal dans la Famille Noire Antillaise*, Paris: Presses Universitaires de France.
Bagley, C. (1971a) 'Mental illness in immigrant minorities in London', *Journal of Biosocial Science*, 3, 449–459.
Bagley, C. (1971b) 'The social aetiology of schizophrenia in immigrant groups', *International Journal of Social Psychiatry*, 17, 292–304.
Bagley, C. and Binitie, A. (1970) 'Alcoholism and schizophrenia in Irishmen in London', *British Journal of Addiction*, 63, 3–7.
Balarajan, R. and Raleigh, V.S. (1992) 'The ethnic populations of England and Wales: the 1991 Census', *Health Trends*, 24(4), 113–116.
Barkan, E. (1992) *The Retreat of Scientific Racism: Changing Concepts of Race in Britain and the United States Between the World Wars,* Cambridge: Cambridge University Press.

Benedict, R. (1935) *Patterns of Culture*, London: Routledge and Kegan Paul.

Benedict, R. (1942) *Race and Racism*, London: Labour Book Services.

Benedict, R. (1946) *The Chrysanthemum and the Sword: Patterns of Japanese Culture*, Boston, MA: Houghton Mifflin.

Bettelheim, B. (1954) *Symbolic Wounds*, Glencoe, IL: Free Press.

Billingsley, A. (1970) 'Black families and white social science', *Journal of Social Issues*, 26, 127–142.

Black Health Workers and Patients Group (1983) 'Psychiatry and the corporate state', *Race and Class*, 25, 49–64.

Brent Irish Mental Health Group (1986) *The Irish Experience of Mental Health in Britain*, London: BIMHG.

Burke, A.W. (ed.) (1984) 'Racism and mental illness', *International Journal of Social Psychiatry*, Special Issue, 30, 1 and 2.

Childs, M. (1993) 'Sterilisation of the mentally incompetent', *Journal of the Medical Defence Union*, 9(1), 17–20.

Cochrane, R. (1977) 'Mental illness in immigrants to England and Wales: an analysis of mental hospital admissions', *Social Psychiatry*, 12, 23–25.

Cochrane, R. and Stopes-Roe, M. (1977) 'Psychological and social adjustment of Asian immigrants to Britain: a community survey', *Social Psychiatry*, 12, 195–207.

Cocks, S.G. (1985) *Psychotherapy in the Third Reich*, New York: Oxford University Press.

Cole, J. and Pilisuk, M. (1976) 'Differences in the provision of mental health services by race', *American Journal of Orthopsychiatry*, 46, 510–525.

Community Relations Commission (1976) *Aspects of Mental Health in a Multicultural Society: Notes for the Guidance of Doctors and Social Workers*, London: Community Relations Commission (CRC).

Davis, K. (1938) 'Mental hygiene and the class structure', *Psychiatry*, 1, 55–65.

Deleuze, G. and Guattari, F. (1984) *Anti-Oedipus: Capitalism and Schizophrenia* (Translation of 1972 French edition), London: Athlone.

Devereux, G. (1980) *Basic Problems of Ethnopsychiatry (Collected Essays)*, Chicago: University of Chicago Press.

Doi, T. (1973) *The Anatomy of Dependence*, Tokyo: Kodansha.

Dowbiggin, I. (1985) 'Degeneration and hereditarianism in French mental medicine 1840–90', in Bynum, W.F., Porter, R. and Shepherd, M. (eds) *The Anatomy of Madness*, Vol. 1, London: Tavistock, pp. 188–232.

Dunn, J. and Fahy, T.A. (1990) 'Police admissions to a psychiatric hospital: demographical and clinical differences between ethnic groups', *British Journal of Psychiatry*, 156, 373–378.

Eagles, J. (1991) 'The relationship between schizophrenia and immigration: are there alternatives to psychosocial hypotheses?', *British Journal of Psychiatry*, 159, 783–789.

Fernando, S. (1988) *Race and Culture in Psychiatry*, London: Croom Helm.

Fernando, S. (1991) *Mental Health, Race and Culture*, London: Macmillan.

Gaines, A.D. (1992) 'Medical/psychiatric knowledge in France and the United States: Culture and sickness in history and biology', in Gaines, A.D. (ed.) *Ethnopsychiatry: The Cultural Construction of Professional and Folk Psychiatries*, New York: University of New York Press, pp. 171–202.

Gay, P. (1987) *A Godless Jew: Freud, Atheism and the Making of Psychoanalysis*, New Haven: Yale University Press.

Geller, J.D. (1988) 'Racial bias in the evaluation of patients for psychotherapy', in Comaz Diaz, L. and Griffith, E.E.H. (eds) *Clinical Guidelines in Cross-cultural Mental Health*, New York: Wiley.

Gilman, S. (1985) *Difference and Pathology: Stereotypes of Sex, Race and Madness*, Ithaca: Cornell University Press.

Gordon, E.B. (1965) 'Mentally ill West Indian immigrants', *British Journal of Psychiatry*, 111, 877–887.

Gorer, G. and Rickman, J. (1962) *The People of Great Russia*, New York: Norton.

Gorkin, M. (1986) 'Countertransference in cross-cultural psychiatry: the example of Jewish therapist and Arab patient', *Psychiatry*, 49, 69–79.

Gould, S.J. (1977) *Ontogeny and Phylogeny*, Cambridge, MA: Harvard University Press.

Harrison, G., Holton, A., Nielson, D., Boot, D. and Gupe, J. (1988) 'A prospective study of severe mental disorder in Afro-Caribbean patients', *Psychological Medicine*, 18, 643–650.

Hemsi, L.K. (1967) 'Psychiatric morbidity of West Indian immigrants', *Social Psychiatry*, 2, 95–100.

Jaspers, K. (1963) *General Psychopathology* (translation of sixth German edition), Manchester: Manchester University Press.

Jones, B.E. and Gray, B.A. (1986) 'Problems in diagnosing schizophrenia and affective disorders among American blacks', *Hospital and Community Psychiatry*, 37, 61–65.

Kakar, S. (1985) 'Psychoanalysis and non-Western cultures', *International Review of Psychoanalysis*, 12, 441–448.

Kareem, J. and Littlewood, R. (eds) (1992) *Intercultural Therapy: Themes, Interpretations and Practice*, Oxford: Blackwell Publishers.

Kiev, A. (1963) 'Beliefs and delusions of West Indian immigrants to London', *British Journal of Psychiatry*, 109, 356–363.

Kovel, J. (1970) *White Racism: A Psychohistory*, London: Allen & Unwin.

Kraepelin, E. (1904) *Vergleichende Psychiatrie*, translated as 'Comparative psychiatry' (1975), in Hirsch, S.R. and Shepherd, M. (eds) *Themes and Variations in European Psychiatry*, Bristol: Wright.

Kramer, B.M., Rosen, B. and Willie, E. (1975) 'Definitions and distributions of mental disorders in a racist society', in Willie, E., Kramer, B.M. and Brown, B.S. (eds) *Racism and Mental Health*, Pittsburgh: University of Pennsylvania Press.

Kuper, A. (1988) *The Invention of Primitive Society: Transformations of an Illusion*, London: Routledge.

Lasch, C. (1979) *The Culture of Narcissism*, New York: Norton.

Leff, J. (1973) 'Culture and the differentiation of emotional states', *British Journal of Psychiatry*, 125, 336–340.

Leff, J., Fischer, M. and Bertelsen, A. (1976) 'A cross national epidemiological study of mania', *British Journal of Psychiatry*, 129, 428–442.

Lind, J.E. (1914) 'The dream as a simple wish-fulfilment in the Negro', *Psychoanalytic Review*, 1, 295–300.

Littlewood, R. (1986) 'Ethnic minorities and the Mental Health Act: patterns of explanation', *Bulletin of the Royal College of Psychiatrists*, 10, 306–308.

Littlewood, R. (1988) 'Community initiated research: a study of psychiatrists' conceptualisations of cannabis psychosis', *Bulletin of the Royal College of Psychiatrists*, 12, 486–488.

Littlewood, R. (1989) 'Cannabis psychosis', *Psychiatric Bulletin*, 13, 148–149.

Littlewood, R. (1992) 'Towards an intercultural therapy', in Kareem, J. and Littlewood, R. (eds) *Intercultural Therapy*, Oxford: Blackwell, pp. 3–13.

Littlewood, R. (1995) 'Psychopathology and personal agency: modernity, culture change and eating disorders in South Asian societies', *British Journal of Medical Psychology*, 68, 45–63.

Littlewood, R. and Cross, S. (1980) 'Ethnic minorities and psychiatric services', *Sociology of Health and Illness*, 2, 194–201.

Littlewood, R. and Lipsedge, M. (1978) 'Migration, ethnicity and diagnosis', *Psychiatrica Clinica*, 11, 15–22.

Littlewood, R. and Lipsedge, M. (1982) *Aliens and Alienists: Ethnic Minorities and Psychiatry*, Penguin, Harmondsworth. Revised edition (1997), London: Routledge.

Lloyd, K. and Moodley, P. (1992) 'Psychotropic medication and ethnicity', *Social Psychiatry and Psychiatric Epidemiology*, 27, 95–101.

McGovern, D. and Cope, R. (1987a) 'The compulsory detention of males of different ethnic groups', *British Journal of Psychiatry*, 150, 505–512.

McGovern, D. and Cope, R. (1987b) 'First psychiatric admission rates of first and second generation Afro-Caribbeans', *Social Psychiatry*, 22, 134–149.

McGovern, D. and Cope, R. (1991) 'Second generation Afro-Caribbeans and young whites with a first admission diagnosis of schizophrenia', *Social Psychiatry and Psychiatric Epidemiology*, 26, 95–99.

McGrath, W.J. (1986) *Freud's Discovery of Psychoanalysis: The Politics of Hysteria*, Ithaca: Cornell University Press.

Mercer, K. (1986) 'Racism and transcultural psychiatry', in Miller, P. and Rose, N. (eds) *The Power of Psychiatry*, Cambridge: Polity Press, pp. 111–142.

Merrill, J. and Owens, J. (1986) 'Ethnic differences in self-poisoning: a comparison of Asian and White groups', *British Journal of Psychiatry*, 148, 708–712.

Miller, P. (1986) 'Psychotherapy of work and employment', in Miller, P. and Rose, N. (eds) *The Power of Psychiatry*, Cambridge: Polity Press, pp. 143–176.

Mitchell, J. (1974) *Psychoanalysis and Feminism*, London: Allen Lane.

Moynihan, D.P. (1965) *The Negro Family*, Washington: US Department of Labour.

Mumford, D.B. and Whitehouse, A.M. (1988) 'Increased prevalence of bulimia nervosa among Asian schoolgirls', *British Medical Journal*, 297(ii), 278.

Obeyesekere, G. (1990) *The Work of Culture: Symbolic Transformation in Psychoanalysis and Anthropology*, Chicago: Chicago University Press.

Parker, R. and Kleiner, S. (1966) *Mental Illness in the Urban Negro Community*, New York: Free Press.

Parmar, P. (1981) 'Young Asian women: a critique of the pathological approach', *Multi-Racial Education*, 9, 17–27.

Pillay, H.M. *et al.* (1984) 'The concepts of "causation", "racism" and "mental illness"', *International Journal of Social Psychiatry*, 39, 129–130.

Pope, H. and Lipinski, J. (1978) 'Diagnosis in schizophrenia and manic-depressive illness', *Archives of General Psychiatry*, 35, 811–828.

'Racism said to be America's chief mental health problem'. *Psychiatry News*, 15 April, 1975.

Rack, P. (1982) *Race, Culture and Mental Disorder*, London: Tavistock.

Rackett, T. (1992) 'White psychiatrists, black masks: on the racial imperative in critical psychiatry', *Economy and Society*, 21, 295–320.

Renfrew, C. (1992) 'World language and human dispersals: a minimalist view', in Hall, J.A. and Jarvie, I.C. (eds) *Transition to Modernity*, Cambridge: Cambridge University Press.

Richardson, E. and Hendrik-Gutt, R. (1981) 'Diagnosis of psychiatric illness in immigrant patients', *British Journal of Clinical Psychiatry*, 1, 78–81.

Rieff, P. (1966) *The Triumph of the Therapeutic*, London: Chatto & Windus.

Roheim, G. (1950) *Psychoanalysis and Anthropology*, New York: International Universities Press.

Royal College of Psychiatrists (1989) *Report of the Special Committee on Ethnic Issues*, London: Royal College of Psychiatrists.

Rwegellera, G.G.C. (1980) 'Differential use of psychiatric services by West Indians, East Africans and English in London', *British Journal of Psychiatry*, 137, 428–432.

Sabshin, M., Diesenhaus, H. and Wilkerson, R. (1970) 'Dimensions of institutional racism in psychiatry', *American Journal of Psychiatry*, 127, 786–793.

Sahlins, M. (1977) *The Use and Abuse of Biology: An Anthropological Critique of Sociobiology*, London: Tavistock.

Showalter, E. (1985) *The Female Malady: Women, Madness and English Culture, 1830–1980*, New York: Pantheon.

Sterba, R. (1947) 'Some psychological factors in Negro race hatred and in anti-Negro riots', *Psychoanalysis and the Social Sciences*, 1, 411–427.

Sulloway, F.J. (1979) *Freud, Biologist of the Mind*, London: Deutsch.

Szasz, T.S. (1971) 'The sane slave: an historical note on the use of medical diagnoses as justificatory rhetoric', *American Journal of Psychotherapy*, 25, 228–239.

Thomas, A. and Sillen, S. (1972) *Racism and Psychiatry*, New Haven: Brunner/Manzel.

Wallace, E.R. (1983) *Freud and Anthropology*, New York: International Universities Press.

Warner, R. (1985) *Recovery from Shizophrenia: Psychiatry and Political Economy*, New York: Routledge and Kegan Paul.

Wessely, S., Castle, D., Der, G. and Murray, R. (1991) 'Schizophrenia and Afro-Caribbeans: a case–control study', *British Journal of Psychiatry*, 159, 795–881.

Willie, C.V., Krammer, B.M. and Brown, B.S. (1973) *Racism and Mental Health*, Philadelphia: University of Pittsburgh Press.

15 Sexual health and ethnicity

K. A. Fenton and Kaye Wellings

Racial categorisation, where classification is based on the individual's physical attributes (e.g. eye and skin colour) has been and is increasingly used as a variable for analysis in epidemiological and social research. Proponents argue that the potential benefits are many, and include the ability to detect variations in health across racial groups, investigate disease aetiology and inform targeted interventions. However, its use has also been criticised (Bhopal *et al.* 1998, Bhopal and Rankin 1999). Racialisation of health and health outcomes tends to be reductionist, attributing observed differences to 'physical attributes' rather than social or economic factors, which may be stronger determinants of the outcome of interest (Wyatt 1991, Bhopal and Rankin 1999). Racial categorisation may also (intentionally or not) reinforce racial stereotypes, and in fields such as sexual health may lead to wariness among communities about the intentions and values of the researchers (Fenton *et al.* 1997). Others argue that given the rich cultural diversity in Britain today, knowing that the prevalence of a particular disease is higher among 'Black' people is of limited use in targeting interventions.

In an effort to overcome some of these limitations, the use of the word *ethnicity*, as opposed to *race*, has been advocated (Wyatt 1991, Bhopal and Rankin 1999). Ethnicity implies that an individual's socialisation is part of a collective (and measurable) identity that is socio-culturally based. Although by no means ideal, it is seen as one method of incorporating and measuring the influence of cultural factors on health experience and outcomes.

Discussions about sexual health and ethnicity, therefore, involve not one but two taboos. Ethnic inequalities in sexual health raise particular sensitivities, with concerns about irresponsible handling of statistical data, racial stereotyping and fears about stigmatising communities (Fenton *et al.* 1997). This perhaps explains the relative lack of data available to us, which limits our ability to explore variation in sexual behaviour and sexual health status with ethnicity. Surveillance data and *ad hoc* research studies in the United States have shown variations in sexual health outcomes between broad ethnic groups ('White'/'African American'/'Hispanic'). Investigation of similar inequalities in Britain is relatively unexplored. This is in part because ethnicity data are generally not collected in routine heath statistics. *Ad hoc* surveys on sexual health outcomes have focused on attenders of sexually transmitted disease (STD) clinics or have examined differences across racial categories (e.g. 'Black', 'White', 'Other').

Some limited data are available from large-scale cross-sectional surveys, for example the National Survey of Sexual Attitudes and Lifestyles (NSSAL) collected data in 1990 and 1991 from nearly 19,000 respondents aged between 16 and 59 in England, Wales and Scotland. Yet this survey suffered a number of methodological problems with regard to ethnicity. These stem partly from classification issues and partly from the size of the sample involved and its implications for analysis. Chief among the problems relating to sample size is the difficulty of adjusting for confounding by socio-economic variables. Self-identification was used to elicit ethnicity, providing a show card from which respondents selected the group they considered they belong to, the categories being those used by the Office for National Statistics (ONS) at the time. The category 'Black' was not disaggregated into Black African and Black Afro-Caribbean. This survey is currently being repeated and the ethnicity classification question to be used in the second survey rectifies this oversight.

Nevertheless, the quantitative data suggest considerable variation in sexual behaviour with ethnicity, most notably in initial sexual experiences and first sexual intercourse. NSSAL data show the ethnic group called Asian to be powerfully protective in terms of early intercourse. Asian women begin sexual experience 3 years later than their Black and White counterparts, with a median age of 21 (Johnson *et al.* 1994). A smaller proportion of women who reported as Asian (11 per cent) had intercourse before the age of 16; among those who self-identified as White the proportion was 19 per cent, and it was higher among those who self-reported as Black, at 26 per cent. These figures are for the total sample for all ages. There has been a progressive decline in age at first intercourse and the proportions were higher for younger respondents in the sample, though the numbers are small. In survival analysis there were significant differences between curves for these groups.

Despite later sexual activity and an increased tendency for sex to take place within marriage where childbearing is generally less problematic, Asian women were more likely to have had an abortion both at some point in their lives, and in the more recent time period of the last 5 years, than White women (Johnson *et al.* 1994). The increased prevalence of termination of pregnancy seems somewhat incompatible with the evidence of delayed first intercourse occurring with marriage in this group. The use of contraception, however, showed a steep gradient by ethnic group. Asian women being considerably less likely to have used contraception in the last year than Black and White women.

More recent population-based analyses of attenders of STD clinics have uncovered evidence of ethnic variations in the prevalence of diagnosed sexually transmitted infections. Lacey and colleagues (1997) recorded details of all residents within the boundaries of Leeds Health Authority who presented with gonorrhoea (culture confirmed) from April 1989 to September

1993 at Leeds General Infirmary, the only STD clinic serving the city. High rates of gonorrhoea were observed among Black men, and younger men were at highest risk with an incidence of 2–3 per cent per year. The neighbourhoods with the highest rates of infection were inner-city areas with high proportions of ethnic minority groups. However, after controlling for age, sex and socio-economic group, Black men and women in Leeds were more than ten times more likely than White men and women, and fifty times more likely than Asian men and women, to have had one or more episodes of gonorrhoea during the study. White men and women were nearly five times more likely than Asians to have had one or more episodes of gonorrhoea during the study period.

Low and others (1997) contacted sixteen departments of genito-urinary medicine (GUM) in Lambeth, Southwark and Lewisham and collected data from eleven departments during 1994–95. Again the highest rates of STD were found among young Black men with incidence rates of 1–2 per cent. Women from Black minority ethnic groups had around ten times the rate of gonococcal infection than that seen in White women. Rates were higher among Black men than among Black women for all age groups except the youngest – aged 15–19 years. Again inequalities in gonorrhoea rates persisted after adjusting for socio-economic confounding; men from Black minority ethnic groups being eleven times more likely than those from White groups to acquire gonorrhoea. Roughly one in ten gonorrhoea episodes reported from departments of GUM in England occurred among residents of Lewisham, Southwark and Lambeth.

Both these studies show membership of a Black ethnic group to be associated with a higher risk of acquiring gonorrhoea, as judged by incidence rates, even after controlling for socio-economic status. By any standards, the differences in disease incidence between the groups give cause for concern. Why are rates so high among ethnic populations in the United Kingdom? There are no known biological reasons to explain why racial or ethnic differences alone should alter the risk for STD or unwanted conceptions. The explanatory factors may be epidemiological or socio-cultural.

From an epidemiological perspective, the association between ethnicity and sexual health may be due to chance, bias or true association. Chance is unlikely to account for the association, given the consistency of findings across research studies. Biases in the design of studies may account for some of the differences. Attenders of STD clinics are more likely to have high-risk sexual lifestyles, increased numbers of partners and to have been previously diagnosed with an STD (Johnson *et al.* 1996). Health-seeking behaviours will also influence who goes to STD clinics and when, which leads to recruitment bias among STD attenders. These factors make STD clinic data unrepresentative of the wider population and may lead to an overestimation of high-risk sexual behaviours if findings are extrapolated to the wider community.

If there is a true association between ethnicity and sexual health outcomes what factors may explain this? The risk of spread of a sexually transmitted infection (STI) within a given population is denoted by the *basic reproductive rate* (R_0), which is dependent upon the transmission probability (β), the rate of partner acquisition (c), and the average duration of infectiousness (D). β and D are the two biological factors within the model. However, all may be influenced by cultural factors.

For example, condoms reduce the probability of disease transmission by providing an effective barrier. NSSAL failed to find significant differences between the ethnic groups in terms of condom use. Nevertheless, the study revealed a tendency, documented elsewhere, for a preference amongst Black men and women for systemic (non-barrier) methods – that is, those not directly related to the act of intercourse (Elam *et al.* 1999). Some have suggested that this may be explained by a cultural tendency to equate virility with fertility and a consequent preference for methods, which are not specifically intercourse related; there was also less tolerance for surgical methods of contraception among either Black or Asian men and women compared with those self-defining as White. The importance of specific cultural practices, for example female and male circumcision and the use of vaginal drying agents, in determining sexual and reproductive health outcomes have been highlighted in ethnographic studies (Brown *et al.* 1993, Tyndall *et al.* 1996). Here, culturally prescribed practices can increase the risks associated with disease transmission. Although such practices are theoretically amenable to intervention, effecting change may be difficult where practices are seen as being a part of a cultural identity.

Variations in sexual health are also explained in terms of the interrelationship between an individual's culture and ethnic background on the provision and use of sexual health services. This in turn may influence the *duration of infectiousness* (D). The stigma of sexually transmitted diseases and of attendance at GUM clinics varies with cultural group (Elam *et al.* 1999), and it may mean that individuals delay accessing these services or taking advantage of available interventions. Negative attitudes towards GUM clinics, clinic staff and doctors have been documented across a variety of ethnic groups (Fenton *et al.* 1999a). Indeed, there is some evidence that, for Asian and African communities, the general practitioner (GP) remains the choice of first call for advice and information on sexual matters. Among Black gay and bisexual men the negative attitudes of clinic staff, insensitivity of clinic doctors and confidentiality concerns have been cited as the main reasons for not attending STD clinics and seeking care outside this sector (Fenton *et al.* 1999b). The attitudes are not without foundation and many inner-city minority communities may be further disadvantaged by the delivery of sub-standard sexual health services and interventions (Monk 1992). Negative attitudes towards minority groups in a society may be reflected in the views of health service providers, and the resultant prejudice and discrimination may serve not only to hinder health service use but also to diminish the benefits received from such use. Negative experiences associated with accessing GUM clinics, such as racism, insensitive or intolerant staff and poor facilities, serve to maintain the stereotypes of STDs afflicting those at the margins of society.

The main behavioural factor influencing disease transmission is the rate of partner change, c, or the rate of acquisition of new partners. Few studies have looked at variations across ethnic groups. Although the total number of reported sexual partners may give some indication of the magnitude of partner change, it is difficult to distinguish between concurrent and sequential partners. Univariate analysis in NSSAL suggested that Black men reported having twice the number of sexual partners in a lifetime than White men did (with medians of eight compared to four respectively), but the number of observations was small and multivariate analysis was not carried out to adjust for confounding factors. However, a twofold increase in the number of partners among Black men seems unlikely to account fully for the tenfold difference in the incidence of disease. Qualitative studies highlight variations across ethnic groups in attitudes towards multiple and concurrent relationships (Elam *et al.* 1999).

Partner selection and the question of 'who mixes with whom' is also an important aspect in the transmission of STDs. People tend to have partners within their own ethnic group, thereby increasing the risk of onward transmission of infection within particular communities. Barlow and colleagues (1997) examined patterns of assortative sexual mixing among GUM attenders, enquiring about the ethnicity of the last sexual partner, and found a close and closed pattern of sexual mixing within ethnic groups.

Taking into account differences in sexual behaviour, the transmission dynamics of sexually transmitted infection, and the widespread deficiencies in appropriate sexual health services, we begin to get a sense of the differential weighting which should be attached to the predisposing factors. Yet anxieties around the tension between these positions may inhibit public health efforts. There are moves on the part of interested groups to improve services. Blackliners, for example, are working with staff to improve services and researchers are evaluating ways of effectively involving communities in sexual health-related research and development initiatives (Fenton *et al.* 1999c). For such interventions to be effective, however, the potential for racism in sexual health services needs to be recognised and addressed across a wide range of agencies and sectors.

From a sociological perspective, ethnic and cultural background have the potential to influence sexual health in a number of ways: how we learn about sexual matters, our attitudes and practices related to sex, our choice of partners, how we relate to and accept sexual health promotion messages and utilise sexual health services. In concert, these influences may either act to place some groups at increased risk of adverse sexual health outcomes, such as infection or unplanned conception, or lead to more protective measures in other groups.

In all communities, cultural norms operate to proscribe certain attitudes and behaviours and to prescribe others. In general, social mores correspond closely with cultural norms. Societies which condone, or have relaxed social attitudes towards, for example, early sexual experience, concurrent sexual relationships or contact with sex workers, are more likely to have higher prevalence of these behaviours (Cleland and Ferry 1996). Where certain behaviours are effectively censured, the impact on sexual health status may well be protective, examples being delayed coitarche and sex within marriage. As STD prevalence in Britain is highest within mid–late adolescence this 'natural intervention' has a potentially protective effect on STD acquisition by reducing the numbers of sexual partners, rate of partner change and the probability of contact with the prevalent pool of infection.

Cultural influences on sexual lifestyles and attitudes are not static however. Complex patterns of sexual lifestyle occur, where communities are in transition and where there is age-related diversity within the group. Young people may, for example, increasingly share the social norms of the community into which they are integrating, while their parents and other older members of the group may retain more traditional norms. Living within a more sexually open society can have immediate effects on an individual's attitudes and lifestyle. In Britain, exposure to a more open society has resulted in increased knowledge about sexual and reproductive health in general, alternative sexual lifestyles and a range of sexual practices, even among first generation immigrants but most markedly among successive generations (Elam *et al.* 1999). For those born in Britain, exposure to individuals from other ethnic backgrounds (including the ethnic majority), to sex education in schools, to ease of access to sexual material and to the onslaught of media interest in sex has opened the discourse on sexual behaviour. Even among cultures where it is currently the norm not to discuss sexual matters, external informal and formal influences will change the manner in which successive generations of young people are socialised regarding sexual matters. Less positively, rapid integration into another culture may lead to discordance between sexual behaviours as currently practised and the cultural norms governing such behaviours. In such cases, behaviours may be more covert and less amenable to preventive intervention and this may have negative implications for sexual health status.

Cultural variations interact with social structural factors. As with other health-related conditions, the socio-economic experience of many ethnic minority communities in Britain places them at a disadvantage as far as sexual health status is concerned. Sexual health promotion in socially deprived or economically disadvantaged areas must compete against other priorities. Immigration concerns, economic survival, child rearing and social integration are often more pressing and immediate concerns for many ethnic minorities. The effect of religion may reinforce cultural influences on sexual behaviour. Among some communities, the influence of religion may be difficult to untangle from that of culture, for example in many Islamic communities. Also, religious dictates may be used to strengthen cultural messages relating to behaviours and practices (Elam *et al.* 1999).

Case study: cross-cultural variations in learning about sex

Research has shown how learning about sex is influenced by an individual's cultural background. It has an impact on the messages individuals receive, the sources which are available and the timing at which the information is obtained. Recently conducted ethnographic research provides complementary data and richer fertile insights into the sexual behaviour of ethnic groups. In-depth qualitative interviews carried out by the exploring ethnicity and sexual health (EXES) team (Elam *et al.* 1999) sought personal attitudes, social norms and cultural mores in relation to sexual behaviour among Indians, Bangladeshis, Nigerians, Ugandans and Jamaicans resident in inner London.

A number of common patterns emerged among Indian and Bangladeshi communities. Cultural and religious influences remain important among Asians, particularly among Muslims, and are particularly effective in dictating modes of deportment and interaction for growing children, proscribing pre-marital contact with the opposite sex, and placing sexual experiences and sexual intercourse firmly within the context of marriage. These beliefs are largely maintained among Asian women and some Asian men in Britain, despite having attended mixed-gender schools and having received sex education in British schools.

Asians born in this country receive school sex education, but the evidence suggests a marked absence of discussion about sexual matters at home. Other adults play an important role in providing information at or near the time of marriage (particularly to the bride to be), but few informal sources of information among young women were reported, especially among those born abroad or among those mixing mainly within their ethnic group in the United Kingdom. The indications are that Bengali women value the health service as a point of contact for information on sexual matters, the GP being the main source.

For young Asian men (Indian and Bangladeshi), especially those in the United Kingdom, relatively freer opportunities for mixing in a multicultural society have provided increased opportunities for learning about sex from peers from other ethnic groups. For those who grow up in the United Kingdom there is also school sex education and access to media coverage of the subject.

There is some suggestion that attitudes towards non-penetrative sexual contacts are changing among younger Indian and Bangladeshi women. This may precede other changes in sexual behaviour. Among young Asian men, this change appears to be more rapid and appears to be driven by the greater exposure to sex in the media, sex education, the prevailing 'youth culture' and, perhaps most importantly, access to opportunities for sexual activity available in Britain. Of course there is a great deal of heterogeneity within the Asian groups and the above comments are generalisations. A strong taboo seems, however, to exist in Asian communities around sex, and opportunities to mix socially are few.

The picture appears to be different for Black Africans and Jamaicans. Among Jamaicans considerable exposure to sexual matters in the family through observing parents and family members cuddling, etc., and through talking about sex in the home was typically reported. They are more likely to receive informal exposure to sex education because they are less protected socially and are more likely to interact outside their ethnic grouping.

Common to all communities was a dearth of information provided by parents. Strongly prohibitive messages, however, were conveyed to women. Pre-marital sex and pregnancy were equated with shame. Yet, ironically, this association is strongest in communities in which information about contraceptive use, or provision, is absent, than in those communities in which sex and contraception are more freely discussed. Parents typically focused on the negative consequences of sexual activity, e.g. STD and HIV infection.

Among Nigerians, Ugandans and Jamaicans older female relatives provided an important role in discussing sexual matters with pubescent girls, though boys were accorded less attention. Living in the United Kingdom has provided a freer environment, introduced new behavioural patterns (e.g. the appropriateness of public displays of affection, such as kissing) and allowed greater access to information through media and literature.

Conclusion

There is no straightforward link between ethnicity and sexual health. Methodological concerns have highlighted the difficulties of applying and interpreting racial and ethnic categorisations in sexual-behaviour research. Ethnicity may well be a proxy marker for other, more important, determinants of health outcomes including social class, economic status and educational achievement. Attempts to adjust for socio-economic status in ecological studies of ethnic variations in sexual health are in their infancy and need refining.

The relationship is also complicated as the prevalence of specific STDs varies across different ethnic groups. Different explanations are needed to account for the increased prevalence of gonorrhoea among Black Caribbeans (Lacey *et al.* 1997, Low *et al.* 1997), genital warts among White British (Catchpole *et al.* 1997) and HIV/AIDS among Black Africans [Public Health Laboratory Service (PHLS) 1998]. Although epidemiological and socio-cultural factors may be significant contributors, the influence of wider contextual determinants, e.g. global HIV and STD pandemics, immigration history and travel to home countries, should also be considered.

Not all ethnic minority groups are at increased risk. The quantitative studies have consistently shown the relatively low prevalence of reported STDs among Britain's South Asian (Indian, Pakistani and Bangladeshi) communities. Qualitative research has highlighted a number of culturally mediated protective behaviours and attitudes including delay in first sexual intercourse and reduction in life-time numbers of partners. Whether these protective effects are maintained over time will be dependent upon the mixing with the ethnic majority, the interplay between the cultures and religious influences.

Finally, ethnic variations in sexual health outcomes reflect larger inequalities in health and must be interpreted in context. Poverty, social inequalities and institutional racism all create and perpetuate inequalities. Maintaining good sexual health necessarily becomes secondary to economic survival for those at greatest risk, particularly among political and economic migrants. Sexual health promotion is made difficult by the need to speak openly and without stigma about what is seen by many as an intensively private matter. Effective intervention will only be achieved through collaboration with at-risk communities, using culturally appropriate mechanisms and allowing for incremental change.

References

Barlow, D., Daker-White, G. and Band, B. (1997) 'Assortative sexual mixing in a heterosexual clinic population—a limiting factor in HIV spread?', *AIDS*, 11, 1039–1044.

Bhopal, R. and Rankin, J. (1999) 'Concepts and terminology in ethnicity, race and health: be aware of the ongoing debate', *British Dental Journal*, 186(10), 483–484.

Bhopal, R., Donaldson, L. and White, B. (1998) 'European, Western, Caucasian, or what? Inappropriate labeling in research on race, ethnicity, and health', *American Journal of Public Health*, 88, 1303–1307.

Brown, J.E., Ayowa, O.B. and Brown, R.C. (1993) 'Dry and tight: sexual practices and potential AIDS risk in Zaire', *Social Science and Medicine*, 37(8), 989–994.

Catchpole, M., Hughes, G., Rodgers, P.A., Brady, A.R., Kinghorn, G., Mercey, D. and Thin, N. (1997) 'Behaviour, Ethnicity and STIs. Results and implications of a survey of STD clinics in England 1994–1997', Paper presented at the International Congress of Sexually Transmitted Diseases, Seville, 19–22 October, Abstract P556.

Cleland, J. and Ferry, B. (1995) *Sexual Behaviour and AIDS in the Developing World*, London: Taylor and Francis.

Elam, G., Fenton, K., Johnson, A., Nazroo, J. and Ritchie, J. (1999) *Exploring Ethnicity and Sexual Health*, London: SCPR.

Fenton, K.A., Johnson, A.M. and Nicoll, A. (1997) 'Race, ethnicity, and sexual health', *British Medical Journal*, 314(7096), 1703–1704.

Fenton, K.A., Chinouya, M. and Davidson, O. (1999a) 'Can community participation and sexual behaviour research be integrated in a meaningful way? The MAYISHA study', Paper presented at the Thirteenth International Society for Sexual Transmitted Disease Research Conference, Denver, 11–14 July, Abstract No. 239.

Fenton, K.A., Elam. G., Johnson, A.M., Nazroo, J. and Ritchie, J. (1999b) '"Let me tell you what needs to be done." Suggestions for improving inner-city sexual health services and health promotion from local ethnic minority communities', Paper presented at the Thirteenth International Society for Sexual Transmitted Disease Research Conference, Denver, 11–14 July, Abstract No. 307.

Fenton, K.A., White, B., Weatherburn, P. and Cadette, M. (1999c) *What are you like? Assessing the sexual health needs of black gay and bisexual men*, Final Project report, Big Up.

Johnson, A., Wadsworth, J., Wellings, K. and Field, J. (1994) *National Study of Sexual Attitudes and Lifestyles*, Oxford: Blackwell Publishers.

Johnson, A.M., Wadsworth, J., Wellings, K. and Field, J. (1996) 'Who goes to sexually transmitted disease clinics? Results from a national population survey', *Genitourinary Medicine*, 72, 197–202.

Lacey, C.J.N., Merrick, D., Bensley, D.C. and Fairley I. (1997) 'Analysis of the sociodemography of gonorrhoea in Leeds, 1989–93', *British Medical Journal*, 314, 1715–1718.

Low, N., Daker-White, G., Barlow, D. and Pozniak, A.L. (1997) 'Gonorrhoea in inner London: results of a cross sectional study', *British Medical Journal*, 314, 1719–1723.

Public Health Laboratory Service (PHLS) (1999) AIDS Centre and the Scottish Centre for Infection and Environmental Health. *AIDS/HIV Quarterly Surveillance Tables. UK Data to End December 1998.*

Tyndall, M.W., Ronald, A.R., Agoki, E. *et al.* (1996) 'Increased risk of infection with human immunodeficiency virus type 1 among uncircumcised men presenting with genital ulcer disease in Kenya', *Clinical Infectious Diseases*, 23(3), 449–453.

Wyatt, G. (1991) 'Examining ethnicity versus race in AIDS related research', *Social Science and Medicine.*, 33, 37–45.

16 Challenges and policy implications of ethnic diversity and health

R. Balarajan

Background

Britain is a multicultural and democratic society. While significant strides have been made in terms of acceptance of its diversity, there are still unmet challenges. Health and social care agencies face the challenge of providing a service that is equitable to all regardless of colour or creed. In this chapter some of the weaknesses in the system are examined. It is argued that providing a service that is inclusive to all communities and responds to changing needs does not require vast expenditure but practical and innovative ways of redistributing resources. As the recently published White Paper highlights, this requires a close partnership between health authorities, local authorities and the local communities. While such a tripartite partnership has not been conspicuously successful, with sufficient support it could be developed into a thriving strategy.

Knowing the people

It is part of the Citizen's Charter in the United Kingdom that purchasers and providers of care should know their client base in some considerable detail. Often the organisational culture in the National Health Service (NHS) has supported 'business as usual', irrespective of evidence to support particular interventions or levels of performance. The subject of ethnicity and health has had a high profile. In recent years, with a commitment to meeting the health needs of ethnic groups coming from the Government, the Chief Medical Officer (CMO) and the NHS Executive, lack of awareness or competing priorities can no longer be advanced as justification for inaction by senior management or professionals responsible for health services.

Social and economic circumstances

Social, economic and cultural profiles vary between and within ethnic populations. A notable example of this heterogeneity is that of housing among those who migrated or whose ancestors migrated from the Indian subcontinent. The proportion of Indians living in owner-occupied housing

(82 per cent) is higher than the average among all people in England and Wales (68 per cent). In contrast, the proportion for Bangladeshis is 44 per cent, with almost 40 per cent living in council housing. Extended families in South Asian households are common. This has its advantages, but it can lead to significant overcrowding, especially among Bangladeshi households. The Fourth National Survey showed that the quality of housing also differs significantly. Whereas the quality of housing among owners is generally better than that of renters for Indians and African Asians, high proportions of Pakistani and Bangladeshi owner-occupied households lack sole access to amenities such as an inside toilet and central heating. Single-parent households are more common among African Caribbeans (16–20 per cent of all households compared with 3–4 per cent among those from the Indian subcontinent and 11 per cent overall), with about 40 per cent of live births occurring 'outside marriage'. This compares with 30 per cent for all women in England and Wales and 1 per cent in women from the Indian subcontinent. Unemployment is unacceptably high among ethnic minority populations – 25 per cent among economically active African Caribbean men aged 16+ compared with 11 per cent for men in England and Wales. The proportion rises to over one-third in African Caribbean men under 25 years of age compared with 18 per cent in their White counterparts. Again, about one-third of Bangladeshi and Pakistani women are unemployed compared with 6 per cent among women nationally. Ethnic groups are more likely to be in lower occupational grades, to have poorer job security and to work unsociable hours. Ethnic populations tend to reside in deprived, congested, violence-prone inner-city areas, which gives a further twist to produce a situation of 'multiple jeopardy'. Whereas concentration in these areas enhances ethnic identity and increases access to political power, in urban areas they are also more likely to face poorer employment opportunities and poorer access to health services.

Cultural context

It is important to be aware of the culture and health beliefs of the different communities. It could be argued that the service should address mainstream issues but remain sensitive to ethnic issues. This may be a pragmatic model for the future but it is not *de facto* an appropriate model to address the existing situation.

Linguistic difficulties

Difficulties in communication among some groups within the South Asian community require a positive approach. The ageing of the first-generation cohorts of these populations means that they will make increasingly greater use of the services than has hitherto been experienced. Many second-generation migrants communicate with their GP in a language other than

English, especially women. Another compounding factor is the gradual retirement of current practitioners from ethnic communities who have held the front line for many years. Newly qualified South Asian doctors often do not speak the languages of their parents or do not practice in these relatively deprived areas. This highlights the need for interpreters and adequate translation services. Currently, these are poorly distributed and in some places members of the family, especially children, act as interpreters.

Use of alternative therapies

Ethnic groups often use alternative remedies, such as acupuncture and herbal remedies, which have not been subject to rigorous scientific testing. Faith and confidence, however, play an important part in the healing process, and it may be necessary to provide support for interventions that people believe in until such time as evidence on clinical efficacy becomes available. Only 15–20 per cent of interventions are based on scientifically measured clinical benefit, and it is clearly important to substitute knowledge for belief and supposition. Refusal to invest in interventions because of non-availability of evidence of a beneficial effect may, however, be harmful and cause distress to patients. This is different from reacting to evidence that an intervention has no beneficial effect.

Low uptake of screening services

There is little awareness in ethnic groups of many major national initiatives, such as cervical screening. This raises questions about the effectiveness and the role of the Health Education Authority. Uptake of cervical cancer screening nationally is about 60 per cent. The uptake in women of Indian subcontinent origin is about half that level, with significant proportions saying that they did not know what a cervical smear is (one-third in Bangladeshi women), or that they had never been recommended to have one (one-third in Pakistani women). This reflects poorly on the outreach of preventive care among sections of ethnic minority women, and there is clearly scope for improvement. Local studies have shown that poor uptake is due more to poor administrative arrangements than to indifference to screening. Muslim women prefer to see a female GP. In fact, a substantial proportion of all women in this country would prefer to see a female GP. Randomised clinical trials or meta-analyses are not needed to make simple pragmatic and low-cost responses to these issues.

Health needs

Chronic diseases such as diabetes and hypertension are excessively prevalent among some ethnic groups. Mortality from diabetes is seven times greater among Bangladeshis than among all people in England and Wales. Although not as extreme, higher prevalence is also a familiar feature among other Asians and in African Caribbeans. Furthermore, these ethnic groups are more susceptible than Caucasians to serious secondary complications such as coronary heart disease, stroke and end-stage renal failure. The difficulty in coming to terms with a life-long disabling disease and the need to comply with treatment for life cuts across the health beliefs and health behaviour of some ethnic groups. Is this worth a trial to see whether a disease management approach might work? Would it help if these communities were supported by dedicated diabetic nurse practitioners? Is there a role for preventive practitioners focusing on such interrelated chronic conditions as diabetes, coronary heart disease and hypertension? As these relatively young populations age, the burden of chronic disease in the communities as well as on the NHS is likely to grow. It is crucial that we look at models of care that will deliver effective intervention in terms of prevention and care in both primary and secondary sectors.

Hypertension is another disease that disproportionately kills and disables people from ethnic minorities. African Caribbeans around the globe are known to suffer disproportionately from hypertensive disease and stroke. Recent research has shown that Bangladeshis in this country also experience high levels of stroke mortality. Conventional measures of socio-economic circumstances do not explain all of this excess. Other factors related to the stress of migration, discrimination and the disproportionate impact of cumulative deprivation are likely to be implicated. Unlike the United States, where there are special screening programmes for hypertension, these are not readily found in areas of Britain with high proportions of African Caribbeans. An opportunistic approach to screening needs to be considered. These are only some of the areas where consensus on the best approach needs to be developed. Consensus conferences may be one way of achieving solutions to some of these key issues.

A striking inequality is the high rate of infant mortality and congenital anomalies among Pakistani infants. There are several likely explanations, the most significant being high levels of consanguinity, low rates of participation in genetic screening and an unwillingness to accept termination when fetal abnormalities are identified. Despite the sensitivity of these issues, working in partnership with the community is essential to tackle this inequality.

There is also the issue of changing lifestyles in ethnic communities, with the attendant health risks. Excessive alcohol consumption among Sikh men and their increased prevalence of cirrhosis of the liver is an example. High levels of smoking among Bangladeshi men which could lead to increasing levels of lung cancer in the future is another.

Strategy for ethnicity and health

The approach to ethnicity and health is patchy and opportunistic. There could be a successful balance whereby within the mainstream, issues are addressed through special projects and programmes, evaluation of which should be part of performance management reviews.

Primary care

Primary care provides the bedrock for most people's health care and is the gateway to other specialist services. The limited information available from studies, however, shows unequal access and dissatisfaction among patients. Most ethnic minority communities live in inner cities where the quality of primary care varies widely and there is a preponderance of 'single-handed' GPs, who often lack the support and facilities of a group practice. People from ethnic minorities, South Asians in particular, consult their GPs more frequently than the general population, but this is sometimes for problems or difficulties unrelated to medical needs. There is a case for developing a more innovative approach with greater involvement of other health professionals, since such broad-based support at the primary care level may appropriately be provided by someone other than the GP.

Community clinics, such as maternal and child health clinics, are often used by ethnic groups. They provide the opportunity to persuade mothers to accept and use preventive services more widely and also to address other issues such as those related to nutrition and other lifestyle habits.

Cross-sectoral work

Services frequently fail to provide satisfaction because of a lack of cooperation between the various agencies involved. While continuity of care is a central feature of primary care, the level of communication and collaboration often falls short of what is desirable. Where such joint working breaks down, inevitably patients suffer. With the high prevalence of diseases such as diabetes and hypertension among ethnic minorities, it is especially important to achieve regular inputs from a range of sources. There is a strong argument for more managed care in such situations in partnership with ethnic communities.

Equitable allocation of resources

Information detailing expenditure on ethnic minorities is not available. Historical spending patterns have often favoured well-endowed areas. For example, in west London, Hammersmith receives much more per capita than Southall or Northolt. The health needs of these two areas are so different that if a zero-based budget approach was adopted a reversal in the order of magnitude of the allocations would be expected. It is important that the allocation of resources to small localities is considered. Although the use of RAWP and subsequent initiatives was meant to achieve equity of per capita funding at the health authority level, allocations at the sub-district level have been straight-jacketed. Purchasers have tinkered at the margins with minor services such as family planning, rather than introduce changes which impact on core specialities or activities.

Over the 3 years of its existence, the NHS Ethnic Unit dispensed around £3 million to health authorities for developmental projects. It was intended to build awareness within the communities because a prerequisite was the participation of community organisations. In many instances, however, the projects do not appear to have brought about changes in the service. Often they were either not completed or adopted by the service organisation and were not evaluated.

Public health strategy

Strategy in certain key areas, such as hypertension, diabetes, coronary heart disease and haemoglobinopathies, should be developed with the help of consensus meetings. At a recent bilateral conference between the United Sates and Britain, on ethnicity and health, a document was signed expressing ministerial intent to explore a range of good practices and is a good example of partnership development.

Ethnicity and health should feature specifically in national initiatives such as 'Our Healthier Nation' and the inequalities agenda. There should be a range of initiatives, key areas and targets geared specifically to the needs of the ethnic population. For example, among Bangladeshis, diseases for which there are national targets (coronary heart disease, hypertension and stroke) are important but other targets are needed for diabetes, oropharyngeal and liver cancers, smoking-related diseases, and maternal and child mortality. The high level of some of these diseases in ethnic groups also means that the levels of the national targets need to be revised.

Health service strategy

Purchasing strategy

Issues related to ethnicity need to be considered in many processes such as resource allocation, primary and secondary care. Primary care purchasers, for example, should reflect on the evidence that patients from ethnic groups are currently under-represented in cohorts of patients receiving secondary care and interventions such as coronary artery bypass grafting, in spite of being more prone to coronary heart disease.

Provider strategy

Standards are important for high quality of care. For example, measures of waiting time, referrals, GP and secondary care need to be monitored, and more resources into communication, health education and preventive measures should be considered. The National Service Frameworks should provide a major advance in this direction.

Intelligence

Intelligence is essential for good management but there is virtually no data that can be used to monitor referrals, outcomes of treatments and whether ethnic groups get the benefit of expensive treatment.

Some progress was made with the inclusion of a question on ethnic origin in the 1991 Census. While this has provided valuable information on the distribution and characteristics of ethnic populations, it cannot be used to produce morbidity, mortality or fertility rates for ethnic groups. Ethnic monitoring of admissions to hospital was introduced in April 1996, but implementation has been slow and coverage is less than 50 per cent nationally. Significant improvements in the completeness and quality of data will be needed before it can be used to examine admission rates, morbidity patterns, etc., among ethnic minority populations. Health is therefore largely measured in terms of mortality for the national targets. However, as ethnic origin is not recorded on death or birth registration certificates (an act of parliament is required to achieve this), such vital parameters of a community's health are available only for the first generation. The result is that we are largely ignorant about the health profile of the 40 per cent or so of ethnic minority people who are United Kingdom-born. Nor is the scene set to change in the near future. As the next census is due in 2001, the opportunity to analyse mortality by ethnicity will be lost until the following census unless urgent steps are taken to introduce ethnic origin on vital registration forms.

Addressing gaps in information needs foresight and commitment from central government to implement linkage of GP and hospital records. Longitudinal studies are the best solutions in the long term but they are also expensive to set up.

Research strategy

We do not need to wait for a gene to be isolated or for ways to be found to engineer its replacement or function. The dramatic decline in coronary heart disease (CHD) mortality in this country over the last decade is a case in point. More applied research, such as that which could help to curb the high burden of morbidity and mortality associated with diabetes, is needed.

Research is, ultimately, only of value if it translates into better experience and outcomes for patients. It is doubtful that the national research and development (R&D) programme or local projects have achieved this. This is partly due to the time needed to transform study proposals into a workable programme. It is also often due to a lack of will and money to complete the development of the business and deal with the objections that inevitably challenge the process of change.

It is essential that the allocation of resources for research match the research needs of ethnic minorities. Ethnic groups provide useful control subjects for studies and contribute to the knowledge base of science, but they have not necessarily benefited from these studies. The selection of researchers and their acceptability to the communities under research is another issue that needs to be considered if the value of the work is not to be compromised.

Training and education

The need to introduce the subject of ethnicity into the medical curriculum has at last been recognised. This should include undergraduate, postgraduate and continuing education of doctors and other health professionals. The benefits in improved doctor–patient relationships and treatment would amply justify the investment of time and resources taken up. The Royal College of General Practitioners (RCGP), along with other royal colleges and the General Medical Council, has a crucial role to play in developing the curriculum and achieving the necessary changes.

Doctors represent only a small fraction of those who care for patients and a similar review of training curricula of other care workers, including those of nurses, social workers, health visitors, should be undertaken.

Eliminating discriminatory practices

Britain prides itself on offering equal opportunities to all, irrespective of race, religion or colour. While these values are adhered to in principle, equality is yet to be achieved in practice. Although there is a range of laws and codes of practice aimed at preventing discrimination, there are many areas where it persists. There is plenty of evidence that the career prospects for people from ethnic minorities are poorer than those of their White counterparts in the NHS. A recent article in the *British Medical Journal* made the point that the NHS would need to treat its staff fairly before it could expect patients to receive equal respect.

It is necessary to appoint senior managers and, more importantly, chief executives and chairpersons of agencies from ethnic minority backgrounds. Until very recently, there had been no known ethnic person in such posts. It is important to break the mould of seeing ethnic representatives only in middle management or in specific roles in the NHS management structure. Regrettably, officers appointed to promote issues such as equality have disappeared under recent cuts in management, often under the pretext that such matters are accommodated within mainstream policies on inequality. A host of issues will no longer be dealt with because there is no one to raise them or do the spadework.

Need for organisational change

It is difficult for the community to understand the business culture of Health Authorities. The level of participation by service-users, be it in policy development, purchasing or providing services, is not one of the strengths of the NHS. It could be argued that the 'corporate' culture of the NHS is neither inclusive nor participatory. Community health councils play a significant role, but they do not have the necessary experience or expertise to address issues related to ethnicity. Councils for racial equality exist but they do not generally feature as stakeholders in the business of health. Alternative approaches, such as a 'consultative body' covering a wider area than just one health authority, would be both cost-effective and facilitate a comparative assessment of services by different agencies. The need for local machinery that reflects local needs and views, backed up by professional support, is conspicuous by its absence. In areas where ethnic minorities are not 'clustered', alternative mechanisms such as a 'commissioner' or equivalent could be tried. Non-executive directors are often expected to take on such roles but conflicts of interest arise and the culture of top NHS management inevitably imposes some constraints.

A related issue is the reluctance of senior management to prioritise ethnic issues. It is only by building specific changes into the performance management agenda that they are likely to get into action plans. Table 16.1 shows what will be necessary for the provision of adequate health care to ethnic minorities.

Table 16.1 Framework for a contract

Individual level
Equal access to primary, secondary and tertiary health care
Ensure equitable outcomes
Information on services available
Effective communication ensured in a consultation
Religious and other cultural issues sensitively addressed
Help desk/line to address queries

Community level
Involvement in purchasing and providing care
Involvement in policy development
Ensure differences within localities are considered in allocation of resources

Staff
Recruitment and retention of suitably qualified personnel from ethnic groups
Equal opportunities to career development
Curriculum development
Cultural competence

Organisational
Intelligence to monitor needs, referrals, access to treatments and outcomes
Research prioritised to community needs
Develop indicators and targets for outcomes
Focus on improving access to primary care in inner cities
Commitment from senior management
Ethnic issues include performance management and action plans

Conclusion

The lack of resources is often an excuse for inertia. Historical patterns of spending determine decisions with little margin to be innovative. There needs to be a mechanism that allows a substantial part of the budget to be held back for zero-based planning, which would allow innovative schemes to be adopted. The suggestions above do not consume more resources but require practical and innovative ways of redistributing the existing resources and, above all, the political will to see the changes through.

References

Balarajan, R. and Bulusu, L. (1990) 'Morality among immigrants in England and Wales, 1979–83', in Britton, M. (ed.) *Mortality and Geography: A Review in the Mid-1980s, England and Wales*, London: HMSO.

Balarajan, R. and Raleigh, V.S. (1997) *Ethnicity and Health. A Management Guide to the NHS*, London: HMSO.

Health Education Authority (1994) *Black and Minority Ethnic Groups in England*, London: Health Education Authority.

Marmot, M.G., Adelstein, A.M. and Bulusu, L. (1984) *Immigrant Mortality in England and Wales 1970–78: Causes of Death by Country of Birth*, Studies of Medical Population Subjects No 47, London: HMSO.

National Institute for Ethnic Studies in Health and Social Policy (1997) *Ethnic Minorities in England and Wales. An Analysis by Health Authorities Based on the 1991 Census*, London: National Institute for Ethnic Studies in Health and Social Policy.

Nazroo, J.Y. (1997) *The Health of Britain's minorities*, Policy Studies Institute.

Rudat, K. (1994) *Black and Ethnic Minority Groups in England: Health and Lifestyles*, London: Health Education Authority.

Index